NATURALISTIC PSYCHOLOGY IN GALEN AND STOICISM

Naturalistic Psychology in Galen and Stoicism

CHRISTOPHER GILL

OXFORD
UNIVERSITY PRESS

OXFORD
UNIVERSITY PRESS

Great Clarendon Street, Oxford OX2 6DP
United Kingdom

Oxford University Press is a department of the University of Oxford.
It furthers the University's objective of excellence in research, scholarship,
and education by publishing worldwide.

Oxford is a registered trade mark of Oxford University Press in the UK
and in certain other countries

Reprinted 2013

British Library Cataloguing in Publication Data
Data available

Library of Congress Cataloging in Publication Data
Data available

ISBN 978-0-19-955679-3

To Karen (1958–2010)
Ross, Jack, Harry, and Ralph

Preface

This book, on the psychological ideas of Galen and Stoicism, is the third of three studies I have written in recent years on ancient psychology, the first two of which were on notions of self or personality in Greek and Hellenistic/Roman culture. The aims and scope of the present book, and its relationship to the two preceding ones, are set out in the first (introductory) chapter. An overview of Galenic and Stoic thinking on psychology, located in the framework of their theories as a whole, is provided in the first section of Chapter 2.

In writing this book, I have had very generous support which I am happy to acknowledge here. In 2003–6, I held a Leverhulme Major Research Fellowship, which enabled me both to complete the preceding book on ancient psychology, *The Structured Self in Hellenistic and Roman Thought* (Oxford University Press, 2006) and to write a first draft of the present book. In 2006–7, my research was supported by the University of Exeter and the Arts and Humanities Research Council Study Leave scheme, which allowed me to complete a final version. I am grateful to two anonymous readers for the Press (at different stages), and also to my colleague John Wilkins, for constructive comments which have helped me to improve this version further. I would like to thank Hilary O'Shea for her advice and support and also all the staff involved at Oxford University Press for their cooperativeness and efficiency.

During the period of my work on this book, the Department of Classics and Ancient History at Exeter has emerged as a leading centre for research on Galen, with John Wilkins and, more recently, Julius Rocca also working on different aspects of Galen's rich legacy of writings. Our collaborative activities have included a two-day research workshop on Galen (2003) and an international conference on 'Galen and the World of Knowledge' (2005), with a volume based on the conference published in 2009 with Cambridge University Press. Another international conference, 'Teleology in the Ancient World: The Dispensation of Nature' (2009), has explored the interplay between ancient philosophical and medical approaches to the idea of natural design. We have also had a large number of seminars on Galen either as part of our weekly Department seminar series or in conjunction with the Exeter Centre for Medical History, with which our work on ancient medicine is increasingly linked. Parts of this book have been presented as papers in these seminars. More recently, I have become involved, with other Exeter colleagues, in the 'Galen in English' project (a series of new translations with introduction and notes, directed by Philip van der Eijk), the first of which will be on Galen's shorter psychological works. Cooperation in this work has been highly informative and congenial. Discussions on Galen with colleagues and other scholars have been immensely helpful to me in working on this book, particularly as sustained study of Galen (as distinct from Stoicism) is a relatively new interest for me.

While writing the book, I have also given papers on Galen and Stoicism at the Southern Association for Ancient Philosophy at Oxford (2005) and a conference on 'Body and Soul' in Hamburg (2007), and also a paper on Galenic psychology at the Institute of Classical Studies, London University. Responses to these papers have been acute and useful. The first two papers have been published, are included in the References at the end of the book (as Gill 2007*a* and 2009), and are cited in footnotes (like my other published work) when their content is close to that of any part of this book.

My wife Karen died during the final stages of the production of this book, after a long illness, though with periods of remission. Throughout this illness she showed a searching energy, a sense of fun and joy in living, and a deep concern for others, rather than herself, that were inspirational to many people. Her qualities have been a source of strength to our four sons and me as we help each other to rebuild our lives. This book is dedicated jointly to them and Karen with great love.

C.G.

Contents

Note on Conventions

Typical references to Galen's works in this book take this form:

Gal. *PHP* V.287–8, 3.10–11, p. 170.9–16 De Lacy
QAM IV.815–16, *SM* 2.73.16–74.21.

Normally, as in these two cases, the first reference (given in Roman and Arabic numerals) is to the standard Kühn edition (1819–33) of Galen's works (unless the work is not included in Kühn). This is followed by a reference (normally in Arabic numerals only) to a modern edition of the work in question. The second reference is to the book, chapter, page or line of the modern edition. Thus, the first reference here is to Book 3, chapters 10–11, p. 170 and lines 9–16 of De Lacy's edition of *PHP.* The second reference here is to *Scripta Minora* (full ref. given below), Book 2, from p. 73, line 16 to page 74, line 21. (The only other references given in a combination of Roman and Arabic numerals are to Kraus's edition of *Mor.* (Kraus 1939).) For abbreviations to Galen's works and the editions or translations cited by name alone, see 'Galen's Works Cited' below. For other commonly used abbreviations, see below.

The abbreviations for other ancient authors and works are normally those used by H. G. Liddell, R. Scott, and H. S. Jones, *A Greek–English Lexicon*, 9th edition (Oxford: Oxford University Press, 1940), or P. Glare (ed.), *Oxford Latin Dictionary* (Oxford: Oxford University Press, 1982). Authors and texts cited are given in full form in the Index of Ancient Passages. All quotations in Greek, Latin, and other foreign languages are translated. Translations are mine, unless otherwise attributed. Texts and translations are based on the most recent Oxford Classical Text (or, where none is available, Budé, Loeb, or Teubner edition), except as indicated. Where quotations are attributed to Long and Sedley (see full reference below), their translation is normally used, sometimes modified as indicated.

All secondary works cited by author and date are included in the References at the end of the book. Internal references are made by section (e.g. 5.2 below), or take this form: 'see text to nn. 13–14 above' (referring to the same chapter) or 'see Ch. 3 above, text to nn. 12–13'. 'He/she' or 'her/him' are used indifferently as indefinite personal pronouns, even when summarizing ancient authors who use only masculine pronouns for this purpose. When translating ancient authors, their practice of using masculine forms for this purpose is retained.

Commonly used abbreviations in this book, which do not appear in this form in Liddell, Scott, and Jones, or the *Oxford Latin Dictionary*, are as follows:

CMG *Corpus Medicorum Graecorum* (multi-volume series of editions of medical texts, normally with translation and commentary, published in Berlin by Akademie Verlag).

LS A. A. Long and D. N. Sedley, *The Hellenistic Philosophers*, 2 vols. Cambridge: Cambridge University Press, 1987 (references are normally to sections and passages).

SM I. Marquardt, I. Müller, G. Helmreich (eds.), *Claudii Galeni Pergameni Scripta Minora*, 3 vols. Leipzig: Teubner, 1884–93, repr. Amsterdam: Hakkert, 1967.

SVF H. von Arnim (ed.), *Stoicorum Veterum Fragmenta*, 4 vols. Leipzig: Teubner, 1903–5, repr. Munich: Sauer, 2004.

Galen's Works Cited

This list includes all Galen's works cited in this book. The list gives (1) the abbreviation used throughout the book, (2) the standard Latin title (though most of the works are in Greek), (3) the English title used here. In some cases, the Latin title is followed by the edition normally cited here (usually in the *Corpus Medicorum Graecorum* Series (*CMG*)); and sometimes the English title is followed by the English translation normally cited here (when this is not identical with the *CMG* edition). The Latin titles and abbreviations used are based on those given in Kollesch and Nickel (1994) or Hankinson 2008*c*, appendix 1 (a very useful list). The English titles used are those given in Hankinson 2008*c*, appendix 2, except in the case of *Aff. Dig.*, *Indol.*, *Mor.*, *Pecc. Dig.*, and *QAM*. For these works I use the English titles adopted in Singer forthcoming. All editions and translations noted here by author and date alone are cited in full in the References. The order of Galenic works listed here is alphabetical, based on the Latin abbreviation used.

AA	*De Anatomicis Administrationibus. On Anatomical Procedures.*
Adv. Jul.	*Adversus Julianum. Against Julian.*
Aff. Dig.	*De Proprium Animi Cuiuslibet Affectuum Dignotione et Curatione. Diagnosis and Treatment of Psychological Affections* (in short, *Psychological Affections*) (Singer 1997*a*).
An. Ut.	*An Animal Sit Quod in Utero Geritur. Is the Embryo an Animal?*
Ars Med.	*Ars Medica. Art of Medicine* (Singer 1997*a*).
Art. Sang.	*An in Arteriis Sanguis. On Whether Blood is Contained in the Arteries.*
Caus. Puls.	*De Causis Pulsuum. Causes of Pulses.*
Foet. Form.	*De Foetuum Formatione* (Nickel 2001). *On the Construction of the Embryo* (Singer 1997*a*).

Hipp. Elem.	*De Elementis ex Hippocrate* (De Lacy 1996). *On the Elements according to Hippocrates.*
Hipp. Epid.	*In Hippocrates Epidemiarum Libri I–VI. On Hippocrates' 'Epidemics'.*
Hipp. Off. Med.	*In Hippocratis De Officina Medici. On Hippocrates' 'Surgery'.*
Indol.	*De Indolentia. Avoiding Distress* (Boudon-Millot 2007*b*).
Int.	*Introductio seu Medicus. Introduction.*
Lib. Prop.	*De Libris Propriis. On My Own Books* (Singer 1997*a*).
Loc. Aff.	*De Locis Affectis. On Affected Parts.*
MM	*Methodos Medendi. On the Therapeutic Method.*
MMG	*Ad Glauconem de Methodo Medendi. Therapeutics to Glaucon.*
Mor.	*De Moribus. Character Traits* (Mattock 1972).
Nat. Fac.	*De Naturalibus Facultatibus. On the Natural Faculties* (Brock 1916).
Nerv. Diss.	*De Nervorum Dissectione. On the Anatomy of the Nerves.*
Opt. Doct.	*De Optima Doctrina. On the Best Method of Teaching.*
Opt. Med.	*Quod Optimus Medicus sit quoque Philosophus. The Best Doctor is also a Philosopher.*
Ord. Lib. Prop.	*De Ordine Librorum Proprium. The Order of My Own Books* (Singer 1997*a*).
Oss.	*De Ossibus ad Tirones. On Bones for Beginners.*
Pecc. Dig.	*De Animi Cuiuslibet Peccatorum Dignotione et Curatione. Diagnosis and Treatment of Psychological Errors* (in short, *Psychological Errors*).
PHP	*De Placitis Hippocratis et Platonis.* (De Lacy 2005) *On the Doctrines of Hippocrates and Plato.*
Plat. Tim.	*In Platonis Timaeum* (Larrain 1992). *On Plato's Timaeus.*
Praen.	*De Praecognitione* (Nutton 1979). *On Prognosis.*
Prop. Plac.	*De Propriis Placitis* (Nutton 1999, Boudon-Millot and Pietrobelli 2005). *On My Own Opinions.*

QAM	*Quod Animi Mores Corporis Temperamenta Sequantur. Psychological Faculties Depend on Bodily Mixtures* (Singer 1997*a*).
San. Tu.	*De Sanitate Tuenda. On the Preservation of Health.*
Sem.	*De Semine* (De Lacy 1992). *On Semen.*
SMT	*De Simplicium Medicamentorum Temperamentis ac Facultatibus. On the Properties of Simple Drugs.*
Symp. Diff.	*De Symptomatum Differentiis. Differences of Symptoms.*
Temp.	*De Temperamentis. On Mixtures* (Singer 1997*a*).
UP	*De Usu Partium* (Helmreich 1907–9). *On the Utility of the Parts* (May 1968).
Ven. Art. Diss.	*De Venarum Arteriarumque Dissectione. On the Anatomy of Veins and Arteries.*

1

Introductory: Galen and Stoicism—Paradoxes and Potential

This introductory chapter sets out in very broad terms the main aims, themes, and argument of the book. I do not try here to offer an introduction to Galen and Stoicism more generally. However, in 2.1 I place Galenic and Stoic thought on psychology within the larger framework of their theories as a whole and I also refer there to general studies of Galen and Stoicism. Elsewhere in the book, I provide the information or background needed to make sense of the topic under discussion at any one time. Here, my focus is on exploring the underlying project or agenda of the book, and thus to give a framework for the detailed treatment of specific topics later on.

This book is a study of Galenic and Stoic ideas about human psychology. More specifically, it examines the *relationship* between Galenic and Stoic psychological thinking. I explore how Galen responds—often very critically—to Stoic ideas and how far those criticisms are justified. I also suggest that, if we get behind Galen's critical reaction to Stoicism, we can see that the two theories have a good deal in common and that they are complementary in important respects. There is a paradox, therefore, in the fact that Galen is so remorselessly critical of a theory with which he has potentially much in common. I think that the two theories could have been fruitfully combined and that the combination would have yielded a more convincing and powerful account of human psychology than either theory offers on its own. The Galenic and Stoic theories, taken separately, are highly illuminating in different ways; but, had they been combined, the outcome might have been the most compelling account of human psychology in antiquity. The combination of the two theories would also have anticipated certain striking features of modern thought about psychology and psychotherapy.

Galen was a major medical practitioner and writer in the second century AD (129–*c*.216); Stoicism originated in the Hellenistic era (from the late fourth to the late first century BC), though it remained an important philosophical tradition until at least Galen's time. Galen left a huge body of works; this book focuses on those Galenic texts that are relevant for psychology, especially *On the Doctrines of Hippocrates and Plato* (*PHP*),[1] while placing these writings in the context of his thought and medical work as a whole. I also give special attention to the Stoic works on psychology that Galen discusses, especially Chrysippus' (lost) treatises *On the Psyche*[2] and *On Passions*. The book is centred more on Galen than on Stoicism, in that it takes its starting-point from Galen's response to Stoicism and the thinking that underlies this response. But, in another sense, the book is equally about both theories; more precisely, it is about the relationship, actual and potential, between them. Although Stoicism continued as an active movement until Galen's time and we have Stoic writings surviving from the first and second centuries AD, under the Roman Empire, Galen directs his attention to Stoicism in its original, Hellenistic form, especially the treatises of Chrysippus, the third head and main theorist of the school (*c*.280–*c*.206 BC). So the relationship being studied here is an asymmetrical one, between a second-century AD medical writer and practitioner and a third-century BC philosophical theory, but, nonetheless, one that is fully alive for Galen and his contemporaries. It is also a relationship that I seek to bring to life for modern readers, by accentuating its importance in the history of ideas about psychology and its implications for modern thought. In this respect, the book is about two kinds of reception, Galen's reception of Stoic psychology and our, contemporary, reception of this reception; and both kinds of response make up the intellectual programme for this book.

[1] For abbreviations for titles of all Galen's works noted in this book, see 'Galen's Works Cited' above.

[2] Here and elsewhere in this book, I normally treat 'psyche' (*psuchē*) as a naturalized English term. As is often noted, the English terms used to translate this term (e.g. 'mind', 'soul', 'personality') are all to some degree misleading in their connotations.

What kinds of topic are treated here? There are three main themes. One is the relationship between bodily form (human anatomy and physiology) and psychological function. A second is the relationship between different psychological functions, especially reason and emotion. A third is the therapy of emotions, a method practised on the assumption that emotions (or at least *some* types of emotion) count as 'sicknesses' and need to be cured. Both Galen and the Stoics have complex and well-developed ideas about each of these themes and about how they are linked with each other.[3] To make full sense of these themes, we need to consider several related topics or questions. One is how Galenic or Stoic thought on psychology and the body fits in with their ideas about the proper methodology of natural inquiry and their philosophy of nature. Another is the sense in which each of these theories sees the human being as (in psychological terms) a unified whole or a collection of independent parts. Another relevant topic is the relationship between the therapy of emotions and medical treatment, including the question how far each of these forms of treatment is directed, wholly or mainly, at the person viewed as a psychological or bodily entity.[4]

The topics outlined are ones that anyone concerned with psychology, in virtually any sense of that term, might be interested in.[5] But what particular reason is there for giving close attention to Galenic and Stoic ideas on these topics—as opposed to any other ancient ideas—either as part of the history of thought on this topic or as potentially relevant to contemporary thought? More specifically, why is the *relationship* between Galenic and Stoic ideas of special significance, as I am suggesting? In essence, my answer to these questions is that these theories, though framed from different standpoints and possessing different strengths and weaknesses, are complementary in important ways that are not always appreciated. Their complementary nature is crucial for their potential interest for modern thought. Although each of the theories prefigures certain strands in contemporary thought about psychology, the combination of the two

[3] See Chs. 3, 4, and 5 below respectively on these topics.

[4] See 2.2–3, 4.4, 5.4 below on these topics.

[5] I set aside the question whether 'psychology' means the same thing in ancient and modern thought (on which see Everson 1991*a*); at any rate, the topics just noted are important ones in both ancient and modern versions of the study of psychology.

theories (had it occurred) would have offered a powerful anticipation of certain striking currents in modern thought.

The complementary character of the two theories derives partly from a shared approach to psychology and partly from the fact that they bring to this area different but compatible conceptual strengths. The common ground between them is indicated, in the first instance, by the term 'naturalistic', which is coupled with 'psychology' in the title of this book. 'Naturalistic', as will be explained later, has a number of meanings in this connection.[6] In the first instance, what I mean is that both theories conceive the human psyche as an integral part of an embodied organism (the human animal) which is seen in turn as an integral part of the natural world. There is a strong contrast with ancient (or modern) versions of mind–body dualism, especially Platonic ones, in which the psyche or mind is seen as belonging to a radically different type of being from the body or from the natural world in general.[7] Each of the two theories has a highly distinctive contribution to make to this shared naturalistic approach to psychology. Galen, in his voluminous writings, especially *PHP*, draws on, and synthesizes, medical (and also much philosophical) thinking on psychology and the body as this had evolved over a period of about six centuries; and for this reason alone he is immensely important for the study of ancient thought on this topic. But he also brings to bear a very cogent method of natural inquiry (one often seen as anticipating modern scientific method), which he applies with special effectiveness to a central question of ancient debate, the location of the 'ruling part' of the psyche or in modern terms, the mind. Galen's demonstration, by methodical examination, that this part is located in the brain, and that it operates through the body by means of the nervous system, is one of the major achievements of ancient medicine and science, and is also crucial in shaping Galen's entire approach to the study of human psychology.[8] Stoicism has no comparable contribution to make to the study of human anatomy or physiology, as this bears on human psychology. Indeed, the Stoics adopted and retained till

[6] See further Ch. 2 below, esp. 2.2–3.

[7] On this type of dualism in Plato and Middle Platonism, see Ch. 2, n. 41 below.

[8] See Ch. 2 below, text to nn. 102–10, 137–40.

Galen's time and beyond views on this topic that Galen attacks as both misguided and ill-supported, above all the belief that the ruling part of the psyche is located in the heart.[9] On the other hand, what Stoicism has to offer is, in the first instance, a highly coherent and fully theorized analysis of all the aspects of psychology treated in this book. These include their accounts of the relationship between different psychological functions, and between those functions and the body (in general terms at least), and related ideas about psychological sickness and therapy. As I bring out in the course of this study, the Stoic accounts are often significantly *more* theoretically consistent and credible than Galen's competing accounts.[10] Thus, these two ancient theories are of interest for modern readers, in part, because they offer two powerful and suggestive perspectives on human psychology, each of which has its own special strengths.

However, there is a more specific reason why the relationship between their theories on these topics is of particular interest and why it makes sense to study the two theories together. This is not simply because Galen himself discusses Stoic ideas on these topics, often critically, and is, indeed, a major source of evidence for their views. The reason is that, on certain key points, as I argue here, their ideas are complementary and could profitably have been combined. Most strikingly, Galen's anatomical account of the workings of the brain and nervous system would have fitted much better with the Stoic (unified) analysis of the functions of the ruling part of the psyche than it does with the Platonic tripartite psyche with which Galen actually tries to combine his anatomical account.[11] Also, the Stoic arguments for a body-based account of the psyche, and their explanation how this is compatible with ideas of agency and responsibility are ones which, I maintain, would also have fitted well with at least some aspects of Galenic thinking about embodied psychology and the management of emotions.[12] In both respects, a combination of Galenic and Stoic ideas could have produced a more powerful and compelling version of the naturalistic conception of human psychology than either theory is able to offer on its own. On aspects of psychology less closely linked with the body, the scope for

[9] See 2.2 below.

[10] See further 3.2–3, 3.5, 4.2–4, 5.2–4 below.

[11] See 3.2–3 below.

[12] See 3.5 below.

collaboration between the two theories is less obvious. Certainly, on the reason–emotion relationship, and on the question how far the human psyche should be conceived as forming a whole or a collection of independent parts, Galen and the Stoics seem very far apart.[13] However, even on this topic, we can ask how far this disagreement was inevitable, and whether, for instance, Galen's account of the role of the brain might have been combined with the Stoic view that the mind (*hēgemonikon*) embraces and integrates rational and emotional functions.[14] On the subject of the therapy of emotions, Galen, at least sometimes, adopts a rather Stoic-style approach, though one that is at odds with the Platonic-style views about psychological functions that he also embraces in this context. Here too, the combination of Galenic and Stoic ideas could have led to a more coherent overall theory.[15] A further, and still more suggestive, combination might have been that of Galen's medical method of treatment, directed primarily at the body, and the Stoic therapy of the emotions, directed at the person as a psychological agent. This would have brought together what are, arguably, the most highly developed and cogent examples of these respective practices in antiquity.[16] Thus, the scope for creating a coherent and effective set of Galenic and Stoic ideas, based on the fact that they share a naturalistic conception of human psychology, was very considerable; and the creation of such a combination would have had very substantial implications for the history of human thought on psychology.

However, in practice, this combination was not created. The Stoics—at least the Hellenistic Stoics—were, obviously, not in a position to produce this synthesis and Galen, though he was in this position, did not do so.[17] On the contrary, Galen's most ambitious and wide-ranging work on psychology, *On the Doctrines of Hippocrates and Plato*, is dominated, at least in Books 2–5, by a thoroughgoing *attack* on Stoic ideas about embodied psychology and psychological functions. Hence, it may seem rather pointless to spend time reflecting on the outcome of a hypothetical, but

[13] See 4.2–4 below. [14] See 4.1 below, text to nn. 25–7.

[15] See 5.2 below, text to nn. 28–76. [16] See 5.4 below, esp. text to nn. 314–26.

[17] See further on the two theories and their attitudes to partnership with other theories 2.1 below, including text to nn. 83–7 on the Stoics of Galen's own time.

unrealized, combination of Galenic and Stoic ideas. It might seem to make better sense to concentrate on Galen's actual intellectual combinations of medical and Platonic (or Aristotelian) philosophical ideas in psychology. Of course, I accept that it is worthwhile to explore those intellectual combinations too, as I do to some extent in this book.[18] But there are several reasons why it is, in my view, worthwhile to go beyond Galen's actual intellectual alliances and to consider other possible ones, as well as to subject to critical examination some of the attempts he does make at such combination.

One reason is that doing so brings out more clearly the degree of conceptual consistency or inconsistency between different aspects of ancient thinking about psychology. As stressed in Chapter 3, there is a rather glaring inconsistency between Galen's anatomically based account of the workings of the brain and nervous system and the three-centre theory of psychological functions that Galen adopts from Plato. There is scope for a much more consistent account, namely between the Galenic theory of the role of the brain and the Stoic theory of the functions of the ruling part of the psyche. The common feature is that both theories presuppose a single, unified centre of psychological activity.[19] The fact that no one in antiquity actually thought of producing this combination of ideas does not make it any less conceptually consistent. A similar point could be made about the other types of combination discussed in this study. The Stoic account of mind–body relations (an explicitly physicalist one) is—arguably, at least—more consistent with Galen's ideas about embodied psychological functions than any account of this topic which he actually offers. Indeed, on both these topics, there are indications of internal tension or contradiction (or of vacillation and ambiguity, in the case of mind–body relations) in Galen's thinking, which could have been avoided by the combination of Galenic and Stoic ideas envisaged here.[20] Similarly, the combination of Galenic-style medical treatment directed at the body and Stoic therapy directed at the person as psychological agent represents a conceptually possible and consistent one, albeit one that was never adopted in antiquity.[21] Hence, exploring these counterfactual combinations of

[18] See e.g. 3.2, 4.3 below, on Galen's use of Platonic (and Platonic–Aristotelian) psychology. [19] See 3.2–3 below. [20] See 3.5 below.
[21] See 5.4 below.

ideas is not a mere exercise in historical fantasy (or the idea of 'what if?') conducted for its own sake. It is a means of analysing the consistency or inconsistency of psychological ideas in a way that goes beyond the combinations we actually find in antiquity, while also, I would suggest, shedding a revealing light on those combinations.

There is a second reason for pursuing these hypothetical combinations and one that relates to our own contemporary perspective on these topics. I suggested earlier that this book can be understood both as a study of Galen's reception of Stoic ideas—and his *possible* reception of them—and also as a modern response to Galen's reception. As I bring out in Chapter 6, some at least of the combinations of Galenic and Stoic ideas envisaged in this book would produce theories that are very close to some modern ones. The most obvious example is the combination of the idea that the mind forms a single psychological centre, combining rational and emotional functions, and the idea that it is located in the brain and operates on the body as a whole through the nervous system. This is, more or less, the standard modern picture, and it is very close to the Galenic–Stoic synthesis that I posit here. Indeed, if we explore the analogy in more detail, certain strands in recent research on the functions of the brain, on the one hand, and in the philosophy of mind and emotion, on the other, are strikingly similar to the kind of Galenic–Stoic synthesis I have in view.[22] The position is rather less straightforward as regards the relationship between modern practices of psychiatry or psychotherapy and ancient medical or philosophical forms of therapy. However, in this area too, there are some suggestive analogues between, for instance, modern medical approaches to mental illness and Galenic body-based medicine, on the one hand, and between modern psychotherapeutic methods and those of Stoic psychological therapy, on the other. More generally, it is instructive to consider in the modern context as well as the ancient one the implications of a combination of Galenic-style medical treatment and Stoic-style psychological therapy.[23] I should make it plain that, in highlighting these actual or potential links between ancient and modern ideas, I am not assuming that modern beliefs are necessarily right or normative, or that ancient ideas are valid only in so far as they approximate to

[22] See 6.2 below. [23] See 6.3 below.

modern ones. My point is the different one that exploring these analogies across cultures and periods helps to bring out the conceptual coherence or psychological credibility of the Galenic–Stoic combinations I posit here. Also, accentuating the analogies underlines the point that these Galenic and Stoic combinations are of more than simply historical interest today, even if those ideas are based on very different methods and assumptions from those of much modern theory and practice.

What does this book add to previous scholarship on Stoicism or Galen? On the whole, the book has more to offer in new interpretation of Galen than of Stoicism, especially in helping to place Galen's thinking on psychology (under the various headings considered here) within the larger framework of ancient thought. But the aim, above all, is to add to our understanding of the *relationship* between the two theories and to reflect on the conceptual implications of this relationship for the historical study of ideas about psychology.

On both theories, the last twenty years or so have been ones of intense scholarly activity, and the book builds on this work. In the case of Stoicism, along with most recent treatments, I assume that their theory of human psychology, for instance as regards emotions, is credible and coherent, though it has often been seen in ancient and modern times as lacking in plausibility or coherence.[24] The book aims especially to advance our understanding of Stoic ideas about embodied psychology, psychological wholeness and partition, and psychological health and sickness, by correlating their thinking on these subjects with that of Galen.[25] The book also builds on recent scholarship, both textual and exegetical, on Galen. I take account, for instance, of some new discoveries: the complete Greek text of *On My Own Opinions* and the recently found *Avoiding Distress*.[26] I also draw on much recent illuminating and acute interpretative analysis of Galen's thought and ideas.[27] However, in writing this book, I have become aware how much fundamental work still needs to be done on Galen, both in making

[24] See 4.2 below. [25] See 3.2, 3.5, 4.4, and 5.3–4 below.

[26] See 3.5 below, text to nn. 219–23, 249–51, and 5.2 below, text to nn. 78–98.

[27] Hankinson 2008*c* offers a useful selection of such work. The survey of Galenic psychology in 2.1 below indicates some of the scholars on whose work I have drawn.

texts and translations more available and in exploring their content and significance. A welcome new development is a series of English translations of Galenic works with commentary, the first volume of which (in which I am involved) will be on the shorter psychological works. Parts of this book can be seen as providing supporting commentary to that volume.[28] More broadly, I hope this book will contribute to making Galen's thought better known among scholars and students of ancient philosophy and Classical studies generally as well as those focusing on ancient medicine. I also hope that it will communicate the intellectual cogency of Galenic and Stoic ideas to readers primarily interested in the history of philosophy or psychology.

One scholar's previous work in this area needs special comment. In two major, path-breaking, books (1996 and 2003*a*), Teun Tieleman sets out both to examine the methodology and background of Galen's critique of Stoic ideas in *PHP* 1–3 and 4–5 and to reconstruct the Stoic theories (on the location of the ruling part of the psyche and on emotions) that Galen criticizes there. More precisely, he aims, in effect, to rescue the Stoic theories from Galen's misrepresentation, a task which is especially important because Galen is such a vital source for the theories.[29] Tieleman's reconstructions of Chrysippus' *On the Psyche* and *On Passions* seem to me highly convincing, and I have drawn fully on these here, though sometimes qualifying aspects of his analysis.[30] Indeed, I do not think it would make much sense for me to write the kind of book attempted here without the pioneering and meticulous mapping of the subject offered by Tieleman. However, there are some salient differences between our approaches. I offer a more broadly based, and in certain respects more speculative, reflection on the conceptual relationship between these two ancient theories of psychology, and on their significance for modern thought.

28 Singer forthcoming, in a planned series whose general editor is Philip van der Eijk. See esp. 3.5 and 5.2 below.

29 The long-term objective of Tieleman's work, and that of other Utrecht scholars, is to supplement or replace the standard collection of sources for Stoicism (*SVF*=von Arnim 1903–5) with source-books based on better methodological and interpretative principles.

30 See 3.2 and 5.2 below; for some qualifications to his interpretations, which in general I accept, see e.g. 4.4 below, text to nn. 234–43, 259–67, 5.4 below, text to nn. 267–89.

As already indicated, I give special attention to the question how far the two theories are intellectually compatible and could, indeed, have been combined (by Galen), a question not addressed by Tieleman. I hope that, taken together, our books on Galen and Stoicism on psychology will be seen as offering complementary analyses which throw new light on both of these, very rich, ancient theories.

It is also worthwhile to correlate my aims in this book with that of my two previous books on ancient psychology (1996 and 2006), of which the present one is in some ways a continuation. Both earlier books were framed as studies of ancient ideas about personality or self; and it was my original intention to present this book in the same way, though in the event I have offered it under the broader heading of 'psychology'. My first book in this area, *Personality in Greek Epic, Tragedy, and Philosophy: The Self in Dialogue* (1996), was devoted equally to literature and philosophy (Plato and Aristotle). It was also focused equally on study of ancient ideas about psychological functions and about interpersonal and communal relationships. A major theme was the contrast between 'subjective-individualist' and 'objective-participant' conceptions of person, coupled with the claim that the Greek archaic and Classical thought expressed the latter—but not the former—conception.[31] My second book, *The Structured Self in Hellenistic and Roman Thought* (2006), as well as treating a later period of ancient thought, was more exclusively focused on ancient philosophy, though it dealt also with the reception of philosophical ideas in Hellenistic and Roman literature (ch. 7). I also deployed there the contrast between 'subjective-individualist' and 'objective-participant' conceptions of person, as part of a critique of the commonly held view that Hellenistic and Roman thought expresses a shift towards a more subjective or individualistic conception of person (ch. 6).

The present book is closely related to the preceding one (2006) in period and in its focus on theoretical ideas, rather than on literature. As brought out shortly, some of my main claims here can be defined, in part, by reference to categories and themes explored in the earlier book. However, the present book is distinctive in its focus on the Galen–Stoicism relationship, in which Galen is treated as a thinker of

[31] See Gill 1996, esp. Introduction and ch. 6.

equal interest, and not just as a source or critic of Stoic ideas, as in my previous work.[32] Correspondingly, this book gives special weight to questions that naturally arise within this relationship, including questions about the interface between bodily form and psychological functions and about how psychological therapy is related to medical treatment,[33] questions which have not had a comparable importance in my previous work. More broadly, the book seeks to correlate ancient medical and philosophical approaches to psychology in a way that goes beyond anything I have attempted elsewhere. Although this book shares a number of themes with its two predecessors (including the study of psychological functions and the question how far human beings constitute psychological wholes),[34] I have not framed the book as a study of 'personality' or 'selfhood'. Although I still retain a strong interest in that subject,[35] I think that the main topics treated here (psychology and the body, the reason–emotion relationship, and the therapy of emotions) are best presented under those headings, rather than as forming part of a study of the self. For related reasons, the contrast between 'subjective-individualist' and 'objective-participant' conceptions of person is not deployed here, though I think that the latter conception is the relevant one for the kind of ideas treated in this book. This book might be seen as providing part of the material for a study of second-century AD thinking on 'the self', though such a study would also probably need, like my 1996 book, to embrace ideas about social and personal relationships and to correlate theory and literature in the period.[36]

I close this introductory chapter by showing how the special character and potential of the Galen–Stoicism relationship can be defined by reference to themes explored in my preceding book on Hellenistic and Roman thought (2006). I suggested there that what is distinctive about Stoic (and, in a different way, Epicurean) thinking

[32] Contrast, to some extent at least, the approach of Gill 2006: ch. 5 (also Gill 1983 and 1998). [33] See Ch. 3, 5.4, and 6.3 below. [34] See esp. Ch. 4 below.

[35] See Gill 2008*b–d*, esp. 2008*c*, which sets out my view of the possible future of this subject.

[36] I do not at present plan to write a book on this subject; for some relevant discussions, see Foucault 1990, Reydams-Schils 2005, Sorabji 2007, Trapp 2007: chs. 4–5.

about human nature and psychology is a striking combination of naturalism, holism, and revisionism. Both these Hellenistic theories combine a naturalistic view of human beings, as embodied animals that form an integral part of nature, with a strongly unified or holistic world-view and conception of knowledge. They also combine these features with certain radical (Socratic or quasi-Socratic) ethical claims and with a tendency to revise or modify categories and ideas which are prominent in the pre-existing philosophical tradition. In all three respects (naturalism, holism, and revisionism), there are salient points of contrast with important features of Platonic or Aristotelian thought. However, there are also aspects of Platonic and Aristotelian thought which may have helped to shape the emergence of these features of Stoic and Epicurean thought.[37] In the post-Hellenistic period (from the first century BC until the second century AD), we can see signs of a reaction against these aspects of Stoic and Epicurean thought, particularly in thinkers influenced by the synthesis of Platonic and Aristotelian ideas that contribute to the intellectual movement we call 'Middle Platonism'. A special target is the Stoic theory of emotions or passions, which reflects their strongly unified or holistic psychological theory. This is the object of intense criticism by thinkers including Plutarch and Galen, who presuppose the Platonic–Aristotelian view that the psyche consists of a complex of rational and non-rational parts, and who see the Stoic account as misguided or inconsistent, rather than as expressing a substantively different conceptual framework.[38] Hence, Galen's critical response to Stoic ideas about the reason–emotion relationship and about the therapy of emotions in *PHP* 4–5 can usefully be located in the broader picture of the intellectual cross-currents in Hellenistic and early Roman Imperial thought studied in my earlier book. This helps us to understand the intensity of Galen's critique of Stoic ideas about emotions and emotional therapy and his failure to acknowledge its distinctive qualities (despite the fact that he sometimes adopts aspects of the Stoic approach to emotional therapy).[39]

One of the themes just mentioned, that of holism, is worth exploring more fully here, using concepts not found in my earlier

[37] See Gill 2006: chs. 1–2. [38] See Gill 2006: ch. 4.

[39] See 4.2 below, also 5.2, text to nn. 31–44.

books, since this offers an illuminating broader perspective on several of the aspects of the Galen–Stoicism relationship treated in the course of this book. It also helps to show that Galen's relationship to Stoic thought is a complex one, involving points of similarity as well as contrast. This underlies the central claim made in this book, namely that a combination of certain features of Galenic and Stoic thought about psychology could have produced a set of ideas which is more powerful than either theory taken in isolation.

One of the topics that arise in the Galen–Stoicism relationship is the question of how to understand the relationship between parts and wholes, for instance, as regards the nature of the human psyche. In discussing this question, it is useful to refer to a general theoretical contrast sometimes drawn in modern philosophy between two different ways of understanding the part–whole relationship.[40] We can identify two patterns of thought, one (atomistic or pluralistic) pattern associated with the idea of 'composition' and the other (holistic) pattern associated with 'structure'. The conceptual difference between the two patterns of thought can be brought out in a number of ways. In the first pattern ('composition'), to put it very broadly, the focus is on the parts and in the other ('structure') it is on the whole. More precisely, the contrast is between seeing the whole as identical with, and defined by, the combination of its parts and seeing the whole as the primary locus of identity, to which the parts are subordinate. In the first pattern ('composition'), the parts are identifiable independently of the whole, and in the second ('structure'), the parts are identifiable only in the context of the whole. In the first pattern, we can say that the whole *has* structure (understood as the combination of its parts), in the other, the whole *is* structure (which gives the parts their identity).

These contrasting patterns of thought can be used in various ways, for instance, to define types or categories of reality or knowledge. I am using them here as a way of characterizing different types of explanation or analysis, which can be applied to the understanding of psychology, the scope of knowledge, or reality in general. More specifically, I use them to identify features of Stoic and Galenic

[40] The rest of this paragraph is based on Gill 2007*a*: 95–6. The formulations that follow are taken from Harte 2002: 158–67, 267–81, an analysis of Platonic thinking about the part–whole relationship.

thought which are either distinctive of one of the theories or held in common with the other theory. For instance, I think there are a number of features in Stoic thought that reflect an intellectual outlook centred on 'structure', rather than 'composition'. On a series of important topics, the Stoics argue for a radically unified or holistic view in a way that runs counter to conventional ideas and standard philosophical distinctions and categories, particularly those of the Platonic or Aristotelian framework. This point applies to the Stoic conception of the human being as (like other animals) a unified psychophysical structure, as distinct from a combination of psyche and body.[41] It applies to their view of the human mind or 'control-centre' (*hēgemonikon*) as a unified locus of psychological functions, including those normally subdivided between reason, emotion, and desire.[42] It also applies to their conception of the spectrum of natural kinds (*scala naturae*), which cuts across standard distinctions between living and non-living entities.[43] The Stoics also adopt in a very strong form an idea prevalent in Hellenistic and Roman thought, namely that complete knowledge consists in a combination, and to some degree synthesis, of the three main branches of philosophy, namely logic, ethics, and physics.[44] Their views about the relationship between the three branches of knowledge have a direct bearing on their radical and revisionist conception of the emotions or passions and of what constitutes a fully 'rational' psychological process or state.[45]

If Stoic thought expresses, in a consistent way, a holistic or 'structure' approach, combined with revision of more familiar ideas and categories, how should we characterize Galenic thought in comparable areas? What we find, I think, is not so much a systematic contrast between the two theories in this respect, but, rather, a mixed or complex position, and one that bears directly on the question raised here, how far Galenic and Stoic thinking is conceptually compatible.

[41] See Gill 2006: 29–46; also Ch. 2 below, text to nn. 218–22, Ch. 3 below, text to nn. 257–77.

[42] See Gill 2006: 75–7; also Ch. 4 below, text to nn. 90–115.

[43] See Gill 2006: 31–2; also Ch. 2 below, text to nn. 206–12.

[44] See LS 26: Gill 2006: 160–2, 199–200; also Annas 1999: 109–12 and 2007.

[45] See Ch. 4 below, text to nn. 116–57, 262–7, Ch. 5 below, text to nn. 272–85. Their ideas on these topics reflect a close linkage between psychology (which, in Stoicism, falls partly under 'physics') and ethics. See also Gill 2005: 454–7.

The area where this contrast in patterns of thought is most strongly marked is that of their respective conceptions of psychological functions in *PHP* 4–5, including a debate about the nature of psychic illness and health, which centres on divergent ways of understanding the relationship between psychic parts and wholes. Galen's bafflement by—or refusal to understand—Stoic thinking on these topics seems to point to a deeper conceptual gulf between the two theories. This gulf seems to derive, at least partly, from the contrast between holistic and atomistic approaches to human psychology.[46] It also reflects Galen's failure—or refusal—to recognize that the Stoic view of emotions as psychic illnesses expresses certain radical (Socratic-style) ethical claims, which run counter to standard ways of thinking about psychological stability or instability and about what psychological illness and cure involve. Galen's reaction against Stoic holism and revisionism makes this aspect of human psychology one on which their conceptual frameworks seem most deeply opposed and antithetical.[47]

However, I do not think this conceptual contrast applies equally to all aspects of Galenic and Stoic thought. There are features of Galen's thinking, for instance, which also express an aspiration towards a thoroughly unified or holistic outlook. For instance, his project of grounding medicine on an encyclopaedic body of knowledge (including much knowledge drawn from philosophy) reflects this approach. So does his comprehensive analysis of the natural universe in terms of mixtures of elements and his systematically teleological account of the organization of the animal body.[48] This point holds good even if the Stoic philosophy of nature is, as suggested later, significantly, *more* holistic than Galenic and involves a more radical revision of traditional categories of thought.[49] Also, Galen's anatomically based account of the role of the brain and the nervous system, arguably, implies a highly unified psychological model. On the other hand, there are aspects of Galen's thinking about embodied psychology that are in sharp contrast with this unified or holistic view, and also with Stoic thinking on the same subject. For the Stoics, the

[46] See Ch. 4 below, esp. 4.4. [47] See 4.2 and 5.4 below.

[48] See below 2.1, text to nn. 6–10, 2.2, text to nn. 91–4, and 2.3, text to nn. 157–73. Galen's aspiration to create his own 'world of knowledge' is a recurrent theme in Gill, Whitmarsh, and Wilkins 2009. [49] See Ch. 2 below, text to nn. 197–212.

hēgemonikon is the unitary centre of a unified psychophysical system. But, for Galen—at least as far as psychological functions are concerned—the *hēgemonikon* is one (dominant) centre in a composite psyche made up of three, independent centres, housed in brain, heart, and liver respectively. For Galen, these are loci for three different types of psychological process (reasoning, emotion, and appetite), whereas for the Stoics these and other psychological processes are, in adult humans, functions of a single, unified, rational centre.[50]

Although Galen, again, rejects, or fails fully to understand, the holistic character of the Stoic conception, this does not, in this case, reflect a radical difference in their way of thinking about embodied psychology. Indeed, as just noted, Galen's anatomically based account of the role of the brain and nervous system implies, precisely, this kind of unified picture of psychophysiological workings. Hence, one can claim that the Stoic account of the role of the *hēgemonikon* is more consistent with Galen's anatomical picture than is the three-centre (Platonic-style) theory that he actually adopts. To put the point differently, there are competing strands in Galen's account of embodied psychology, especially as presented in *PHP* 1–3, which might have been resolved if Galen had been prepared to adopt a Stoic-style unified psychological model rather than a Platonic tripartite one.[51] Thus, the broad contrast between holistic and atomistic (or 'structure' and 'composition') conceptual frameworks can be used to highlight tensions within Galen's own psychological theory as well as points of conflict between Galenic and Stoic thinking. The contrast also helps us to see the force of the suggestion that at least some Galenic and Stoic ideas could have been combined in a way that would have benefited both of these theories. Thus, this contrast brings out both the potential for combination between Galenic and Stoic ideas and the paradoxical fact that Galen devotes so much energy to rejecting a theory with which he has, in certain key respects, much in common.

[50] See 3.2–3 below. [51] See, again, 3.2–3 below.

2

Galenic and Stoic Psychology: Two Versions of Naturalism

2.1 GALENIC AND STOIC PSYCHOLOGY: PROJECTS AND PARTNERS

So far, I have set out the claims to be made in this book in very general terms. In this chapter, I locate these claims in a more specific, and historically grounded, survey of the two theories and of their relationship. This survey sets the scene for the more detailed discussion of key aspects of Galenic and Stoic psychology (in Chapters 3–5) that carries the main argument of the book. I first consider where the topic of psychology sits in the larger framework of Galenic and Stoic thinking. Also, since my claim is that the two psychological theories could have been profitably combined, I discuss how far, and in what way, each theory was, in fact, open to partnership (explicit or implicit) with other approaches. Second, I compare the theories in two respects, their thinking about the methodology of natural inquiry and the philosophy of nature (2.2–3). This comparison identifies important features of their relationship and provides crucial background for subsequent chapters, especially Chapter 3, on Galenic and Stoic thought about psychology and the body. The comparison also reinforces the claim made here, that the Galenic and Stoic theories have in common a naturalistic approach to psychology, and more generally, by contrast with some other ancient theories, especially that of Plato or thinkers in the Platonic tradition. This shared naturalism of approach renders more surprising, and regrettable, Galen's lack of interest in exploring intellectual partnership with

Stoicism, though here and elsewhere, I also consider explanations why Galen has such a critical or reserved attitude towards Stoicism.

First, then, where does the study of psychology sit within the two theories and what is their respective attitude to partnership with other theories? In this respect, as in some others, their approaches can be seen as contrasting but complementary. In Galen's writings, 'psychology' is not an obviously relevant subdivision,[1] but is, none the less, a topic that is relevant in various ways to his wide-ranging medico-philosophical project.[2] In fact, I think that Galen's most distinctive and original contributions to psychology arise out of key features of this project, namely his anatomically based study of the role of the brain and other bodily organs and his analysis of the physical basis of body and matter generally. 'Psychology' has a more explicit and securely defined place in Stoic theory. One might expect this to be the case since Stoicism is a philosophical system in a much more straightforward sense than Galen's thought is. Stoic thinking about psychology reflects what have been recognized since antiquity as striking features of their philosophy, namely its analytic coherence and systematic character, combined with great conceptual boldness and a fondness for paradox. Stoicism is much less impressive than Galenic thought in the empirical study of anatomy and of the physical basis of psychological functions. These differences between the two approaches contribute towards making them complementary. Stoicism would have gained by drawing on the anatomically based results of the work of Galen and his medical predecessors, and Galen would have profited by deploying the more fully theorized and internally consistent approach to psychology of Stoicism, as well as its unified or holistic account of psychological processes. Was it ever possible, in fact, for this kind of partnership to have occurred? As explained later, Galen was much more open to intellectual alliance than Stoicism seems to have been at any period, including Galen's lifetime. Hence, Galenic engagement with Stoic ideas was more likely than Stoic engagement with Galenic ideas, though in psychology, at least, this engagement actually occurred only to a limited extent.

[1] For Galen's own reviews of his writings, see *On My Own Books* (*Lib. Prop.*), *The Order of My Own Books* (*Ord. Lib. Prop.*). See also n. 3 below.

[2] On this project, see Nutton 2004: 230–47, also discussion below and 2.2 below.

Galen, unlike Aristotle or Stoic thinkers such as Chrysippus, did not write a full-scale treatise *On the Psyche*, that is, a work that sets out in analytic form a set of theorized claims about the psyche.[3] Also, Galen consistently refrains from expressing a view on certain questions which were central for such discussions, notably that of the nature or 'substance' (*ousia*) of the psyche, meaning whether it is physical or non-physical in nature and mortal or immortal. Galen maintains that these questions, along with a number of other major cruces of ancient theory, belong to purely speculative philosophy, rather than the kind of medically directed inquiry he is engaged in.[4] However, relevant Galenic works (especially *PHP* and *QAM*) do express views on related topics which fall squarely within the scope of treatises on the psyche from Aristotle onwards. These include the question whether the psyche has parts or not, the location of the ruling part of the psyche, and the functions of the psyche. Also, as Tieleman stresses, Galen uses concepts and distinctions that are central in the post-Aristotelian theory of psychology, especially the distinction between the capacities (*dunameis*) of the psyche and its parts (*merē* or *eidē*); 'parts' were conceived by Galen as spatially and physically distinct, whereas 'capacities' were only distinct in function. In these and other ways, Galen's terminology and thinking seem to show the influence of post-Aristotelian summaries of doctrines (what we call 'doxography') and of contemporary philosophical writing on this topic, especially in the Platonic tradition, even though he did not write a formal treatise on the psyche.[5]

Galen's seemingly cautious or ambivalent attitude towards the topics that had become typical of the theoretical study of the

[3] We now know, from the newly rediscovered text of *Prop. Plac.*, that Galen wrote a book *On the Psyche* (*Prop. Plac.* ch. 7, Boudon-Millot and Pietrobelli 2005: 179.26–9). But this seems to be a critical discussion of Chrysippus' identification of psyche with (physical) *pneuma*, also referred to in the same context (see also 3.5 below, esp. text to nn. 266–70). See also the Latin version of *Prop. Plac.* ch. 7, in Nutton 1999: 80, where Galen refers to the same work but without a title. The work cited does not seem to be a full-scale treatise *On the Psyche*, like that of Aristotle or Chrysippus.

[4] Other such questions, according to Galen, include whether the universe was created, whether there was a void outside the cosmos, and whether god is corporeal. See e.g. *PHP* V.766–7, 9.6.21–22 De Lacy, V.780, 9.7.9–11 De Lacy, *Prop. Plac.* 2.1–3, 3.1–4 Nutton. See further Donini 2008: 185–6, Hankinson 2008*a*: 178–80.

[5] Tieleman 1996: 8–12, 2003*a*: 61–88, 2003*b*; also Mansfeld 1990: 3141–3.

psyche reflects his general stance towards philosophy. Was Galen, at bottom, a philosopher or a doctor? This is not a question that allows an easy or unequivocal answer. On the one hand, in his youth, he studied with the four main philosophical schools of the time (those of Plato, Aristotle, Epicureanism, and Stoicism).[6] He also studied philosophical as well as medical texts in his long and elaborate education and throughout his life; and his own review of his writings (*On My Own Books* or *Lib. Prop.*) reports that he produced what seem to be purely philosophical texts, especially on logic or methodology.[7] On the other hand, after his decision, at the age of 16, to devote himself to medicine, he seems to have thought of himself as, primarily, a doctor.[8] The distinctive approach to medicine that he adopted is one that draws, to an exceptional extent, on a huge range of types of learning, including that derived from philosophy (above all, logic). But Galen also stressed, more than some other theoretically minded doctors in his day, the importance of taking full account of practical experience, and also of keeping in mind the fundamentally practical objective of the art of medicine. Hence, although Galen aims explicitly at creating a combination or synthesis of medicine and philosophy,[9] this is, typically, conceived as harnessing philosophical knowledge to medical objectives. Hence Galen's relegation of certain topics, such as the question of the 'substance' of the psyche, to the sphere of purely philosophical speculation, is consistent with his presentation of medicine as his overriding project. Even so, Galen takes a very generous view of the scope of philosophical material that in some way contributes to medical objectives or is compatible with his role as a doctor, including much that falls under the heading of 'ethics' in Hellenistic and Roman philosophy. Hence, in *PHP* 4–5, he extends the discussion to include the nature of

[6] Galen lived from 129/130 to 210–217. (All dates relating to Galen in this book are AD, unless otherwise indicated.) His education in philosophy and medicine extended from 143 to 157 at least. On Galen's life and works, see Boudon-Millot 2007*a*: xi–lxxx, Nutton 2004: 216–29, Hankinson 2008*d*.

[7] See *Lib. Prop.* XIX.39–48; a major loss is his 15-book work on logic, *On Demonstration.*

[8] See *Aff. Dig.* V.41–2, *SM* 1.31.23–32.11, *Ord. Lib. Prop.* XIX.9.59, *SM* 2.88.13–17. See further Nutton 2004: 216–23, Boudon-Millot 2007*a*: xxi–xl, Hankinson 2008*d*: 3–4.

[9] See e.g. Galen's essay, *The Best Doctor is also a Philosopher* (*Opt. Med.*), I.53–63.

emotions and the reason–emotion relationship; and his work on this topic provides material for later essays on the therapy of emotions, normally seen as falling within the province of philosophical writing.[10]

The most striking case where Galen's medical expertise is used to inform his understanding of psychology is his use of anatomy to confirm the role of the brain and nervous system, rather than the heart and veins or arteries, as the basis of intelligence, motor functions, and perception. Galen's expertise in anatomy was, apparently, developed in his lengthy period of medical education (146–57), which included a four-year stay at Alexandria (153–7). This was the place where the third-century BC doctors, Herophilus and Erasistratus had made their path-breaking discoveries of the role of the brain and nerves;[11] and anatomical work had been revived there in the second century AD, particularly by Marinus.[12] During this period, Galen produced a first edition of the treatise, *Anatomical Procedures* (*AA*), which, in its final form, records some of Galen's own work on the brain and nerves.[13] Galen, presumably, continued this work on his return in 157 to his home city of Pergamon, when he took up a public appointment as doctor to the gladiators, involving surgery on injured gladiators. His expertise in surgery and mastery of anatomy were shown on his arrival in Rome in 162 by a series of spectacular public demonstrations, centred on the proof that the centre of higher psychological functions is located in the brain.[14]

Galen's use of sustained and careful observation of animal anatomy, combined with logical analysis and systematic reasoning, to confirm the role of the brain and nerves is widely regarded as his outstanding contribution to medical inquiry, and one that prefigures modern scientific experimental method.[15] Galen's writings *PHP* 1–6 and *UP* (*On the Utility of the Parts*), of which Book 1 was written in

[10] See Chs. 4–5 below.

[11] On these discoveries, made in part through human vivisection (on condemned prisoners provided by Ptolemy), see Solmsen 1961: 184–97, von Staden 2000: 87–96.

[12] See May 1968: 23–38, Rocca 2003: 2–4, 31–46, 2008: 243–4; Galen acknowledges fully his debt to Marinus' 20-book treatise on anatomy, *Lib. Prop.* XIX.25–30.

[13] *AA* II.651–706, XI.4, 11.

[14] Galen recounts these displays in *On Prognosis* (*Praen.*); see Rocca 2003: 6–11, 2008: 244–5.

[15] See further text to nn. 101–10, 137–40 below.

Galen's first visit to Rome (162–6), seem to have been conceived, in large measure, as show-cases for Galen's anatomical discoveries.[16] More precisely, he saw them as contexts in which he could use his anatomically based knowledge to inform—or even to transform—major philosophical debates such as that between heart-centred and brain-centred views of human psychology and between teleological and non-teleological conceptions of the human body.[17] Throughout his subsequent career, Galen consistently presents the role of the brain and nerves, established by his inquiries, as the feature of human psychology about which he is most confident, by contrast with his agnosticism about other central philosophical questions about the psyche.[18]

A second important case of the influence of medical inquiry on Galen's thinking on psychology is that of the philosophy of nature. Galen, especially in his second stay in Rome (169–75), developed what we might call a 'biological' view of natural reality. A crucial feature is the idea that physical matter should be understood in terms of the 'mixtures' (*kraseis*) of elements or opposites (hot, cold, dry, wet), and that these mixtures form the basis of the 'humours' which make up the organic systems of animal bodies. The animal body, in a related line of thought, is conceived as a coherent structure of organs, each of which has its own utility or function (*chreia*) and natural faculty or capacity (*dunamis*).[19] This conception of the body as an organic system underlies important features of Galen's medical practice, including his systematization of earlier medical work on drugs, diet, nutrition, and also on the management of health by 'regime' (*diaita*) or controlled life-style, in which the idea of health as a well-balanced mixture of elements plays a central role.[20] This biological

[16] Both texts were dedicated to Boethus, an influential Roman politician and supporter of Galen (Rocca 2003: 7–8, esp. n. 45).

[17] Cf. Rocca 2003: 17–21, 46–7.

[18] See e.g. *PHP* V.454–5, 5.4.2–3 De Lacy, V.600–1, 7.3.2–3 De Lacy; *Prop. Plac.* 3.2–4 Nutton, and ch. 3, Boudon-Millot and Pietrobelli 2005: 173.18–174.3. See also 2.1, 3.1 Nutton (and ch. 2, Boudon-Millot and Pietrobelli 2005: 172.31–173.2, ch. 3, Boudon-Millot and Pietrobelli 2005: 173.16–18), on the topics Galen does *not* claim to know about). See also n. 4 above on topics on which Galen disowns knowledge; and see further Ch. 3 below, text to nn. 208–23.

[19] See further text to nn. 163–72 below.

[20] See further on 'mixture' in Galen's medical practice (including regimen) and his thinking on food and drugs, van der Eijk 2008: 291, 293–5, 298–300, Vogt 2008: 306–10.

conception of matter and natural entities is presented by Galen as being sharply opposed to the mechanistic analysis of natural reality offered by atomists such as the Epicureans. Galen's thinking on this topic is closely related to his strongly teleological world-view, according to which each bodily organ has its own inbuilt purposive structure.[21] These ideas are set out in a series of works written in Galen's second visit to Rome, including *On Mixtures* (*Temp.*), *On the Natural Faculties* (*Nat. Fac.*), and Books 2–17 of *On the Utility of the Parts* (*UP*). They also lie behind the works on pharmacology, foodstuffs, and regimen produced in this period and subsequently.[22]

The line of thought just outlined constitutes a more speculative line of inquiry, based on a longstanding tradition spanning ancient medicine and philosophy, than the anatomically based study of the role of the brain and other animal organs discussed earlier. However, like his anatomical work, it expresses Galen's distinctive emphases in medicine on combining logic-based systematization of information with practice-based observation. This strand in his thought also has implications for his understanding of human psychology. In a broad way, it underlies his picture of bodily workings in *PHP*, which is closely linked with the analysis of psychological functions in Books 1–3 and 6.[23] It also underlies his thinking on the humoral basis of human mood and character, which forms a relatively minor strand in Galen's thinking, though it was an influential one in the later European history of thought.[24] More importantly, it forms the basis of the late work, *Psychological Faculties Depend on Bodily Mixtures* (*QAM*), in which Galen comes closest to offering a theoretical account of the relation between body and psyche.[25] Although this aspect of Galen's thinking is less impressive, to modern eyes, than his anatomical work, which anticipates modern scientific experimental method, it is a very important part of his medical–philosophical

[21] See further text to nn. 157–62 below.

[22] For a useful outline of the chronology of Galen's life and works, see Singer 1997*a*: l–lii. For detailed treatment, see Ilberg 1889–97. See also n. 6 above.

[23] The four elements are also discussed in detail in *PHP* V.662–702, 8.2.1–6.56 De Lacy, as an example of common ground between Hippocrates and Plato.

[24] See further Gill 2008*a*: 104–6; the classic study of the history of European thought on humours (esp. black bile) is Klibansky, Panofsky, and Saxl 1964.

[25] See Knuuttila 2004: 94–6, Gill 2008*a*: 106–8; and see further 3.5 below.

project, and one that generates certain distinctively Galenic views on psychological questions, especially in *QAM.*

These ideas represent the clearest cases where his unfolding medico-philosophical project shapes his ideas on psychology. However, they do not exhaust the scope of Galen's writings on topics that bear on psychology. In *PHP* 4–5, Galen engages in debate with the Stoics, especially Chrysippus, about the relationship between reason, emotion, and desires in a way that does not derive directly from his medical thinking or practice, though it is related to the argument about bodily organs and psychological functions in *PHP* 1–3. Galen here adopts Platonic–Aristotelian views about psychic parts and ethical development that are in sharp and explicit contrast to Stoic theory on these subjects. Subsequently, Galen produces a large number of works on ethical topics, of which those surviving in some form include *Psychological Affections* (*Aff. Dig.*), *Character Traits* (*Mor.*), and the recently discovered *Avoiding Distress* (*Indol.*). These works mostly reflect the Platonic–Aristotelian approach found in *PHP* 4–5, though this is sometimes (rather awkwardly) combined with lines of thought that show Stoic influence.[26]

This strand of Galen's thought differs in several ways from those outlined earlier. As already indicated, there is little direct linkage between Galen's medical techniques and practice and the claims and subject matter of these writings. Indeed, it is not quite clear why Galen thinks he is well-qualified to write on ethics and ethical psychology, though he, evidently, regards this activity as related to his larger medical objectives. Also, this aspect of his work is, significantly, less innovative or original in approach than the more medically based work on human psychology (the findings based on his study of anatomy or physiology, for instance). One recurrent theme is the idea that qualities of character are innate in human children and in animals, a theme that is sometimes explicitly linked with Galen's thinking on the physical basis of psychological characteristics. But, as brought out later in this book, this theme is not entirely consistent with other (mostly Platonic–Aristotelian) dimensions in Galen's thinking about ethical development that he adopts in these

[26] See Chs. 4–5, below; on the mixture of philosophical influences in *Aff. Dig.*, see 5.2, text to nn. 32–76.

works.[27] Also, as already noted, it is not clear that the picture of human psychology Galen argues for in *PHP* 4–5, centred on the idea of distinct and competing sources of motivation, is consistent with the anatomically based analysis of psychological functions offered in *PHP* 1–3. The Stoic, unified or holistic, analysis of psychological functions, arguably, fits his anatomically based account of the role of the brain and nervous system better than the tripartite theory he adopts from Plato.[28] Hence, although Galen, in this aspect of his psychological thought, is as critical of Stoic ideas as he is in *PHP* 1–3, this is another area where Galen might have benefited from adopting, rather than rejecting, Stoic ideas and approaches. For one thing, Stoic theory in this area has an internal coherence that Galen's thinking, at least partly, lacks. Also, Stoic thinking about emotions and the therapy of emotions has much greater psychological plausibility than Galen allows.[29] If Galen had been prepared to take Stoic ideas on these topics more seriously, he might have been able to develop a more coherent set of ideas—and ones more consistent with his anatomical discoveries—than we actually find in his writings.

But is Galen open in principle to intellectual alliances of this kind, and could this openness have been extended to Stoicism? In fact, much of Galen's writing in this area, and in others, involves explicit or implied intellectual collaboration. *On the Doctrines of Hippocrates and Plato*, for instance, is presented as designed to bring out shared or cognate ideas (including ones that bear on psychology and the workings of the body) in Plato and Hippocrates.[30] Much of *QAM* takes the form of citing or referring to previous medical and philosophical writings in support of the thesis, which also serves as the title of the work, that 'the faculties of the soul follow the mixtures of the body'.[31] Also, when Galen comes close to stating a formal position of his own on this topic he does so, for the most part, through restatements of earlier ideas, especially those in the Aristotelian tradition.[32] Some of the most distinctive features of Galen's philosophy of nature, including its teleological and biological approaches, are presented

[27] See 5.2 below, esp. text to nn. 113–17, 122–36.
[28] See 3.2–3 below.
[29] See 4.2 and 5.3 below.
[30] See 3.3 below and 4.1 below, esp. text to nn. 30–1.
[31] See Lloyd 1988: 15–18 and 3.5 below.
[32] For some examples, see text to nn. 214–15 below.

as constituting an intellectual consensus among thinkers including Hippocrates and philosophers such as Aristotle.[33] Even where there is no explicit acknowledgement of influence or partnership, we can often detect the strong underlying presence of philosophical categories or terminology, particularly those of Aristotle or a fusion of Platonic and Aristotelian ideas.[34] Outside *PHP* 1–5 and certain other contexts, such as *QAM*, ch. 11, where anti-Stoic polemic is very marked, Galen is quite prepared to include the Stoics within the areas of consensus he claims, for instance, on the idea that matter consists of a mixture of elements or opposites rather than atoms. So the possibility of intellectual partnership is a very real one for Galen, and one that can, in principle, be extended to Stoicism.[35]

Why is intellectual collaboration of this type such a marked feature of Galen's writings? A number of partly overlapping factors seem to be at work. Galen's overall project of using philosophy to inform and deepen medical practice makes it natural for him to present his work as a combination of both techniques; *PHP* is an obvious and striking example. Also, Galen's alliance, explicit or implicit, with some of the greatest figures from the earlier philosophical tradition, as well as with Hippocrates, the pioneer of ancient medicine, is surely designed to give his ideas and practices greater credibility, by contrast with his medical competitors. This way of formulating his thought also reflects the fact that Galen wrote many commentaries, in a style ranging from private notebooks to more finished and published writings, on Hippocratic and philosophical works, especially those of Plato and Aristotle. His practice as a commentator (or note-taker) and as a medical thinker merges and overlaps; indeed, given his huge written output and the pressure of time under which he must have worked, this is hardly surprising.[36] Galen's collaborative

[33] See text to nn. 193–201 below.

[34] On Aristotelian influence, see text to nn. 48–58 below; on Platonic–Aristotelian thinking about psychological parts, see Ch. 4 below, text to nn. 33–4, Ch. 5 below, text to nn. 12–18, 43–54, 102–17.

[35] See 2.3 below, text to nn. 193–205.

[36] See *Lib. Prop.* XIX.33–8 (Galen's commentaries on Hippocrates and Erasistratus), XIX.46–7 (his commentaries on Plato, Aristotle, and the Stoics, the latter all on Stoic logic). See further on Galen as a commentator, especially on Hippocrates, Manetti and Rosselli 1994, Flemming 2008, and von Staden 2009.

mode also fits in with other, well-marked, features of the philosophical and cultural life of the period. From at least the first century BC onwards, writings in the Platonic tradition especially often adopted a stance of partnership, often embracing Aristotelian or Peripatetic ideas and sometimes Stoic ones as well (or instead).[37] In his massive learning and readiness to allude to this learning or to express his own thoughts by such allusions, Galen is typical of the broader literary culture of his day, that of what modern scholars call 'the Second Sophistic'. He is typical of his broader culture too in his preference for older, 'classic', thinkers, with whom he identifies, as contrasted with contemporary or even more recent figures, including those of the Hellenistic era.[38] In spite of this, it is extremely likely that Galen actually draws many of his medical and, perhaps, philosophical ideas from more recent, even very recent writings, although he sometimes draws a discreet veil over the exact extent of his indebtedness.[39]

Galen's readiness to ally himself with earlier thinkers or to formulate his ideas in the form of versions of earlier ideas needs to be taken together with other, less evident, features of his work. His account of the ideas of previous thinkers (including those with whom he identifies) is often highly selective or incomplete, and is sometimes positively misleading. This reflects the fact that Galen is not writing as a historian of earlier medical or philosophical thought—even if modern scholars necessarily have to use his extensive writings as sources to try to construct this kind of history. Galen refers to the views of other thinkers, at least outside the commentaries, and sometimes within them, as a way of carrying forward his own distinctive medico-philosophical project, with its own complex set of claims, themes, and priorities. For instance, Galen's version of Plato is, to a large extent, narrowly focused on

[37] See further Dillon 1977 (1995); also Dillon and Long 1988.

[38] On Galen and the 'Second Sophistic', see von Staden 1997*a*; on Galen's relationship to his broader literary and intellectual culture, see Gill, Whitmarsh, and Wilkins 2009; on the tendency in thought of this period to idealize earlier figures and to see them as a source of 'ancient wisdom', see Boys-Stones 2001, esp. chs. 6–7.

[39] On the latter point, see Lloyd 2008: 40–1 (also on his attitude to contemporaries generally), and von Staden 2009 on the artful mixture of reticence and display in his references to Hellenistic commentaries on Hippocrates.

the account of embodied psychological functions in *Timaeus* 69–72 and some other passages which seem to imply a physical basis for psychological states.[40] This version drastically elides the psyche–body dualism that forms a central part of Plato's thought (especially in the *Phaedo*) and of later Neoplatonism. This kind of dualism is stressed by many Platonists in the period from the first century BC to the second century AD (so-called 'Middle Platonism').[41] Galen himself in *QAM* acknowledges this side of Platonic thought, and distances himself from it.[42] Even more strikingly, Galen's version of Hippocratic thought is also highly selective, and Hippocrates is used as a virtual alter ego for Galen in his self-presentation as a doctor.[43] A related feature of Galen's practice is that his intellectual alliances are not necessarily consistently maintained and vary considerably according to the thesis he maintains in any given work. Thus, as just noted, Galen embraces certain aspects of Platonic thought in *PHP* and in parts of *QAM*, while also distancing himself from other characteristic Platonic positions elsewhere in *QAM*.[44] As brought out later in this chapter, this practice also applies to his relationship to Stoicism. Despite his intense, even virulent, rejection of Stoic ideas in *PHP* and sometimes elsewhere, he is quite prepared to cite them as supporters on topics where their thought converges, including the nature of the elements and the influence of bodily states on psychological ones.

These aspects of Galen's practice reflect the fact that he is, as it is sometimes put, an 'eclectic' in his philosophical ideas; he explicitly

[40] See further Lloyd 1988: 18–24 (on *QAM*), Tieleman 1996: xxviii–xxxi (on *PHP*), Gill 2006: 296–8, 308–11 (Galen's reading of Plato's *Timaeus* and *Republic*); also De Lacy 1972 and Chiaradonna 2009. On Galen as commentator on Plato, see *Lib. Prop.* XIX.46 and Flemming 2008: 327.

[41] See further on psyche–body dualism (in Plato), Robinson 2000, (in Plato and Neoplatonism) Gerson 2002, in Middle Platonism, Dillon 1977 (1995): 174–8 (Philo of Alexandria), 202–8, 211–14 (Plutarch), 290–3 (Albinus, here identified with Alcinous). On Alcinous, see also Dillon 1993: chs. 23–5 (pp. 31–4, with commentary on pp. 147–60). On Plutarch's dualism, see also Gill 2006: 228–9, 284–5.

[42] See 3.5 below, text to nn. 238–41.

[43] See Tieleman 1996: xxxi–xxxiv, Lloyd 2008: 40, Flemming 2008: 334–6, 339–40.

[44] See *QAM* IV.780–2, 789–91, 805–7, 809–14 (more 'physicalist' aspects of Plato's thought on psychology) contrasted with 785, 787 (the Platonic claim that the psyche is non-bodily).

refrains from affiliating himself with any existing school and is indeed quite dismissive of the validity of this kind of allegiance.[45] Eclecticism has sometimes been thought to be characteristic of philosophical thought in Galen's period, and, more broadly, of the whole period from the first century BC to the second century AD, sometimes called the 'post-Hellenistic' period of philosophy. But, more recently, scholars have stressed the point that most thinkers of this time signal their allegiance to a specific philosophical school or tradition, even if they interpret this affiliation in a rather generous or inclusive way. Platonists in this period are particularly open to engagement with other traditions, a stance sometimes characterized as 'syncretism'.[46] Galen is sometimes associated with the Platonism of this period (which we call 'Middle Platonism'); though it has recently been shown that his positions, when closely examined, are not characteristic of Platonism in this period.[47] Galen is, in fact, rather exceptional in his age in the degree of his intellectual eclecticism or independence; and this reflects his distinctive, and largely exceptional role, as one aiming to harness certain philosophical ideas to an unfolding medical project. Hence, despite his recurrent adoption of (a highly selective version) of Platonic ideas, there is no reason in principle why he could not have allied himself to Stoicism as well or instead, if he had chosen to do so.

It is instructive, in this connection, to review Galen's attitude to Aristotle. This relationship forms a striking parallel, in certain respects, to his understanding of Stoicism. Also, considered from another standpoint, Aristotle's importance for Galen helps to explain why Galen does not, for the most part, feel the need to ally himself with Stoicism.

As some recent scholarship has underlined, Galenic thought is strongly indebted to Aristotle's ideas, methods, and terminology. This is the case, for instance, in the two areas on which, later in this chapter, Galenic and Stoic thought are shown to have significant links, namely the methodology of natural inquiry and the

[45] See e.g. *Aff. Dig.* ch. 8 V.42; also M. Frede 1987: 281–5, Donini 1992: 3497–3502, Hankinson 1992.

[46] See Dillon and Long 1988, also (on 'post-Hellenistic' philosophy and the appropriation of earlier ideas) Boys-Stones 2001, esp. chs. 2–3, 6–7.

[47] See Chiaradonna 2009; also De Lacy 1972: 27–9.

philosophy of nature. Central to Galen's methodology is the systematic application of logical reasoning to information based on empirical observation of natural bodily structures. Galen comments in detail on most of Aristotle's logical works, and his own account of logic and its application owes a good deal to Aristotle, though the method he adopts is not uniformly or exclusively Aristotelian.[48] Galen is also wholly familiar with Aristotelian works, such as *Parts of Animals* and *Generation of Animals*, which represent the most comprehensive attempt before Galen to examine the bodily forms of animals and their modes of reproduction. The key features of Galen's philosophy of nature, a firmly teleological approach and a biological conception of nature (centred on the idea of the elements as the basic constituents of matter), are both anticipated and strongly influenced by Aristotelian thought.[49] Aristotle (at least, to a large extent) assumes that psychological functions are those of naturally embodied animals; and Galen comes close in *QAM* to adopting a version of Aristotle's account of the psyche as the 'form' of the body.[50] The points just outlined are also ones on which Galenic and Stoic thought also converge, though Galen does not always acknowledge this resemblance. Galen also, typically, adopts the ideas that the psyche consists of rational and non-rational parts and that ethical development depends on a combination of (a specific kind of) inborn nature, social habituation, and rational choice. These ideas represent a fusion of Platonic and Aristotelian thought in ethical psychology, of a kind that is found in a number of Middle Platonic thinkers in the first and second centuries AD such as Plutarch.[51]

Although Galen sometimes acknowledges the pervasive influence of Aristotle on his thought, he does so less than one might have expected. In his most important work on psychology, *PHP*, the figures selected as his intellectual prototypes are Hippocrates and

[48] See *Lib. Prop.* XIX.47 for his commentaries on Aristotle (all on logical works); also Moraux 1984: 689–91, Morison 2008, esp. 70–5, Tieleman 2008: 51–3.

[49] See Moraux 1984: 729–35, Kovačić 2001 (see index, 'Antike Autoren', under 'Aristotle'), Hankinson 2008*b*: 214–15, 219–20; see also text to nn. 157–205 below.

[50] See 3.5 below, text to nn. 229–37.

[51] See e.g below 4.3, text to nn. 189–91, 5.2, text to nn. 52–6.

Plato, not Aristotle. In his writings on the philosophy of nature, Galen sometimes presents Hippocrates as his main predecessor in formulating a teleological picture of nature or in explaining matter in terms of the elements, though Aristotle had provided a much more fully articulated account of these topics and one that was, probably, more influential on Galen's thought.[52] Also, Galen's positive references to Aristotelian ideas are counterbalanced by vigorous criticisms of Aristotle, and his followers, for errors of fact and reasoning. Galen singles out for special criticism Aristotle's failure to grasp the role of the brain and nerves in exercising cognition and motor functions, as well as his mistake in seeing the heart as the central point of the nervous system.[53] In fact, the heart-centred view of embodied psychological functions is retained in the Aristotelian school throughout this period, and is strongly reaffirmed by the important Aristotelian commentator, Alexander of Aphrodisias, a younger contemporary of Galen.[54] Galen also criticizes Aristotle for his failure to go further than he does in applying the teleological analysis of bodily parts.[55] As Philip van der Eijk underlines, Galen's criticism of Aristotle on these points reflects his view that Aristotle should have known better than to make these mistakes. It is precisely because Aristotle is treated as a serious and relatively systematic predecessor to Galen in using dissection of animals to support his analysis of natural forms that he is subjected to higher standards of criticism than other thinkers, including Hippocrates and Plato.[56]

Why is Aristotle treated by Galen in this, apparently rather unfair, way? The probable answers are, in different ways, illuminating for understanding Galen's (generally rather negative) relationship to

[52] See e.g. *Hipp. Elem.* I.447–53; also Hankinson 2008*b*: 217–20, van der Eijk 2009: 266–9; see also Jouanna 2003: 255–61, and Flemming 2009: 72–9, on Galen's attribution to Hippocrates of an essentially Platonic–Aristotelian (teleological) conception of 'nature' (*phusis*).

[53] See e.g. *PHP* V.200–10, 1.8.1–10.20 De Lacy. On Aristotle's thinking on psychophysiology (which is much less dogmatic than Galen implies), see van der Eijk 2000.

[54] Alex. Aphr. *De An.* pp. 94.7–100.17 Bruns, e.g. 94.17–20, cf. Arist. *GA* 2.4, 740^{a}18–23. See further Tieleman 1996: xxvi and 73–6.

[55] See e.g. 1.11–15, 449, 451–3 Helmreich; also van der Eijk 2009: 274–6.

[56] See van der Eijk 2009.

Stoicism. One, very important, factor is surely the significance for Galen of the disagreement with Aristotle—and the Stoics—about the location of the ruling part of the psyche. Galen's establishment of the role of the brain and the nerves, as noted earlier, was regarded by him as the key outcome of his anatomical inquiries, and it serves as the centre-piece of his argument with Aristotle and the Stoics in *PHP* 1–3. The fact that Aristotle, despite his expertise in animal anatomy, failed to identify the proper roles of the relevant organs is, clearly, a factor militating against a more general identification between Galen and Aristotle or the Aristotelians and one that applies on similar grounds to the Stoics.[57] A further consideration suggested by van der Eijk is that Galen is, paradoxically, *too* close to Aristotle, in many respects, for Galen to claim an explicit allegiance. The very fact that Galen is so strongly indebted to Aristotle in a series of ways makes it more difficult for him to acknowledge this bond and to maintain his chosen stance of intellectual independence—and originality. Although Galen is not so greatly indebted to Stoicism, the fact that he is close to this theory too, and in rather similar ways, may also lead him to understate his kinship to Stoicism, especially since he has a specific, and substantial, ground of disagreement with both of the theories. The third factor suggested by van der Eijk is that Aristotelianism in Galen's day represented a more cohesive and determinate position than allegiance to Plato or Hippocrates, and thus left less room for the kind of generous, even idiosyncratic, interpretation that Galen offered in the case of Plato and Hippocrates.[58] As brought out later, Stoicism in Galen's day seems to have shown a similar cohesiveness of approach, and is thus also resistant to the kind of selective identification with other thinkers that Galen favours. Hence, in several ways, Galen's reasons for not linking himself too closely with Aristotle, despite their intellectual closeness, may have implications for understanding Galen's relatively cool relationship to Stoicism.

[57] See further 3.2, 3.4 below.

[58] See van der Eijk 2009: 279–81. On Galen's tactical reasons for preferring Plato to Aristotle as a prototype, at least in *PHP*, see Singer 1991: 55.

There is a further possible implication of Galen's relationship to Aristotle for understanding his attitude to the Stoics, though one that points in a rather different direction. I have suggested that it is rather paradoxical that Galen is so negative towards Stoicism, despite the fact that both theories have in common with each other (by contrast with much of Plato's thinking and contemporary Platonism) a shared naturalism of approach that has a relevance for several topics including psychology. Hence, Galen's decision in *PHP* to ally himself with Plato, coupled with his resolute rejection of Stoic ideas, seems surprising, even taking into account the disagreement with Stoicism over the location of the ruling part of the psyche. However, Galen's closeness to Aristotle has a bearing on this topic. If Galen had wanted to turn to a thinker other than Plato—and one who shared his naturalism of approach—he would surely have been more inclined to turn to Aristotle than the Stoics. As just indicated, most of the points on which Galen is close to the Stoics are also ones on which he is equally close—or closer—to Aristotle. There are also other topics, notably the part-based theory of the psyche, on which Galen's thinking comes close to Aristotle's, but diverges from Stoicism. So, if Galen had wanted to find a thinker whose world-view is more naturalistic (or at least more consistently naturalistic) than Plato,[59] he did not need to turn to Stoicism to find one. Indeed, on many points, including the adoption of a teleological view of animal bodies (in *UP*) or of a physicalist (or near-physicalist) position on the nature of the psyche, Galen *does* turn to Aristotle, rather than Plato, or the Stoics.[60]

The fact that Aristotle was a more plausible alternative than the Stoics, for Galen, as a naturalistic alternative to Plato does not negate the point stressed in this book that Galen also has much in common with Stoicism, and that his thought would have gained (like theirs) by closer engagement between the two theories. Although Galen may not have seen much potential for engagement in this relationship, I think there are strong grounds for taking a different view, and I argue for this thesis in this book. Hence, consideration of Aristotle sheds light on Galen's attitude towards Stoicism without diminishing the

[59] As noted earlier (text to n. 40 above), Galen focuses on the more naturalistic aspects of Plato's thought, ignoring much that points in a quite different direction.

[60] See text to nn. 49–50 above.

interest and significance of this attitude for the study of psychological thinking in antiquity.

Where is the study of psychology located within Stoic philosophy, and what scope does this allow for intellectual partnership with other approaches, such as Galen's? In the first instance, we need to mark certain general differences between Stoicism and Galenic thought, bearing on the extent to which each of these constitutes a theoretical system. By the end of his life, Galen seems to have seen his writings and his ideas as forming a connected whole.[61] But, viewed from the outside, it seems more plausible to see his work as an unfolding series of (theoretical and practical) projects, with certain recurrent themes and an increasing number of internal connections.[62] Stoic philosophy probably also emerged, during the lifetime of the founder Zeno (334–262 BC), in a gradual way that involved both external influences and debate with intellectual associates. Although, after his death, the writings of Zeno became the basis of the school's distinctive teachings, different heads of the school, down to the last recorded head, Panaetius (*c.*185–*c.*110 BC), seem to have formulated the core principles and themes in slightly different ways. However, the third head, Chrysippus (*c.*280–*c.*206 BC), seems to have played a crucial role in setting out the doctrines of the school in a more systematic and internally coherent way.[63] Unfortunately for historians of Stoicism, only fragments and indirect evidence survive from the Hellenistic period when the school, based at Athens, was a fully functioning institution. Although some complete Stoic writings survive from the first and second century AD, much of our evidence for Stoic philosophy derives from summaries, comments, and criticisms from post-Hellenistic, non-Stoic writers such as Cicero, Diogenes Laertius, Plutarch, and Galen himself.[64]

[61] Thus, in two late works, he sets out his writings in an ideal reading order (*Ord. Lib. Prop.*), and summarizes his main doctrines (*Prop. Plac.*).

[62] On the question how far Galen's writings express a unified or a developing position, see Singer 1997*b*.

[63] See Sedley 2003.

[64] On the nature of our sources for Hellenistic philosophy, including Stoicism, see Mansfeld 1999. For extended extracts on Stoicism from these sources, see von Arnim 2004 (=*SVF*), first published in 1903–5 and still the standard source collection, and, translated into English, Inwood and Gerson 1997: part 2, and Inwood and Gerson 2008. See also Long and Sedley 1987 (texts, translations, and commentary, in 2 vols.), sections 26–67. (Hereafter cited as LS, normally referring to section and passage.)

The summaries of doctrines, especially those provided by Diogenes and Stobaeus, in all likelihood, overstate the schematic character of the theory. None the less, it does seem that, from Chrysippus onwards, Stoic philosophy had a high degree of systematicity, perhaps more than any other ancient theory. To this degree, a comparison between Galenic thought (which is, in any case, intertwined with his medical practice) and Stoic philosophy is not, exactly, a like-for-like comparison, though this fact does not diminish the interest of the comparison or the extent to which the two approaches may be similar, or complementary, in ideas and attitude.

In the form in which it has reached us, Stoicism, as a body of theory, is subdivided into logic, ethics, and physics. This became, in the course of the Hellenistic and post-Hellenistic periods, a common way of subdividing ancient theories; in the case of Stoicism, it is coupled with a strong stress on the internal coherence of all three branches with each other.[65] 'Psychology' as a distinct subject seems to fall primarily under physics (the study of nature) in Stoicism; but psychological topics are discussed in all three branches, in ways that exhibit certain recurrent concepts and themes.[66] Three key Stoic notions are those of 'impression' (or 'appearance' or 'presentation', *phantasia*), 'assent' (*sunkatathesis*), and 'impulse' (*hormē*). Another recurrent feature of Stoic thought is the use of the 'wise person' or 'sage' (*sophos*) as a norm; the wise person's state of mind and character is, typically, conceived as one of coherent unity or structure. These notions are deployed in different branches of philosophy to analyse key Stoic ideas. For instance, in the study of logic, understood as including the theory of knowledge, the acquisition of knowledge, seen as a primarily empirical process, is analysed in terms of 'assent' to 'impressions' (the latter concept embraces both perceptions and beliefs). The state of mind of the wise person is also taken as normative for the possession of knowledge and achievement of

[65] On this as a general feature of Hellenistic (and post-Hellenistic) thought, see Algra *et al.* 1999: xiii–xvii; on the Stoic system and the aspiration to link these three branches closely with each other, see LS 26. On Galen as adopting this standard tripartite division (though not in the same systematic way), see Lloyd 2008: 42–3, Hankinson 2008*b*: 210–11.

[66] See esp. LS 39–41 (on gaining knowledge), 53 (on the psyche), and 65 (on passions or emotions).

truth.[67] In ethics, the same notions, combined with that of 'impulse' or 'motivation', *hormē*, are used to analyse features of human life that have evaluative significance, including those of action, emotion, and development. The state of mind and character of the wise person is used in this area too to provide a normative framework for understanding these aspects of human life.[68] Stoic physics studies the psyche (treated as a natural entity) within the framework of study of nature as whole and of its causal principles. Topics treated in works such as Chrysippus' *On the Psyche*, which falls within physics, include the nature of the psyche, and of its ruling part, for which the Stoics coined the notion of 'control-centre', *hēgemonikon*, and the operation of psychological functions such as impression, assent, and impulse. Stress is laid, in this part of the study of psychology, on the physical nature of the psyche, and on the relationship between psychological functions and bodily organization and operation.[69] Galen is a key source for an important part of the argument of Chrysippus' *On the Psyche* and also for his *On Passions*, which falls within the branch of ethics.[70]

As noted earlier, two salient features of Stoic philosophy, taken as a whole, are its holism (analysed earlier in terms of a 'structure', rather than 'composition', approach) and its radical revisionism, in comparison with conventional and preceding philosophical thought.[71] These features are evident in Stoic thought on psychology and are highly relevant for comparison with Galen's thinking, and for understanding Galen's response to Stoicism. For instance, the three notions by which Stoic theory analyses human action and emotion, 'impression', 'assent', 'impulse' (all taken to be 'rational'

[67] See LS 39–41; also Frede 1999*c* (on Stoic epistemology) and Long 1996: ch. 4 on the wise person as a norm in logic.

[68] See LS 57, 62 C (Cic. *Fat.* 39–43), 65. See further Inwood 1985: chs. 3, 5, 6, Long 1999: 572–84, Brennan 2003, Graver 2007: 35–60.

[69] See LS 53; also Annas 1992: 37–70, Long 1996: ch. 19, 1999: 560–72, Graver 2007: 15–34. Gourinat 2005 attempts to reconstruct the contents and order of subjects in Chrysippus' *On the Psyche*, as does Tieleman 1996: part 2, with much more detailed examination of the evidence. On typical topics on psychology within 'physics', see *SVF* 2.773–911 (references in *SVF* are to fragments unless otherwise indicated).

[70] On Galen studied as a source for *On the Psyche*, see Tieleman 1996 (esp. 134–8), and for *On Passions* Tieleman 2003*a*.

[71] See Ch. 1 above, text to nn. 38–46; also, presented in slightly different terms, Gill 2006: 29–46, 75–100.

processes in adult humans) imply a strongly unified or holistic conception of these processes. A crucial point is that assent (saying 'yes') to the content of a rational impression, for instance, 'that it is appropriate to act or feel in a given way', is taken necessarily to produce a motive ('impulse') to act or feel in this way.[72] This form of analysis unifies (or replaces) the dual roles of 'desire' (*orexis*) and 'thought' (*dianoia*) or 'belief' (*doxa*) in the Aristotelian explanation of action.[73] The Stoic analysis also assumes that the human psyche operates in a highly unified way and not as a composite of the two or three independent, and potentially conflicting parts ('reason', 'spirit', or 'appetite'), as is maintained by Plato and Aristotle. Galen tends to presuppose the Platonic or Aristotelian way of understanding these processes and finds the Stoic (holistic and revisionist) conception unfamiliar and unconvincing.[74]

Other aspects of Stoic thinking on psychology, which also exhibit this combination of holism and revisionism, are especially relevant to the claim made here, that Galenic and Stoic thought could have been combined to the advantage of both theories. One innovative and characteristic feature of Stoic thought is a highly unified conception of the psychological centre (*hēgemonikon*), seen as the organizing centre of perception and bodily movement, and also as the seat of both rational and emotional functions. This idea of the control-centre is consistent with the Stoic account of emotions and desires, which are conceived as unitary responses (analysed in terms of impression, assent, and impulse), rather than as responses of a separate, non-rational part of the psyche.[75] As argued later, the Stoic view of the *hēgemonikon* is one that Galen would have done well to adopt, since it is much more consistent with his anatomically

[72] See Brennan 1998: 22–9, 2003: 260–9, Gill 2006: 138–44, Graver 2007: 24–9. For sources, see *SVF* 3.377–420 and LS 65 A–F.

[73] In this respect, the Stoic analysis is even more unified in its picture of human psychology than Aristotle's, which is often seen as offering a cognitive account of emotions and motivation generally. A further point of difference is that aspects of motivation seen by Aristotle as distinct in kind ('dialectical' and 'physical') form part of a single, unified analysis in Stoicism. See Arist. *De An.* 1.1, 403^{a}29–^{b}1; also Brennan 2003: 275–9, Gill 2006: 142, 247–8, Graver 2007: 16–17, 31–2.

[74] See Chs. 4–5 below.

[75] On the linkage between these two innovative features of Stoic thought, see Long 1999: 570–2, 580–3.

based account of the role of the brain and the nervous system than the tripartite psychology he adopts from Plato. The Galenic account of the role of the brain could also have been consistently combined with the Stoic unified view of emotions, desires, and other psychological processes. In other words, two unified or holistic features of the two theories could have been combined, to the mutual advantage of both theories.[76]

As brought out later, there are various reasons why Galen in fact strongly rejects both these aspects of the Stoic theory. But one important factor is, probably, the combination in Stoicism of radical forms of holism combined with revisionism. The Stoics not only dispense with the division between rational and non-rational parts of the psyche found in Platonic and Aristotelian thought, a division whose validity Galen assumes. They also couple this move with certain highly revisionist claims, including the idea that only the wise person is wholly consistent and integrated in state of mind and character, and that all non-wise people (meaning, virtually everyone) are more or less incoherent, or, as they sometimes put it, 'sick' or 'diseased'. A separate but related claim, which also runs counter to much preceding ancient thought about ethical development, is that all human beings are constitutionally capable of developing to the point of achieving perfect wisdom, even though in practice hardly anyone does so.[77] Galen reacts strongly against claims of this kind, which he sees as perverse and misguided, and as being in conflict with his own assumptions about psychological health and sickness and about the basis of ethical character. It is likely that the combination of holism with radical revisionism in Stoic ideas of this kind reinforces Galen's rejection of Stoic ideas about psychological unity which he might—conceivably—have viewed more favourably if they had not been coupled together in this way.[78]

How far were the Stoics, as distinct from Galen, open to partnership or engagement with the ideas of other theories? The answer varies somewhat according to the period of Stoicism being considered;[79]

[76] See 3.2–3 below. [77] See Gill 2006: 256–64.

[78] See 4.2, 4.4, 5.3–4 below.

[79] For an outline chronology of the Stoic school in the Hellenistic period, see Dorandi 1999: 50–1. For its history in the Hellenistic and Roman Imperial eras, see Sedley 2003 and Gill 2003.

but, on the whole, the Stoics are not very open to the kind of partnership that formed a standard part of Galen's procedure. The origins of Stoicism, in so far as we can reconstruct these, involved a good deal of influence from other schools, notably from Polemo, then head of the Academy, and Stilpo, a 'Megaric' teacher with a Cynic approach. Also Plato's *Timaeus* was particularly influential on their thought about physics either directly or as mediated by Polemo. The philosophical positions of Zeno, the founder of the school, seem to have emerged in part through debate with Aristo of Chios, an intellectual associate, though one who developed sharply different views on several subjects and who subsequently distanced himself from Zeno and his school. However, as noted earlier, it seems that, after the death of Zeno, his writings were taken to constitute the nucleus of the school's philosophy, though these were subsequently reformulated and refined by successive heads of the schools and leading Stoics, above all, Chrysippus.[80] Chrysippus' extensive writings, in particular, gave the theory a comprehensive and systematic character, with a strong focus in internal consistency. After the work of Zeno and Chrysippus, Stoic philosophy seems to have remained largely stable and not open to substantial influence from other schools throughout its subsequent history. There was a long period of debate in epistemology and ethics in the third century BC, during which Stoics responded to criticisms by Academic (Platonic) Sceptics, especially Arcesilaus and Carneades. However, this seems to have taken the form of reformulation of the original Stoic positions to defend them against Sceptical criticism, rather than substantive alteration of Stoic ideas as a result of engagement with their critics.[81]

Although the later Hellenistic period brought changes in other ways, Stoic thought does not seem to have altered significantly in this respect. The last head of the school in the Hellenistic period, Panaetius, like his pupil Posidonius, gave more attention to the relationship between Stoicism and other theories, notably that of Plato and Aristotle. Indeed, Galen asserts, repeatedly and emphatically, that in psychology Posidonius abandoned the Stoic unified approach and adopted the Platonic tripartite psychology instead.

[80] See Sedley 2003: 9–18; also Sedley 2002 and Gill 2006: 17–20. The 'Megarics' are a minor Socratic school (Dorandi 1999: 47).

[81] See LS 40–1, 64, 70.

However, as a number of scholars have argued in recent years, close inspection of the relevant evidence indicates that this is a gross exaggeration on Galen's part, and one that reflects the polemical needs of Galen's critique against the Stoic view. A more plausible view is that Panaetius and Posidonius, like an earlier Stoic, Antipater, discussed the relationship between Stoic ideas and those of other theories, especially Plato's, more explicitly than had been the case in the earlier Hellenistic period. Among other factors, this reflects a more general move towards commentary on earlier philosophers, especially Plato and Aristotle, in the late Hellenistic period, which seems to have had some impact within the Stoic school. However, it is not clear that this shift brought with it any modifications of real substance, as distinct from recognition of ideas in common between Stoic and (especially) Platonic thought.[82]

The same point seems also to hold good for Stoicism in the first and second centuries AD. Although this is sometimes seen as a rather uncreative phase of Stoic thought, it is, in fact, the only period from which we have whole treatises from Stoic thinkers (or at least substantial sections of them) on, for instance, astronomy, natural phenomena generally, theology, and the foundations of ethics. Although comparison with earlier Stoicism is not easy, given the lack of complete treatises from this period, we seem to have a continuation of the Hellenistic practice of independent formulation of ideas within a conceptual framework set by Zeno and Chrysippus.[83] Much Stoic writing in this period is in the area of practical ethics, by thinkers including Seneca, Epictetus, and the emperor Marcus Aurelius, for whom Galen served as doctor. Their writings (or, in Epictetus' case, reported teachings) are non-technical in style; and those of Seneca and Marcus at least have sometimes been seen as expressing a more eclectic version of Stoicism, and as showing the

[82] For the views outlined here, see Cooper 1998, Tieleman 2003*a*: 198–287, 2007, Gill 1998, 2006: 266–90 (also on phases of Hellenistic debate, Gill 2006: 136–7, 213–14, 281–3). On the relationship between Stoicism and Plato (or Platonism) more generally, see Bonazzi and Helmig 2007.

[83] The main surviving Stoic treatises from the first and second centuries AD are Cleomedes' *Caelestia* (*Meteōra*), Seneca's *Natural Questions*, Cornutus' *Summary* (*Epidromē*) *of the Traditions of Greek Theology*, and (substantial portions of) Hierocles' *Elements of Ethics*; for an outline, see Gill 2003: 38–40.

influence of Epicureanism in Seneca's case and of several theories, including Plato's, in Marcus' case. Seneca and Marcus were, it is true, leading Roman politicians in their day and neither were Stoic teachers in a formal sense. Even so, the extent to which their writings express an eclectic outlook has often, I think, been overstated; and even Marcus' *Meditations* can be seen as reflecting a determinately Stoic approach, although this is sometimes couched in an idiom which evokes other theories or attitudes.[84]

Galen's own evidence for Stoic thought and teaching in his day confirms the impression of a school concerned to maintain its own integrity of approach. It is clear that Stoics in Galen's day still referred in detail to the writings of Zeno, Chrysippus, and other Hellenistic heads, on questions such as the location of the ruling part of the psyche (the *hēgemonikon*) in the body. This adherence to the original Stoic teachings on this question goes some way towards explaining Galen's exhaustive critique of those texts (and his close examination and citation of them) in *PHP* Books 2–3.[85] Hence, though I shall argue here (3.2) that Stoicism could consistently have adopted the brain-centred account of embodied psychology offered by Galen (and, before him, by the third-century Ptolemaic doctors), this is not how things seemed to Stoics in Galen's own day. Some of Galen's references to Stoic thought (especially outside polemical contexts such as *PHP* 2–5) present them positively as part of a larger tradition of medical and philosophical thought going back to Aristotle and, beyond him, to Hippocrates.[86] It is less clear whether the Stoics of his day would have thought of their ideas in this way. Galen tells us of two Stoic thinkers of the Roman Imperial period, Aeficianus and Simias, who found in Hippocrates the idea of perception as a basis for cognition. However, this seems to be another instance of Stoic thinkers finding in earlier thinkers support for their own views, rather than a more full-hearted kind of engagement with another theory.[87] Taken overall, then, Galen seems to have been

84 See further Gill 2003: 40–50, 2007*b* and *c*; also Annas 2004, Cooper 2004: 309–34.

85 See Gal. *PHP* V.240–6, 2.4.50–5.30 De Lacy; also Tieleman 2009: 288–9.

86 See text to nn. 197–201.

87 Gal. *Hipp. Off. Med.* XVIIIB.654, cf. *Ord. Lib. Prop.* XIX.58; Aeficianus belonged to the generation of Galen's teacher in Smyrna, Satyrus. See further Tieleman 2009:

much more open to intellectual partnership than the Stoics, either in his own day or previously. Although, I shall argue, closer engagement would have benefited both theories, Galen—despite his massive opposition to Stoicism on certain points—is more likely to have recognized this point than the Stoics.

2.2 METHODOLOGY OF NATURAL INQUIRY

In this and the following section, I explore two aspects of the theories which constitute a crucial part of the background for understanding their distinctive approaches to psychology. These aspects (methodology of natural inquiry and philosophy of nature) are also important for bringing out the sense in which their approaches to psychology can be described as 'naturalistic'. I also aim to bring out respects in which their thinking on these subjects is cognate or complementary, whether or not this is recognized by Galen in his responses to Stoic thought. I also highlight certain larger conceptual differences between the two theories, relating especially to holism and revisionism, which bear on their respective ideas on psychology. The features considered here are especially relevant for understanding Galenic and Stoic thinking on psychology and the body, discussed in Chapter 3. But there are also important links with the ideas on ethical psychology examined in Chapters 4 and 5, as well as the concluding comparison with modern thought in Chapter 6.[88]

The question of the sense in which both theories adopt a 'naturalistic' approach to psychology is explored more fully in the next section.[89] But one obviously relevant point, evident in Chapter 3, is that a key part of both approaches to psychology is the study of the embodied psychological functions of human beings and other animals, considered as integral parts of nature. It is also clear, especially

293–4, and compare the approach of Stoics to other theories outlined in text to n. 82 above.

[88] For instance, the significance of differences regarding holism and revisionism comes up again in 4.4, 5.4, and 6.3, and the shared 'naturalism' of the theories is important for the comparison with modern thought in 6.2.

[89] See text to nn. 213–25 below.

from Galen's critique of Stoic thought in *PHP* 2–3, that both theories apply specific methods of inquiry, directed at understanding psychological functions conceived as being those of natural entities. However, by contrast with the philosophy of nature, where Galen stresses points of convergence with Stoicism,[90] his attitude to the Stoic method of inquiry is uniformly critical, at least in *PHP* 2–3, where it is examined in most detail. There are a number of reasons for this consistently negative response. One is that Galen, understandably, regards his own method as much better conceived, especially as regards questions such as the physical location of the ruling part of the psyche. Another is that Galen, it would seem, misunderstands or misrepresents the nature and rationale of the Stoic method of inquiry. However, his negative attitude should not lead us to overlook some important common or complementary features in the two theories. Stoic theories on logic and causation, along with those of Aristotle, seem to have made an important contribution to the formation of Galen's distinctive method, but Galen does not acknowledge this contribution, at least in *PHP* 2–3. On the other hand, his view that his own method of natural inquiry is superior to that of Stoicism is certainly justified in most respects. Since both theories, in key respects, share a naturalistic approach to psychology, there is no reason in principle why the Stoics could not have adopted Galen's methods or his main findings, for instance, on the location of the ruling part of the psyche. In practice, for chronological and other reasons, outlined earlier, the Stoics did not adopt this method and were unlikely ever to do so. But this does not negate the point that their theory would have benefited from doing so.

I begin by offering a general account of Galen's method of natural inquiry, which he saw as providing crucial support for his medical techniques. We need to relate this method to Galen's specific stance in relation to medical practice in his day, about which Galen is our main source. From the fifth century BC onwards, there had been a continuing debate between those who saw medical practice as dependent on theoretical inquiry into

[90] See text to nn. 196–201 below.

nature and those who presented it as an independent method, based on experience and a more or less codified set of techniques. In Galen's writings, these approaches are characterized as those of Rationalists or Dogmatists, on the one hand, and Empiricists, on the other, with the Methodists maintaining a third, in some ways intermediate, position. The Methodists advocated using a relatively simplified set of medical techniques, which were, however, based on certain theories about the nature of illness and about medical methodology. Galen tells us that he was attracted, at an early stage, to Empiricism; but his mature writings reflect an independent position, which seeks to combine the best features of Rationalist and Empiricist practice. On the one hand, he is ready to draw on the experience-based findings of Empiricist doctors, and also sometimes the work of Methodist doctors such as Julius Soranus, despite his virulent criticism of Methodism as an approach. On the other hand, he adopts the core Rationalist thesis (which he thinks has not been actually taken far enough by Rationalist doctors) that medical practice must incorporate a systematic understanding of natural reality if it is to respond effectively to new and unpredictable circumstances. This position underlies Galen's massive programme of inquiry and systematization of knowledge in fields including anatomy, physiology, nutrition, and pharmacology, which he sees as underlying his own therapeutic practice, and which he thinks should inform all proper medical practice.[91]

Galen's stance regarding medical practice is linked with a distinctive position as regards the acquisition of knowledge. Debate between the main medical schools was intertwined, in Hellenistic and Roman thought, with responses to the two main forms of scepticism current in philosophy at this time. These consist in scepticism about the possibility of gaining knowledge at all and scepticism about the possibility of producing credible and coherent theorized accounts of knowledge. Empiricism and to some extent Methodism seem to be directly influenced especially by the latter type of scepticism.[92] Galen, in his mature thought, takes up a resolutely non-sceptical position,

[91] See M. Frede 1985: xx–xxxiv, 1987: 243–78, Hankinson 1991*c*: xxvi–xxxiii, Nutton 2004: 230–47, van der Eijk 2008; on Methodism, see Tecusan 2004: 7–21.

[92] See M. Frede 1985: xxvi–xxx, 1987: 248–9, 252–60, 276–8.

which aligns him with Rationalist or Dogmatist doctors as well as many previous philosophical theories. On the central question of the criterion of knowledge, Galen repeatedly asserts that there are two criteria, reason and perception (or experience), a claim that is linked with his aim of bridging Rationalist and Empiricist approaches in medicine. Galen insists that both reason and perception provide independent access to certain kinds of truth, for instance, theoretical principles on the one hand and particular observed facts on the other. In a related move, he maintains that perception is in principle capable of grasping, in pre-theoretical form, the same ideas and truths that can be understood in analytic form by reason. But Galen also insists that medical practice, which he sees as allied with natural inquiry, depends on close integration of systematic and ordered rational analysis with accurate perception-based observation.[93] As he sometimes puts it, medicine depends on a combination of 'reason' (*logos*) and 'testing' (*peira*).[94] It is this combination that constitutes what we (moderns) might call Galen's 'scientific' method and which is also crucial for making sense of what I am calling his 'naturalistic' approach in psychology.

In examining this method, it is best to begin with its 'rational' side, which is associated by Galen, to an extent unique in ancient medical practice, with formal logic, which formed an integral part of his studies from adolescence. Logic is presented as vital for the doctor because it enables him—broadly put—to distinguish truth from falsehood and (in Platonic terms) to cut up reality, like a skilful butcher, 'at the joints'.[95] But how does it do this; and how is logic integrated with the work of perception? It sometimes seems as though Galen has in view a single, determinate role for logic. For instance, he sometimes stresses the function of logic in using—but going beyond—perception in identifying the 'indication' (*endeixis*) of underlying connections in reality. This idea seems to draw particularly on the Stoic conception of logical

[93] See M. Frede 1987: 289–97, Barnes 1991: 76–8, Hankinson 1991*b*: 25–6, 1992: 3512–13; see e.g. *MM* X.36.

[94] See Hankinson 1992: 3517–18; see e.g. *MM* X.29–32. See further Hankinson 2009: 219–22.

[95] See Barnes 1991: 61, referring to *MM* X.18; also Barnes 1991: 65–6, Hankinson 1991*b*: 21–2, referring to *MM* X.123 and Pl. *Phdr.* 265e.

proof as revealing by deduction a non-evident conclusion or as offering an 'indicative sign'.[96] Galen also sometimes presents as exemplary the use of logic as a type of 'geometric' method, that is, one which offers demonstrations by going back to certain primary principles or starting-points (*archai*), which can be compared to the geometer's reliance on the definition of mathematical figures.[97] But it is misleading to think that Galen has in view a single determinate role for logic in medicine or natural inquiry. Rather, as Jonathan Barnes underlines,[98] Galen thinks that logical argument, in some more or less fully articulated form, should be integrated with perception-based observation at each stage of medical practice and of the natural inquiry which informs this practice. By looking at some of the procedures Galen has in mind, we can chart the integration of logic with observation and gauge the extent to which this is comparable with ideas about 'scientific' method. We can also see the links between Galen's method of inquiry and the two other strands identified here as the basis of his naturalistic approach to psychology.

First, here are two examples of the 'axiomatic' method of proof, as analysed by Barnes on the basis of Galen's *On the Therapeutic Method (MM)*. This method consists in deducing derivative truths ('theorems') from first principles ('axioms'). This had formed part of logical method from Euclid and Aristotle onwards, but Galen is unusual in applying it to an empirically based practical technique, that of medicine.[99] One application is a case where a man has an abdominal wound and the protruding intestines have swollen. Galen's reasoning focuses on establishing the cause of the swelling and thus inferring possible forms of treatment, including warming the swollen intestine with a warm sponge. Barnes analyses Galen's deliberation into a series of deductions from axioms whose validity Galen assumes. These axioms include: (1) 'elemental opposites "cure" or remove one another', and (2) 'heat and cold are elemental

[96] See M. Frede 1987: 293, Barnes 1991: 98–9, Hankinson 2009: 209–10; see e.g. *MM* X.126.

[97] This method is also characterized as 'analysis', i.e. working back to axioms or premises. See Hankinson 1991*b*: 18–20, 2009: 222–5, Barnes 1991: 66–7; also *MM* X.33–4.

[98] Barnes 1991: 99–100.

[99] Barnes 1991: 66–7.

opposites'. Galen's reasoning also includes a premise that seems to be based on observation (3) 'coldness of the air is causing swelling of the entrails'. From these premises, Galen infers that the removal of cold will cause the swelling to subside, and that the application of heat will bring about this removal.[100] A second example, treating hollow wounds, shows how Galen's use of the axiomatic method is combined with responses to observable variations in the patient's condition. The relevant axioms include the ideas that every type of unnatural hollowness requires filling and that the generation of flesh, like the generation of anything else, requires a material (here, blood) and a technician (here, the correct mixture of the four primary qualities underlying the hollowed area). A further relevant axiom is that all change of quality is accompanied by the production of two sorts of waste matter, from which Galen infers that two drugs are needed (a drying and a cleansing agent) to counteract pus and filth in the wound. His preparation of the strength of the drugs takes into account two factors based on observation, the state (for instance, the moisture) of the wound and that of the patient's body. Galen contrasts the procedure illustrated in this way with that of the other medical schools of his day. That of the Methodists and Empiricists is limited to applying pre-determined routines and methods. Rationalist theory is limited to considering states of organs, whereas Galen's method extends to the more basic level of the uniform ('homoeomerous') parts of the body, such as flesh and blood. The distinctive strength of his method, as Galen himself sees it, lies in the combination of precisely formulated logical method, including the use of axioms, with perception-based observations, interpreted in the light of his logical reasoning.[101]

Another example takes us straight into a question central for the concerns of this book. Galen used his distinctive combination of logical reasoning and observation to settle (as he saw it) a key issue in ancient debate about embodied psychology, whether the ruling part of the psyche is located in the heart or the brain. The core functions of the ruling part are taken by Galen to be perception, volition, and the activation of movement. In logical form, Galen's

[100] Barnes 1991: 91–2, based on *MM* X.414–15.
[101] Barnes 1991: 100–2, based on *MM* X.173–86.

argument centres on identifying an appropriate middle term, which will determine whether the organ in question has, as a unique or distinctive attribute, the characteristic relevant for acting as the base for the functions of the ruling part. Galen assumes that the relevant middle term and distinctive attribute is that of being the beginning or source (*archē*) of the nerves. He offers proof of the claim that only the brain meets this criterion by a set of empirically based observations conducted by vivisection of animals. In particular, Galen demonstrates that cutting the laryngeal nerves, which start in the brain, paralyses the speech-functions, even though the pulse, which starts in the heart, and other automatic functions remain intact. The Stoics, by contrast had claimed (on the basis of the proximity of the heart to the wind-pipe and thus the speech-functions) that the heart housed the ruling part of the psyche.[102] Galen's argument is supported by observation of the effects of cutting links to other organs, notably the heart and the liver, which are taken by Galen to be the source of other internal systems (arteries and veins) but not of the nerves, which is the vehicle for activating volition, movement, and controlling speech-functions.[103]

From a modern standpoint, it is plausible to characterize this procedure as a set of 'experiments', and to say that this is one of the closest ancient analogues to modern 'scientific' method. Galen's procedures do, indeed, exhibit certain features that align them with modern scientific experiments. These include the attempt to eliminate factors irrelevant to the question being investigated and to take account of the effect of the impact on the body of the intervention involved in the procedures. Galen also stresses the repeatable character of the process.[104] This impression is supported by the fact that, at least as regards his account of the role of the brain as the source of

[102] On this Stoic argument, see nn. 139–40 below, and Ch. 3 below, text to nn. 49–52.

[103] See Tieleman 2002: 260–8, 2008: 55–9, referring esp. to *PHP* V.228, 2.4.5–6 De Lacy, V.232–7, 2.4.25–39 De Lacy, V.655, 8.1.22–4 De Lacy. See also Hankinson 1991*a*: 218–29. Galen's procedures used (non-human) animals, who do not, of course, 'speak' in a human sense, but who do vocalize in analogous ways; but Galen notes that a human being wounded in this way also loses speech-functions, *PHP* V.231, 2.4.21–2 De Lacy.

[104] *PHP* V.604, 7.3.13 De Lacy; see also Debru 1994: 1750–2, Tieleman 2002: 266–8.

the nerves, Galen's picture corresponds largely with that which can be established by modern scientific methods, as Julius Rocca has shown in a path-breaking study, which systematically correlates the modern picture of the brain with that offered by Galen.[105]

However—setting aside contemporary debate about the precise nature and truth-status of 'scientific' method and experiment[106]—there are a number of salient features that distinguish Galen's approach from that of modern science. One concerns the form of reasoning involved. Whereas we might now think in terms of a hypothesis, auxiliary hypothesis, and a test implication (which is the basis for the experiment), Galen seems to conceive the proof in terms of deduction from primary principles or axioms.[107] It is true that, here and elsewhere, Galen gives an integral role in the proof to precisely formulated observations. However, he is quite ready to combine what we should see as the results of properly conducted experiments with other considerations, based on common experience, as Galen interprets this.[108] Also, polemical and *a priori* considerations play a substantial role in shaping the arguments within which he deploys observation and the conclusions he draws from his observations.[109] Further, as has often been stressed, the concept of 'experiment' is not a firmly defined one in ancient thought. The concept of 'testing' (*peira*), which Galen adopts, partly following Empiricist practice, is broader and less technical than 'experiment', though it does give a significant role to observation with a precisely defined function.[110] Given these reservations, it is probably best to see Galen's study of the brain as a reflection of his characteristic methodology, combining logical reasoning and observation, rather than as an early example of

[105] See Rocca 2003; also 2008: 247–56.

[106] For challenges to prevailing orthodoxy on scientific method, see e.g. Kuhn 1962, Feyerabend 1975.

[107] Tieleman 2002: 262. On the logical form of the arguments involved, see Barnes 1991: 84–7, Morison 2008: 75–83; also Barnes 2003, which attempts to match the reasoning involved with recognized ancient types of argument.

[108] Tieleman 2002: 269, referring to *PHP* V.357–8, 3.8.35 De Lacy.

[109] On this as a general characteristic of what we think of as ancient 'science', see Lloyd 1979: 151–2, 1991: 72–3.

[110] Tieleman 2002: 257–8, 268 n. 47.

scientific experiment, though some features of his work strikingly prefigure the latter method.

Galen's logico-empirical method is also closely linked with his thinking on causation. Galen, typically, operates with a threefold causal schema; the central thought is that events are to be explained by reference to the *combination* of these causes. The three types are antecedent (procatarctic) causes, preceding causes, and sustaining or containing (synectic) causes. The antecedent cause is a salient external event or factor, the preceding cause is the effect of an external event on an internal state, and the sustaining cause is the determining factor in the resulting event. For instance, exceptional heat in the theatre (antecedent cause) may produce an overheated state (preceding cause) in a person with a disposition tending towards excessive heat, and may thus activate the specific feature of the internal state (synectic cause) that produces fever.[111]

Galen's theory of causes, like his logico-empirical method, forms part of his adoption of a distinctive stance within medical practice in his day. Galen's deployment of a causal framework of this type aligns him with the Rationalist or Dogmatist approach in medicine. Characteristic of this approach is the belief that well-grounded connections can be made between external factors, the internal workings of the body, illness, and treatment, and that these connections can appropriately be analysed in causal terms. The Empiricists and Methodists, influenced in differing degrees by ancient forms of scepticism, reject this type of approach. The Methodists offer a highly codified system of treatment centred on constriction and relaxation, and refuse to engage in speculation about possible antecedent causes or internal states.[112] The Empiricist position is more complex, and appears ambiguous, in both acknowledging and denying the significance of antecedent causes. However, what seems to underlie this position is the belief that there are certain recurrent patterns in illness and treatment, which can be recognized by experience and by drawing analogies between experiences. To this degree, typical antecedent factors for illness can be tracked; but these are treated (in a way that anticipates Hume's scepticism about causes) as event-patterns, known by experience, rather than as part of a causal framework

[111] See Hankinson 1994: 1764–7, 2003: 31–46.

[112] Hankinson 1994: 1759–60.

of explanation, based on theory and inference. Hence, as Galen suggests, an Empiricist and Dogmatist treatment of a bite from a rabid dog might, in practice, be much the same, though the Dogmatist therapy would be based on the assumption that causal analysis is valid and that it can be linked with an account of the internal workings of the body.[113] Galen also defines his approach by contrast with others, including the followers of Erasistratus, who deny the significance of antecedent factors at all. Galen argues that antecedent causes are important, but that a connection needs to be made between antecedent causes and the patient's disposition. As in the example cited earlier, heat in the theatre may be an antecedent cause of fever, but only in the case of patients with a tendency to overheating, in whose case we can also trace the appropriate preceding and synectic causes.[114]

Galen's thinking about causation is thus closely integrated with his logical–empirical medical method. By contrast with Methodist and Empiricist medicine, Galen aims at establishing, through a combination of observation and logical inference, objectively grounded causal links that enable effective treatment of a disease.[115] His method also depends on locating causal analysis in the context of an account of nature that is also, as Galen maintains, objectively grounded. Core features of this account, explained in the next section, are a conception of natural capacities and functions as expressing natural teleology and a view of matter as composed of mixtures of basic elements or opposites. For instance, in considering the causes of changes in the pulse, Galen presents as causes the capacities and functions of the pulse, as well as the combinations of heat and cold which have an impact on the operation of the pulse.[116] More broadly, Galen aims to interpret causal connections in the light of the teleological function of bodily organs and their

[113] The Empiricist position can also be defined in terms of sign-theory. They reject *analogismos* (inference from evident to non-evident) and *endeixis* (indication of what is non-evident), while relying on *epilogismos* (reasoning based on experience-based patterns): Hankinson 1987*a*: esp. 330–9. See also Hankinson 1998: 37–43.

[114] Hankinson 1994: 1760–4, 1998: 30–5, 45–8, 2003: 61–2.

[115] See Barnes 1991: 93–102.

[116] The former are presented as synectic and the latter as procatarctic causes. See Hankinson 2003: 43–6, discussing *Caus. Puls.* 1.1, IX.1–3.

material basis in appropriate mixtures of elements. Galen's causal theory both serves as a link between his logical–empirical method and his philosophy of nature and depends on those other strands in his medical thought.

These distinctive elements in Galen's method (his use of logic and causal theory) are strongly informed by Stoic thinking, along with Aristotelian ideas. This is so in spite of the fact, brought out later, that Galen is highly critical of the Stoic method of natural inquiry, particularly as applied to the question of the location of the ruling part of the psyche.[117] Galen's early studies with Stoic and Aristotelian teachers seem to have centred on logic.[118] His own practice in the treatises draws on the logical forms used in both systems and seems, eclectically, to combine them, though he also evolved his own type of analysis.[119] In certain respects, as Hankinson has stressed, the Stoic form of proof is more crucial for Galen's distinctive medical approach than the Aristotelian. Both forms of argument draw out the consequences inherent in the premises. But a salient part of the Stoic definition of proof is that it 'reveals by deduction a non-evident (*adēlos*) conclusion on the basis of agreed premises', and that it deploys for this purpose an 'indicative sign' (*sēmeion endeiktikon*).[120] As noted earlier, *endeixis*, 'indication' of non-evident conclusions from indicative signs was one of Galen's most characteristic forms of argument. Galen's use of this form of argument reflects his conviction that medical practice must rest on reconstructing the (non-evident) inner workings of the body, if it is to track effectively the basis of illness and cure.[121] It would seem, then, that the Stoic version of proof helped Galen to formulate a

117 For these criticisms, see text to nn. 136–40 below. Galen is also very critical of Aristotle for his alleged mistakes on the same question (text to n. 53 above).

118 Galen studied with (unnamed) pupils of the Stoic Philopator and the Peripatetic (Aristotelian) Aspasius. See *Aff. Dig.* V.41, *SM* 1.31.23–32.5, *Lib. Prop.* 11, XIX.43, *SM* 2.119.2–9. On the logical focus of his Stoic studies at this time, see Tieleman 2009: 284–6.

119 See Barnes 1991: 69, 71, 2003, on Galen's eclectic mix of Aristotelian logical forms and on his tendency not to specify or analyse the logical form of his own arguments. Morison (2008: 70–1, 105–13) maintains that Galen also introduced a form of analysis not found in either Aristotelian or Stoic analysis, namely that of 'relational' syllogisms.

120 Hankinson 2009: 209, referring to Sextus, *PH* 2.135; also, on the indicative sign, see Allen 2001: 170–88.

121 See M. Frede 1987: 293, also text to n. 96 above.

central feature of his logico-empirical method, as well as providing an important part of his equipment for argumentation.

There are also strong general similarities between Stoic theory and Galen's thinking on causation. As Michael Frede points out, in Galen's theory, as in much later ancient thinking about causes, the Stoic, rather than the Aristotelian, approach is dominant. The focus is on the explanation of events in terms of causal sequences, rather than on the analysis of the categories of the factors involved, which is central for Aristotle.[122] Galen's famous proof of the role of the brain as the location of the ruling part of the psyche depends on identifying a 'cause' in a distinctively Stoic sense, namely as a specific body which brings about an action or sequence of events.[123] Also, as in the Stoic theory, a crucial point is that explanation must take into account both external (antecedent) factors and the (internal) disposition of the person affected in order to explain a specific event. This comes out clearly in Galen's explanation, cited earlier, why one person (but not others) becomes fevered in a hot theatre.[124]

Although the Galenic theory is indebted to Stoic ideas in these respects, there are also salient differences. For one thing, the operation of this Stoic-style causal schema presupposes some ideas with a strongly Aristotelian character, including the idea that organs have a natural function or purpose and correlated natural capacities or potentialities.[125] Also, despite the general similarity between Stoic and Galenic thinking on causation, there are significant differences in terminology or analysis. For instance, the second Galenic category, the 'leading' cause, does not figure in Stoic sources, even though it identifies a factor (the initial impact of

[122] M. Frede 1987: 125–8, 143–6. Aristotle's causal analysis is couched in terms of a combination of formal, final, efficient, and material factors (which define the categories of the factors involved), whereas the Stoic account focuses on what Aristotle would call the 'efficient' cause.

[123] On this feature of Galen's proof, see Hankinson 1991*a*: 222; on causes as bodies in Stoicism, see LS 45; see also text to nn. 101–3 above.

[124] On the Stoic theory of causation, see LS 55; also Hankinson 1999: 483–97, Bobzien 1999. On Galen's explanation of fever, see text to nn. 111, 114 above.

[125] Hankinson 1998: 16–20, 2003: 46–57. The main relevant Aristotelian ideas are those of a 'final' cause (end or purpose) and the distinction between potentiality and actuality, as applied to natural entities. See also, on this combination of a Stoic approach and Aristotelian categories, Hankinson 2003: 54–7, 2008*b*: 225–30.

external circumstances on the internal state) which Stoic theory might reasonably have identified.[126] Also, Galen's use of the idea of a containing (synectic) cause is different from the Stoic use: it is deployed as part of the explanation of change rather than the analysis of the factors involved.[127] In addition, Galen does not adopt one very important use of the Stoic causal theory, namely to define the special character of (adult) human agency and responsibility by reference to the distinctive disposition and mode of response of humans as rational animals. This is a form of explanation that Galen might have found useful in *QAM* ch. 11 in particular.[128] Despite these differences, it seems very likely that Stoicism made a powerful contribution to Galen's method, particularly in underlining the importance for medicine of examining the causal interplay between external (antecedent) factors and internal disposition.

A third point of contact between Galen and Stoicism is worth noting, before turning to Galen's critique of Stoic methodology of natural inquiry. This relates to the theory of knowledge or epistemology. Galen claims to have been drawn at an early age towards scepticism about the possibility of knowledge; and there remain some seemingly sceptical or at least non-dogmatic strands in his thinking, notably his refusal to take a stand on certain theoretical questions and his refusal to commit himself to any one philosophical school.[129] However, he is strongly convinced of the possibility of gaining knowledge, for instance, in natural inquiry.[130] The criteria of knowledge for Galen, as outlined earlier, are perception and reason, taken either separately or in combination.[131] At one point, he suggests, in a rather breathtaking claim, that this conception of knowledge underlies sharply differing accounts of knowledge

[126] See Hankinson 1994: 1764–7, 1987*b*: 87–92, 1999: 490–1, 2003: 41–6. Thus, Galen's threefold pattern may go back to the medical writer Athenaeus of Attaleia, rather than Stoicism, though Athenaeus too had Stoic links.

[127] Hankinson 1987*b*: 82–3, Bobzien 1999: 229.

[128] This point was crucial for the Stoic combination of determinism and (adult) human responsibility; see LS 62, esp. C, and Bobzien 1998: ch. 6. On *QAM* ch. 11, see Ch. 3 below, text to nn. 294–304.

[129] *Lib. Prop.* XIX.39–40. See M. Frede 1987: 282–3; also text to nn. 4, 45 above.

[130] See further Hankinson 2009: 206–8.

[131] See text to nn. 92–4 above.

including the Stoic idea of the 'cognitive impression' (*phantasia katalēptikē*) and Academic (sceptical) thought about plausible or examined impressions.[132] He also suggests, in a distinct but related comment, that the use of these criteria is inbuilt in nature, and that it underlies the ability of non-human animals to recognize friend and foe and defend themselves as well as the forms of knowledge constructed by humans on the basis of this natural capacity.[133] Galen's sweepingly inclusive view reflects the kind of 'consensus' approach to philosophical issues we find in Antiochus (a member of the Academy in the first century BC) and in much later Platonic thought between Antiochus and Galen. Indeed, Galen's thinking on knowledge and its attainability may reflect Antiochus' specific views on these subjects.[134] However, the relevant point to note here is that, in spite of his full-scale onslaught on Stoic methodology of natural inquiry in *PHP* 2–3, Galen is still prepared to see the Stoics, alongside other thinkers, as sharing, in broad terms, the same conception of knowledge and its criteria as himself. In fact, the two points identified by Galen—the ideas that knowledge depends on a combination of reason and perception and that human beings are naturally adapted to acquire knowledge[135]—are, on any view, substantive features of Stoic epistemology and themes shared with Galen. There is no reason, in this case (by contrast with Galenic thinking on logic and causation) to see Stoicism as especially influential on the formation of his own thought. But Galen's comments, despite their broad-brush character and polemical context, show that his outspoken disagreements with Stoicism coexist with recognition of significant common ground on questions relating to the methodology of inquiry.

[132] *PHP* V.778, 9.7.3–4, p. 586.16–23 De Lacy. This inclusive claim is the more surprising since the Academic Sceptics consistently questioned the validity of Stoic theory about knowledge, especially the Stoic idea of a 'cognitive impression' (see LS 40–1).

[133] *PHP* V.723, 9.1.11–13, p. 542.7–20 De Lacy, V.725–6, 9.1.19–23, p. 544.8–21 De Lacy. [134] Hankinson 1992: 3511–12, 1997: 161–6, 206–13.

[135] On the combination of empiricism and rationalism (esp. the role of preconceptions, *prolēpseis*) in Stoic theory of knowledge, see M. Frede 1999*c*: 320–1. On the close linkage in Stoic theory between ideas about natural development (conceived as 'appropriation') and about acquiring knowledge (for instance, of the good), see Jackson-McCabe 2004.

I turn now to Galen's criticisms of Stoic methods of natural inquiry, and to the question how far they do justice to Stoic practice, in so far as we can reconstruct this. I focus on the arguments about the location of the ruling part of the psyche in *PHP* 1–3. On both topics, I draw on Tieleman's pioneering and comprehensive treatment (1996). The nub of Galen's critique is that the Stoics, especially Chrysippus, his main target, *fail* to deploy the kind of distinctive logico-empirical method that Galen has developed and applied so effectively to this question. More precisely, he criticizes Stoic methods on two grounds, both related to his own practice: the construction of an appropriate logical framework for the inquiry and the use of empirical observation in conjunction with this logical framework. A particular ground of criticism is that the Stoics fail to draw proper distinctions between four different kinds of premises of argument and use the premises in an undiscriminating and unsystematic way. The four kinds of premise are demonstrative (*apodeiktikon*) or scientific (*epistēmonikon*), dialectical, rhetorical, and sophistical. Galen distinguishes between these premises in this way. Scientific premises refer to the essence (*ousia*) of the object under investigation and are deployed with a view to reaching well-grounded conclusions. Dialectical premises refer to what are, at least, real attributes of the object under investigation, even if they do not refer to its essence; they are used with a view to philosophical training and intellectual challenge rather than reaching definite conclusions. Rhetorical premises, characterized as merely 'persuasive' (*pithanon*), constitute a broad group, including widely held opinions, comments taken from poets and other philosophical writings, and arguments from etymology. Sophistical premises are those dependent on features of language, such as ambiguity or verbal analogy, rather than on the real features of the object in question. Galen's schema for analysing premises is basically Aristotelian, though it may reflect some more recent influences. Galen's complaint is that the Stoics fail to observe these distinctions and that their arguments rely unduly on rhetorical and sophistical premises, as well as mixing all these types together.[136]

[136] Tieleman 1996: 12–23, referring e.g. to *PHP* V.221–2, 2.3.8–11 De Lacy, V. 227–8, 2.4.3–4 De Lacy.

These distinctions are preliminary to Galen's main ground of criticism of Stoic method, which centres on their claim, shared with Aristotle and his followers, that the heart, rather than the brain, is the seat of the ruling part of the psyche. He focuses both on the alleged defects in the logical form of their arguments and their failure to use relevant observation-based evidence. The first move, he argues, should be to establish the essence of the ruling part, which is widely agreed to be the source or centre of perception and motivation (*hormē*). The second is to determine what this source is, which can only be done effectively, he argues, by anatomical dissection.[137] This framework provides the basis for Galen's own argument, set out in syllogistic form in *PHP* V. 649–50, 8.1.3–5. This is that the ruling part is located where the nerves have their source (*archē*); since dissection shows that this is the brain, the brain is the location of the ruling part. Galen demands of those who hold the main competing view that the location is the heart (especially Stoics and followers of Aristotle), that they should construct an argument of similar type and effectiveness. They should show that the attributes of the heart, which need to be established by sound observation, are appropriate for demonstrating that it is the seat of the ruling part.[138] Galen considers, and argues against, a series of claims that might be considered as attempting to offer this type of demonstration. These claims are based on considerations about the relationship of the heart to the brain, about the physical structure of the heart, and about the functions of the heart.[139] Galen gives special attention to the Stoic argument, first formulated by Zeno, that the fact that speech, the vehicle of rational discourse, passes through the windpipe (near the heart) shows that the heart, rather than the brain, is the seat of the ruling part of the psyche. It is against this claim that Galen

[137] *PHP* V.219–20, 2.3.4–7 De Lacy; cf. Tieleman 1996: 23–6.

[138] *PHP* V.219–20, 2.3.4–5 De Lacy, V.227–8, 2.4.3–6 De Lacy: cf. Tieleman 1996: 28. On this argument, see also Morison 2008: 75–83, referring to *PHP* V.240–62, 2.5.1–97 De Lacy.

[139] See Tieleman 1996: 39–55. The latter two claims are supported by (1) Aristotle's statement that the heart has a large number of nerves which function as the origin of movement (Arist. *PA* 3.4, 666^b14–16, Gal. *PHP* V.278–9, 2.8.26–8 De Lacy); and (2) Chrysippus' argument that the heart is widely seen as the source of the emotions (and thus, of reasoning too, on Stoic assumptions), *PHP* V.268, 2.7.6–8 De Lacy.

mounts his powerful counter-argument for the brain, based on the systematic observation of the results of cutting the links between the larynx and the brain or the heart respectively. It is this demonstration that leads Galen to conclude that, even in this case, where the Stoic argument is appropriately formulated, it is open to disproof by methodical empirical observations, notably those based on Galen's own anatomical research.[140]

Galen's critique of Stoic methodology seems, on the face of it, an effective one. But does Galen provide a reliable account of the Stoic argument for the location of the ruling part of the psyche and of Stoic methodology in general? Tieleman maintains that Galen's account is profoundly misleading, but that we can extract from Galen's treatment, taken with other evidence, a more credible interpretation. In particular, he thinks we can reconstruct from *PHP* 2–3 the main line of argument in Chrysippus' treatise *On the Psyche*. Galen, as noted earlier, complains that the Stoics present the four different kinds of premises (scientific, dialectical, rhetorical, and sophistical) 'all jumbled together, one after the other'.[141] Tieleman thinks this is a misleading report of a distinctive methodology of inquiry. The underlying premise of the method, which can be paralleled in other aspects of Stoic theory, is that people in general have a natural capacity for grasping, up to a point at least, the truth about their psychological nature.[142] But philosophy also has a vital role to play in what the Stoics called the 'articulation' (*diarthrōsis*) of concepts and beliefs. 'Articulation' is not just a matter of reporting or summarizing conventional ideas; it represents a process of critical assessment of received ideas and of using them to construct theorized analyses of a given subject. In fact, Tieleman suggests that we can reconstruct from Galen's reports of Chrysippus' theory a progressive analysis of increasingly suggestive popular beliefs, leading from common beliefs to the implications of ordinary language and then to beliefs presented in poetry. Finally, the Stoic method presents fully

[140] Tieleman 1996: 43–4, referring to *PHP* V.231–9, 2.4.20–9 De Lacy; see also text to nn. 101–3 above.

[141] *PHP* V.220–1, 2.3.9, esp. p. 110.19 De Lacy, trans. De Lacy.

[142] A similar view is held as regards knowledge of the good, linked with Stoic ideas about innately formed ideas (*prolēpseis*) and the naturalness of development as 'familiarization' or 'appropriation' (*oikeiōsis*); see Tieleman 1996: 166–8.

argued theories, which offer a more complete and credible account of ideas that are expressed in more informal and less reliable form in popular beliefs.[143]

Tieleman suggests that this interpretation of Stoic method enables us to make sense of apparently puzzling or inconsistent features of Chrysippus' treatment of psychology. For instance, in passages cited by Galen, Chrysippus sometimes states that our inner perception or awareness does not yield definite knowledge about the location of the psychological functions, especially the ruling part of the psyche. As he sometimes puts the point, it is only 'as if' we had an inner awareness of the role of the heart as the seat of emotions such as anger.[144] Galen accuses Chrysippus of equivocation: Chrysippus claims that the role of the heart is something we perceive, implying that we have a good empirical basis for this belief, but Chrysippus also qualifies this claim and denies that such inner perception yields knowledge.[145] There might also seem to be a contradiction between these qualifications and the stronger claims sometimes made by Stoics about the idea that the heart is the seat of the ruling part. For instance, there is no sign of this type of qualification in connection with the formal arguments by Zeno and Chrysippus, based on the proximity of the heart to the functions linked with speech and the expression of rational thinking.[146]

Tieleman argues that there is no real inconsistency here, but rather the working out of the Stoic method of the 'articulation' of concepts and beliefs. The Stoics regard the expression of the common belief that emotions (at least) are located in the breast as a valuable indicator of what they see as the truth about the location of the 'control-centre' (*hēgemonikon*). On the other hand, they do not think that this is a matter on which (inner) perception can yield certain knowledge (or in Stoic terms, 'cognitive impression' (*phantasia katalēptikē*)). But they do think that such knowledge is in principle available, and that fully theorized arguments (such as the speech

[143] See Tieleman 1996: 264–73 (an overview of the method), also 160–2, 166–8, 200–3, 220–1.

[144] *PHP* V.291–2, 3.1.25–9, esp. pp. 172.24, 174.3 De Lacy; also V.288–9, 3.1.15, esp. p. 170.24 De Lacy.

[145] *PHP* V.267–70, 2.7.4–13 De Lacy; cf. Tieleman 1996: 147–50.

[146] For these arguments, see *PHP* V.241–3, 2.5.8–20 De Lacy.

argument) point towards a true account of the matter.[147] Tieleman also suggests that, in defining the epistemic status of beliefs on this matter, and others, the Stoics used the notion of the 'plausible' or 'persuasive' (*pithanon*) as a key criterial idea. Although this notion is normally associated in the Hellenistic period with the sceptical Academy, Tieleman argues that it was also an important idea for the Stoics. The use of this term by Stoics in connection with the arguments on the location of the ruling part should not be taken as implying that the Stoics concede that their arguments are *merely* plausible. Although the Stoics did think that some of the beliefs they cite in support of their theory (for instance, commonly held views) were merely plausible, they also used 'the plausible' as a broad concept that could embrace also true beliefs based on valid arguments.[148] On this basis, Tieleman argues that the methodology of the Stoic argument for the location of the ruling part of the psyche is much better conceived and more systematically carried through than Galen argues and that it is a more tenable alternative to the Galenic account than we might otherwise suppose.

Tieleman's analysis of Galen's critique and his reconstruction of the Stoic theory seem to me highly convincing. What implications does his discussion have for the theme of this section, the relationship between Galenic and Stoic methodology, and for the larger question raised in this chapter, about the extent to which the two theories have a shared naturalistic approach? What emerges clearly from Tieleman's account is that the Stoics have their own distinctive method of inquiry, based on determinate epistemological and procedural assumptions, and not—what you might suppose from reading *PHP* 2–3—that their work simply represents a failed or incompetent version of Galen's method. However, Tieleman's account has a further implication, which has a special importance for my concerns here. Although the Stoics have a distinct and credible method of inquiry, it is not obvious that it constitutes a method of *natural* inquiry, at least by comparison with Galen's method. It seems more appropriate to say that the Stoics have a *general* method of inquiry, which could be applied to different

[147] Tieleman 1996: 174–6, 264–73.
[148] Tieleman 1996: 255–87, esp. 269–70.

branches of knowledge or to various topics. The method is centred on the 'articulation' of existing beliefs and concepts and on determining what has a 'plausible' or convincing claim to truth. In this instance, the method is applied to a question that belongs to natural inquiry, the location in the body of the ruling part of the psyche. But it is not clear that the method, either in general or in its deployment in this case, is specially framed to deal with questions relating to the natural world.

In Galen's case, by contrast, the logico-empirical method, outlined earlier, does seem to be specifically directed to natural questions, at least to certain kinds of natural question. The main difference between the two approaches lies in Galen's use of systematic observation, used in conjunction with logical analysis to determine the questions for investigation raised and the inferences that follow from these observations. In particular, Galen's method was deployed in connection with observation of the animal body, including dissection of living and dead bodies, with a view to reaching conclusions about the workings of the human body, a topic that was central for Galen's medical concerns. Anatomy was a special area of attention, and one on which Galen thought he could claim to have made a distinctive and important contribution, especially regarding the question of the functions of the brain and nervous system. His observation-based work in anatomy informed his teleological analysis of the body in *On the Utility of the Parts* in a way that he, at least, saw as validating the design-based view of the body by contrast with alternative accounts. There is more scope for argument about whether Galen was able to support in this way his account of the 'first principles' of nature, that is, his analysis of matter in terms of the elements.[149] Certainly, we do not find in this connection the same kind of focused and effective use of the logico-empirical method that we find used to establish the location of the ruling part of the psyche. But in those areas where the method was applied, with definite, even impressive, results, it does seem right to say that Galen's method was, in a determinate sense, a method of *natural* inquiry.

[149] For a searching discussion of Galen's claims to have reached knowledge on this subject, see Hankinson 2009, esp. 233–8.

Galen notes that Chrysippus did not claim any special expertise in anatomy.[150] By contrast with, for instance, Aristotle and some of his followers, or the Ptolemaic doctors, Herophilus and Erasistratus, and Galen himself, the Stoic school is not known to have engaged in independent, observation-based anatomy, or, as far as I am aware, in other areas of empirical natural inquiry. This does not mean that the Stoics ignored the results of anatomically based research. They seem to have drawn especially on the anatomical work of Praxagoras (late fourth century BC), who, like Aristotle, saw the heart, rather than the brain, as the source of the nerves. Diogenes of Babylon, in his treatise, *On the Ruling Part of the Psyche*, seems to have offered a detailed account of the Stoic view of the function of the heart, probably formulated against the background of Praxagoras' work.[151] But here, as in other areas of natural inquiry, the Stoic contribution appears to have consisted in the systematization and analysis of the findings and accounts of other thinkers, including those whose work was more directly based on observation. This kind of contribution is consistent with the method of inquiry reconstructed by Tieleman, which gives a special emphasis to the 'articulation' of the concepts and beliefs of others, rather than on independent, observation-based investigation. This method includes discrimination between different kinds of expression of ideas, for instance, between commonly held opinions and theorized philosophical arguments about the location of the ruling part of the psyche.[152] So it is consistent with this method for them to construct theories on the basis of observational findings and theoretical accounts based on these findings, even if Stoic thinkers did not themselves contribute to such research.

Is there any reason why, in principle at least, the Stoics could not have adopted Galen's observation-based findings and incorporated them in their account of embodied psychology? I can see no reason why they should not have done, if circumstances had been different and they had had access to Galen's ideas when Stoic theory was in

[150] Gal. *PHP* V.187, 1.6.13 De Lacy.

[151] Tieleman 1996: part 1, ch. 4; also pp. 189–95. Diogenes was head of the Stoic school in the early to mid-second century. For some indications that the Stoics also responded to the arguments for the competing brain-centred view, see Ch. 3 below, text to nn. 33–7.

[152] See Tieleman 1996: 264–73.

its formative stages, that is, in the late fourth and third centuries BC. As brought out shortly, both theories share a similar philosophy of nature, in certain respects, and also share a 'naturalistic' conception of the psyche, by contrast, at least, with Platonic psyche–body dualism. In other respects too, including their thinking about logic, causation, and theory of knowledge, the theories also have substantial common ground. Thus, I can see no reason in principle why the Stoics, if this had been possible, should not have adopted Galen's logico-empirical method of natural inquiry. To put the point in more qualified form, they could have seen this method as the best available one for certain kinds of natural inquiry, including inquiry about the relationship between anatomical structures and psychological functions. As I argue in Chapter 3, the combination of Galen's anatomically based account of the role of brain and nerves and the Stoic unified account of the ruling part of the psyche would have made up a theory that is more credible and coherent than either account taken in isolation. If the Stoics had adopted the Galenic methodology of natural inquiry, this would have been the first step towards adopting the Galenic account of the brain and nerves; and, conceptually at least, this seems to me entirely possible.

2.3 PHILOSOPHY OF NATURE

The second topic on which I discuss shared or complementary ideas in Galenic and Stoic thought is the philosophy of nature. I focus on two aspects of their thinking: a teleological (design-centred) and a 'biological' conception of nature. I suggest that these add up to a coherent outlook which one might call 'high naturalism'. As well as exploring their common ground on this topic, and the extent to which Galen acknowledges this, I highlight certain broader differences in the way that the two theories conceive these ideas. I also indicate how these differences bear on their respective accounts of the nature of the psyche and on how Galen responds to the Stoic account (at least in *QAM*). This section, together with the preceding one, is designed to support the claim, made in Chapter 1, that Galen and the Stoics share a naturalistic approach to psychology. This shared view underlies the paradox, stressed in Chapter 1, that Galen is intensely critical, especially in *PHP* 1–5, of an approach to psychology with which he has, on the face of it, a good deal in common.

In what sense do the two theories have a shared naturalism of approach? In the first instance, both theories avoid or reject what one might call a non-naturalist or idealist idea of psyche. In the Hellenistic era and in Galen's day, the most prominent example of the latter idea is Platonic psyche–body dualism, as presented in some Platonic dialogues (notably the *Phaedo*) and as adopted by much later Platonism. For this approach, the psyche, more specifically the 'mind' (*nous*) or rational part of the psyche, is a non-natural (non-physical) entity that is only temporarily and contingently related to the body.[153] The Stoics explicitly reject this type of position and argue for the physicality of the psyche and psychological processes. Galen refuses to take a formal view on the question of the physical or non-physical nature of the psyche, which he regards as a purely speculative philosophical question that does not fall within the scope of his medically oriented natural inquiry. But in *QAM*, the Galenic work that comes closest to being a theoretical study of this question, Galen is highly sceptical about the credibility of Platonic psyche–body dualism. His central thesis there, 'that the capacities (or faculties, *dunameis*) of the psyche follow the mixtures (*kraseis*) of the body', while it is not, at least formally, a physicalist claim, comes very close to being such a claim.[154] *QAM* also adopts a naturalist approach to psychology, in that it analyses psychological processes in terms of an idea (mixture of elements) that is fundamental to Galen's philosophy of nature. Also, in other treatises that discuss questions related to psychology, including *PHP* and *Foet. Form.*, Galen treats psychological processes as embodied functions of humans and other animals, and presents the Stoics (plausibly) as doing the same.[155] So, on the face of it, there is a strong case for maintaining that Galen and

[153] See n. 41 above. [154] See further 3.5 below.

[155] In Galenic works of (practical) ethics, such as *Aff. Dig.* or *Mor.* (see 5.2 below), there is little or no reference to the embodiment or physicality of psychological functions; but this reflects a difference of focus, rather than the adoption of a non-physicalist view of psychology.

the Stoics share a naturalist approach to psychology, at least as defined by contrast with Platonic psyche–body dualism.

However, we can also make a stronger, and more positive, claim about Galenic and Stoic thought about nature, namely that this expresses what could be called 'high naturalism'. The salient features of this kind of naturalism are a teleological (design-centred) view of nature and the idea that natural entities have an inherent source of life and inbuilt capacities related to their character and structure; this could be described as a 'biological' conception of nature. The contrasting view, which we might call 'low naturalism', is that the universe as a whole and its contents, including animals, are products of random processes, more specifically, of the mechanical interaction of material objects. The 'high–low' contrast, incidentally, is designed to reflect the Galenic and Stoic view of the contrast, and not my own evaluation. The concept of 'nature' (*phusis*) is an important, even programmatic one, in both theories; and the term is used by them in connection with this type of naturalism.[156] I consider first Galenic, and then Stoic, versions of these ideas, and then discuss how far Galen recognizes this degree of common ground between his approach and the Stoic one.

In Galen's case, we can see, especially in works written around the same time as *PHP*,[157] the explicit adoption of the positions that I am associating with 'high naturalism'. In *On the Utility of the Parts* (*UP*), Galen takes a teleological approach to the study of anatomy, and explicitly links this stance with that of Plato's *Timaeus* and Aristotle's biological works. At the same time, he criticizes thinkers such as Anaxagoras or Epicurus, who present anatomical structure as the random outcome of mechanical processes, or who see the use of bodily parts as an adaptive response by humans and other animals to physical parts that have been formed randomly. In *On the Natural Faculties* (*Nat. Fac.*), Galen identifies, or rather constructs, a debate

[156] On the idea of 'nature' (*phusis*) in Galen, see the comprehensive study by Kovačić 2001, esp. ch. 2 on the theory of elements and physiology, and ch. 5, on teleology and the *scala naturae*; see also Moraux 1981 and Jouanna 2003. 'Nature' as a normative idea in Stoicism spans ethics and physics; for relevant aspects of their theory of the universe, see LS 44, 46–7, 54, and White 2003.

[157] *UP* 1 was written during the same period as *PHP* 1–6 (i.e. 162–6) and *UP* 2–17, *PHP* 7–9, and *Nat. Fac.* during 169–75.

between those who do or do not accept the (in modern terms) 'biological' picture of natural entities and processes that he advocates. Galen identifies this picture with the views of Hippocrates, as well as Plato, Aristotle, and the Stoics. The intended contrast is with those who see natural processes as the outcome of mechanical, material processes, namely Epicurus (again) and some later thinkers including Erasistratus and Asclepiades of Bithynia. In both works, Galen can be seen as defining a kind of 'high' naturalism, by contrast with what is—from a Galenic perspective—the 'low' (mechanistic or materialist) naturalism linked with thinkers such as Epicurus.

I now consider these two strands in Galen's thinking more closely, beginning with the teleological world-view, which Galen holds in a particularly strong form. Galen rejects the idea that there are any features of the natural world that are not subject to explanation in purposive terms.[158] He also rejects the idea that explanation in terms of mechanism or necessity can be combined with teleological analysis.[159] Galen does not only see purpose as built into nature but also assumes the existence of a creator or, more precisely (using the terms of Plato's *Timaeus*), a craftsman or demiurge, though one who operates within the normal causal processes of nature, unlike the Jewish God.[160] Galen's teleological programme is not, however, directed at explaining the universe as a whole or the functions of different natural kinds, considered in relation to each other or to the larger cosmic structure. His primary concern is with the animal, and especially human, body, though this is viewed as an integral part of the natural world. In particular, he sets out to show that each part of the body is perfectly designed to fulfil its own distinctive function and thus to play its role within the body's overall structure. This is

[158] Thus, in *UP* 1.272–6 Helmreich (May 1968: 260–3), Galen argues for the functional effectiveness of the gall bladder, which Aristotle saw as useless (*PA* 4.2, 677^{a}12–19). Galen expands the range of teleological explanation by including aesthetic considerations, e.g. as regards facial and pubic hair; see Hankinson 1989: 215–17, Sedley 2007: 240–1, on *UP* 2.154–5 Helmreich (May 1968: 530–2).

[159] See Hankinson 1989: 211–12, 214–15. Erasistratus is a special target for criticism in these respects, though Galen seems also to be indirectly criticizing Aristotle (see von Staden 1997*b*). On Aristotle's teleology, see Gotthelf and Lennox 1987, part 3, and Johnson 2005.

[160] Hankinson 1989: 219–20; for the contrast with the God of Moses (as Galen puts it), see *UP* 2.158–9 Helmreich (May 1968: 532–4).

the theme of Galen's main, and massive, teleological work, *On the Utility of the Parts.* Here, Galen draws freely on his own anatomical investigations and those of his medical predecessors.[161] Although the teleological approach is presented as inherently defensible, it also serves a heuristic or hypothetical function, in providing a theoretical framework, and a show-case, for Galen's anatomical and physiological study of the human body.[162]

This teleological approach is seen by Galen as closely linked with what one might call his 'biological' conception of natural kinds. This conception consists of a complex of interrelated ideas.[163] Galen maintains that the core principles of matter consist of the elements (hot, dry, cold, wet), and not atomic (indivisible) units. The elements are all capable of being 'mixed' with each other and in this sense of forming a natural continuum; their mixtures form the basic material for all living entities. The elements, in various combinations, form the basis of the four humours in this way: blood (hot and wet), yellow bile (hot and dry), black bile (cold and dry), and phlegm (cold and wet). The humours, in turn, provide the basis for the 'uniform' (homoeomerous) material such as flesh, ligament, vein, artery, and nerve, from which bodily organs are made. It is from these uniform materials that the three main organic systems in the animal body are constructed, seen as centred on the brain, heart, and liver. The transformation of the elements is taken to underpin natural processes of different kinds. For instance, the assimilation of nourishment by the uniform (homoeomerous) parts enables the production of bones and nerves. This framework also explains attraction and repulsion, expressed, for instance, in magnetism and the curative effect of medicines on bodily tissues.[164] More generally, the principle of the complete transformation of elements underlies Galen's understanding of the animal body as a system of interlocked natural processes. Thus, as von Staden puts it, we can see 'digestion, respiration, the pulse, voluntary motor

161 May 1968: 9–43.

162 This is not to suggest that Galen's teleology is presented as merely a heuristic strategy; as stressed by Hankinson 1989: 210–11, it constitutes a substantive claim.

163 On these ideas, see Moraux 1984; 736–42, Kovačić 2001: 89–125, Debru 2008, Hankinson 2008*b*: 210–25.

164 See Kupreeva 2004: 76–84, esp. 82, referring to *Nat. Fac.* X.28, 1.12.

activity, and cognition as continuously interactive components of a larger biological system'.[165]

The main features of this theory of bodily composition are summarized by Inna Kupreeva in these terms:

> a) [the] corporeal principle of things is matter, continuous and changeable throughout; (b) all physical bodies are constituted by the four elements [hot, cold, dry, wet] as described by Aristotle [and Hippocrates]; (c) all living bodies are constituted by the four humours which are analogous to the elements; (d) all the elements change into each other and interact with one another; (e) complex physical properties of bodily organs are all determined by their physical constitution, down to the level of the elements making up their texture.[166]

This framework of ideas is presented in a systematic form in *On Mixtures* (*Temp.*).[167] In *On the Natural Faculties*, Galen defends them, as a set of controversial claims, against what he presents as an opposing, mechanistic conception of nature, associated by him especially with Erasistratus and Asclepiades of Bithynia, as well as Epicurus.[168] Galen's theory rests on two main theoretical assumptions. One is that only a conception of matter as forming a continuum, in which the elements are capable of complete exchange and transformation, can support the idea of nature as a source of animation and internal organization. The opposing view that matter consists of atomic (indivisible) units, whose combination provides the basis of living and non-living entities, Galen regards as untenable. In modern terms, the salient thought seems to be that only reference to a complete (chemical) fusion of elements is adequate to explain the idea of the organic or biological properties of living or natural entities.[169]

165 See von Staden 1997*b*: 199.

166 Kupreeva 2004: 77; also May 1968: 44–5, Hankinson 2008*b*: 210–23.

167 Another important work for this topic is *On the Elements according to Hippocrates* (*Hipp. Elem.*), also written in the period 169–75.

168 See esp. *Nat. Fac.* X.26–30, 1.12. See von Staden 1997*b*, and 2000: 105–16; also Vegetti 1999, underlining the speculative theoretical project of *Nat. Fac.* and the tendentious presentation of other thinkers.

169 See also Hankinson 2008*b*: 213: 'What is ruled out . . . is what one might call the supervenience of generically different properties: any supervenient properties must be similar in general type to properties actually disposed of by the elements they supervene upon.'

A second assumption underlying Galen's theory is that the animal body constitutes an internally coherent structure, in which each of the component parts and organs has a natural activity (*energeia*) and function (*chreia*), and also a natural faculty or capacity (*dunamis*) for performing this activity as part of a larger system. These natural capacities are those of generation, growth, and nutrition; these are associated with more basic (natural) capacities of attraction, retention, assimilation, and repulsion. Galen insists that these natural capacities cannot be reduced simply to mechanical principles. As R. J. Hankinson puts it, for Galen, the 'great mistake of earlier physicians like Erasistratus and Asclepiades was to think that the fluid dynamics of the body can be reduced to [mechanical] principles like that of *horror vacui*'.[170] Galen acknowledges that the idea of a natural faculty is, to some degree, a provisional one, and not a complete or definitive analysis of an organ in its anatomical or physiological nature or in its role as a cause. However, the importance of deploying the idea of a natural faculty or capacity, like that of function, is that it fits with the teleological, non-mechanical, conception of nature to which Galen is committed. The processes of living entities such as human beings are conceived as forming a coherent system of functions that are correlated with the (teleologically informed) anatomical structure of each natural kind.[171] As Galen puts it, near the start of *Nat. Fac.*:

as long as we are ignorant of the true essence of the cause which is operating, we call it a *faculty* [or 'capacity', *dunamis*]. Thus we say that there exists in the veins a blood-making faculty, as also a digestive faculty in the stomach, a pulsative faculty in the heart, and in each of the other parts a special faculty corresponding to the function or activity of that part. If, therefore, we are to investigate methodically the number and kinds of faculties, we must begin with the effects (*erga*); for each of these effects comes from a certain activity (*energeia*), and each of these again is preceded by a cause.[172]

[170] Hankinson 2008*b*: 223. See also von Staden 1997*b*, which argues that Galen radically misrepresents Erasistratus and understates his commitment to natural teleology.

[171] On the idea of natural faculties or capacities, and its importance for Galen, see May 1968: 49–50, Vegetti 1999: 388–91, Tieleman 2003*b*: 144–51 (in connection with psychology), Debru 2008: 270–1, Hankinson 2008*b*: 223–25.

[172] *Nat. Fac.* X.9, 1.4, trans. Brock 1916.

Thus, Galen's ideas about natural faculties, and about the elementary basis of matter, are closely linked with his teleological world-view. Both themes form part of a conception of nature as a source of providential organization and animation, by contrast with an understanding of nature in terms of mechanical processes and fortuitousness.[173]

Could Galen have found similar ideas in Stoic philosophy and how far does he acknowledge the Stoics as previous exponents of (what I am calling) 'high naturalism'? There is a good deal in Stoicism, I think, that prefigures Galenic thought on these topics, as Galen recognizes, at least as regards the 'biological' view of natural kinds. Their shared adoption of this kind of naturalism reflects, in part at least, the impact of one, very important, shared influence. This is Plato, especially the Plato of the *Timaeus*. As some recent scholarship has underlined, Plato's *Timaeus* was a work of immense influence in the Hellenistic and post-Hellenistic eras.[174] Although dialogues such as the *Phaedo* served as a potent influence on those drawn towards psyche–body dualism, the *Timaeus*, arguably Plato's most 'one-world' dialogue, had a powerful appeal for those seeking to formulate a naturalistic view of the universe and its contents. I have suggested elsewhere that, in the context of the early Hellenistic age, Stoicism may have emerged, in part at least, as a form of 'naturalized' Platonism.[175] It seems likely that Plato's *Timaeus*, perhaps mediated through the teaching of the early Academy, played a special role in shaping Stoic thinking about the fundamental principles of physics.[176] Plato's *Timaeus* seems also to have served as a paradigmatic expression for salient features of the 'high naturalism' adopted by both the Stoics and Galen. Most important here is Plato's view of the universe as providentially shaped. One aspect of this view is the picture of the human body as a teleologically designed structure, and of psychological functions as physically located in, and interlocked with, this structure.[177] The influence of this picture on Galen, especially in its linkage between the structure of human anatomy and psychological

[173] On this linkage, see Hankinson 2008*b*: 225–9.

[174] See e.g. Reydams-Schils 1999 and 2003.

[175] Gill 2006: 15–16.

[176] See Sedley 2002, also Dillon 2003: 168–74.

[177] See Pl. *Ti.* 69c–72d.

functions, is explicit in *PHP*.[178] But I have also suggested elsewhere that it may also have helped to shape the Stoic picture of the human (and animal) body as an integrated psychophysical structure, in spite of the obvious contrast between Plato's tripartite psyche and the Stoic unified conception of psyche.[179] Other notable features of the *Timaeus* that may also have promoted what I am calling 'high naturalism' include the idea of a world-psyche that is systematically integrated with the world-body.[180] This may have helped to promote the belief, important for both the Stoics and Galen, that animation or vitality is inbuilt in the natural universe.[181]

As these comments indicate, there is a good deal in Stoicism that anticipates both aspects of Galen's version of 'high naturalism'. But how close, to be more precise, are their two versions and how far does Galen acknowledge the resemblance? I begin with the question of the teleological world-view. In comparing the Galenic and Stoic versions, it is useful to refer to Hankinson's analysis of types of teleology. In his terms, a teleological framework should be seen as 'genuine' if the end-states (the outcome of the design) are conceived as being integral to the explanation of the process of generation and not simply as a way of characterizing processes that can be explained in other ways. A framework is 'without gaps' if all relevant features are explained in this way, as distinct from being explained as incidental, mechanical, or necessary by-products or concomitants of the design. The framework is 'directed' if the explanations make reference to consciously intended purposes.[182] These distinctions enable us to relate Galen's version of teleology to those of Plato (in the *Timaeus*) and Aristotle (especially in his *Parts of Animals*), to which Galen responds explicitly. By these standards, all three of these ancient teleological approaches are 'genuine'. The approaches of Plato and Galen are also 'directed' (both refer to a craftsman-god or demiurge), while only Galen's view is wholly 'without gaps'.[183] The Stoics offer another well-known ancient version of teleology. Their version is 'genuine', like the others,

[178] See Ch. 3 below, text to nn. 120–39; also Gill 2006: 296–8.

[179] Gill 2006: 16–17, 298–304.

[180] Pl. *Ti.* 32a–37c.

[181] See LS, vol. 1, p. 319, on Stoicism; on the relevant Galenic ideas, see text to nn. 163–9 above.

[182] Hankinson 1989: 208–10, 214–15.

[183] See further Hankinson 1989; also 1988.

though not 'without gaps', as explained shortly. Their approach is 'directed' in that the Stoic god is the source of purposive planning but their god is immanent in natural processes and is not a Platonic or Galenic independent craftsman.[184]

In his masterwork on natural teleology, *On the Utility of the Parts*, Galen does not refer explicitly to the Stoic version, although he discusses extensively the ideas of Plato and Aristotle, as well as non-teleological frameworks, which he criticizes.[185] This silence on the Stoics might seem surprising, especially as, like Galen, they offered a teleological account of the human body, to judge from Cicero's account of Stoic theology in *On the Nature of the Gods* (*N.D.*) book 2.[186] Also, Galen, like the first-century Stoic Epictetus, cites the beard as a providential index of maleness (and we have evidence that Epictetus' teachings were known to Galen). But Galen's comments do not highlight the link with Stoic thought on this point.[187]

Why does Galen not seek support in this prominent version of natural teleology, as he does with other features of the Stoic philosophy of nature, noted shortly?

He may, quite simply, not be familiar with the relevant Stoic texts, though he must have known their views in outline.[188]Also, his disagreement with the Stoics about the location of the ruling part of the psyche (and thus about their account of the respective functions of brain and heart), might have deterred him from exploring their teleological picture of the human body in general.[189] However,

[184] See LS 46, 54. On all three versions of natural teleology, see Sedley 2007: chs. 4, 6–7; on Galen's teleology, see Kovačić 2001: ch. 5.

[185] Although some extracts from *UP* are cited as *SVF* 2.1135–7, 1139, these do not contain explicit references by Galen to Stoicism.

[186] Cic. *N.D.* 2.133–50.

[187] Cf. Gal. *UP* 2.153–7 Helmreich (May 1968: 529–32) and Epict. *Diss.* 1.16.9–14. Galen wrote a lost work *In Defence of Epictetus against Favorinus*, though this centred on epistemology (it was anti-sceptical), not on providence; see Gal. *Lib. Prop.* XIX.44, *Opt. Doct.* I.41. See further Flemming 2009: 79–81, who also underlines Galen's reticence about Stoic thinking on providence, and Tieleman 2009: 293, on Galen's reference to Epictetus.

[188] On the limitations of Galen's reading and close study of Stoic treatises, and his apparent reliance on doxographical reports, see Tieleman 2003*a*: 51–8, 61–5, 80–8, and 2009: 296–7.

[189] *UP* 1 was written at the same time as *PHP* 1–6 (162–6), and the rest of *UP* was written during the same period as *PHP* 7–9 (169–75).

Galen's disagreement with Aristotle on the same subject did not have the same effect; he refers extensively to Aristotle's teleological approach to animal anatomy.[190] Another possible reason for Galen's reticence might lie in differences between the two versions of teleology, both on specific points and in their overall focus. The Stoics, like Plato's *Timaeus*, accept that the achievement of natural purpose may entail certain necessary by-products that are not inherently desirable. For instance, Chrysippus, like Plato, thinks that the special functions of the head (centred for the Stoics on sight) entail having more delicate, and thus, fragile bones. Galen, by contrast, in his account of the bones of the head, as in other respects, sees bodily construction as ideally suited for function.[191] Other differences in the Stoic version of the teleological world-view include a focus on the teleological character of the universe as a whole, not just the body, and on the idea of animal species as beneficial for each other.[192] However, Galen's differences from Plato or Aristotle on such points do not prevent him from making extensive references to their ideas on this subject.

Galen's lack of reference to Stoicism on natural teleology and his contrasting readiness to cite them in support of his ideas on the elements may both be tactically motivated. As Mario Vegetti points out, there are salient differences between these two aspects of his thinking, which probably affect the way Galen refers to other theories, including Stoicism.[193] Galen's thinking on natural teleology has a secure basis, as he supposes, in his detailed and systematic work on animal anatomy. Also, Galen's teleological views have widespread

[190] See e.g. 1.4–12 Helmreich (May 1968: 69–75); see further Moraux 1985 and van der Eijk 2009: 266. On Galen's attitude to Aristotle in general (and its relevance for understanding his response to Stoicism), see text to nn. 48–60 above.

[191] See *SVF* 2.1169–70 (= LS 54 Q, esp. (2)) (= Gel. 7.1.1–13, esp. 7), cf. Pl. *Ti.* 75a–d. On the question of the kind of imperfection involved in such cases, see Sedley 2007: 118–21. On the providential function of sight, in Stoic theory, see Cic. *N.D.* 2.140, 145. Contrast Gal. *UP* 1.476–80 Helmreich (May 1968: 409–12) on the thick and thin membranes around the brain and the (positive) functions these fulfil in the body's structure.

[192] See e.g. LS 54 A–E, H–J; and N–P. Although Galen's teleology has a cosmic dimension (e.g. in *UP* Book 17), the main focus is on the design displayed in the animal (esp. human) body.

[193] See Vegetti 1999, esp. 383–6, 391–2, 395.

support among major earlier thinkers, notably Plato and Aristotle, even if he thinks they do not go far enough in design-centred explanation of bodily forms. Galen thus has no special need to cite the Stoics as well, especially as he has a low opinion of their anatomical expertise, in addition to the other points of disagreement just noted. Relevant too, though in a more generalized way, may be certain broader conceptual differences between Galen and Stoicism reviewed shortly, which have a bearing on their respective versions of the philosophy of nature.[194] Galen's account of the elements (and their 'mixtures') is more speculative and less securely supported by empirical investigation than his teleology, though Galen still believes that his ideas are fully defensible.[195] Hence, Galen is keen to recruit the Stoics, as well as Hippocrates and Aristotle, to support his point of view. However, Galen's attempt to create a consensus on the elements involves some blurring of differences between the theories, as well as a highly inventive presentation of Hippocrates.[196] However, regardless of Galen's reticence on Stoic natural teleology, this subject, together with their thinking on the elements, constitutes a solid area of common ground between the two theories, which could have been explored more fully, had Galen chosen to do so.

By contrast, Galen is quite ready to include the Stoics in a supposed consensus about the elements as the first principles, and does so in three different works.[197]

For it was Hippocrates who first of all introduced the doctrine of the Hot, the Cold, the Dry, and the Wet; later Aristotle gave a demonstration of it. Chrysippus and his followers took it over ready-made, and did not indulge in futile strife, but say that everything is blended (*kekrasthai*) from these things, and that they act and react upon each other, and that nature is

[194] See text to nn. 206–12 below.

[195] See further Hankinson 2008*b*: 210–17, 222–3, 345–6, also Hankinson 2009: 233–8.

[196] On the inventive treatment of Hippocrates on the elements, see Hankinson 2008*b*: 211–14, 217–18. See also Jouanna 2003, Flemming 2009: 72–3, on Galen's creative attribution of a providential view of 'nature' (*phusis*) to Hippocrates.

[197] The three works cited below, like *UP* 2–17 (and *PHP* 7–9) were written during 169–75; so Galen's different treatment of the Stoics in this connection, by contrast with that of natural teleology, is not explained by chronological considerations.

constructive (*technikēn phusin*); and they accept all the other Hippocratic doctrines, except in one small matter in which they differ from Aristotle.[198]

Thus, the well-blended individual must enjoy a combination of heat and moisture in his nature, and good balance in fact consists in nothing other than the domination of these two qualities... The same appears to be the opinion of the philosopher Aristotle, of Theophrastus, and subsequently also of the Stoics.[199]

Hippocrates was the first of all the doctors and philosophers we know who undertook to demonstrate that there are, in all, four mutually interacting qualities (*poiotētas*), and that to the operation of these is due the genesis and destruction of all things that come into and pass out of being... [and] that all these qualities undergo a complete blending with one another (*kerannusthai... holas di' holōn*). As to the question whether we are to suppose that the substances (*ousias*) as well as their qualities (*poiotētas*) undergo this complete blending, as Zeno of Citium afterwards declared, I do not think it necessary [to discuss this here].[200]

The main features of Galen's conception of matter, outlined earlier, are the four elements, seen as capable of transformation into each other, which form the basis for the humoral composition of living bodies and for the capacities and functions of their organs. This theme is closely linked, in Galen's mind, with his teleological approach to bodily structures. The element-based conception of matter is seen as a necessary underpinning of the idea of organic entities as coherent (designed) wholes and complexes of inherent or natural faculties and functions.[201]

How credible is Galen's inclusion of the Stoics as supporters of this set of ideas? In several respects, the Stoics seem to fit rather well into Galen's schema. As well as holding a version of the theory of the four elements (hot, cold, dry, wet), they also maintain that the elements are capable of complete interpenetration, more precisely of 'total blending' or 'mixture' (*krasis*). They also link this theory of the interpenetration of elements with the idea that living things have inherent vitality and the capacity for other, more complex,

198 *MM* X.16, 1.2.10, trans. Hankinson 1991*c*. See also X.18, 1.2.13, linking 'Plato, Aristotle, and Chrysippus'.

199 *Temp.* I.523, 1.3, trans. Singer 1997*a*: 208.

200 *Nat. Fac.* II.5, 1.2, trans. Brock 1916, modified.

201 See text to nn. 157–73 above.

functions.[202] Galen's attempt to assimilate Stoic theory on this subject to that of Aristotle is rather more problematic. The Stoic theory of total blending was highly controversial and was strongly criticized by followers of Aristotle.[203] Galen alludes to this criticism in the passage from *Nat. Fac.* just cited, and sometimes modifies his own account in the light of this criticism.[204] However, in *Nat. Fac.* Galen presents this difference between Aristotle and the Stoics as relatively unimportant in comparison with the broader contrast between element-based and atomic conceptions of matter.[205] For the purposes of this contrast, the Stoic theory might, in fact, be seen as even more serviceable than the Aristotelian equivalent because the idea of total blending embodies the principle of mutual transformation of elements in the strongest possible form. To this degree, Galen's co-opting of the Stoic theory seems highly justified. Taken together with the resemblance just noted between Galenic and Stoic thought on teleology, this similarity supports my suggestion that the two theories (along with some other Greek theories) can be seen as adopting a specific kind of naturalism ('high naturalism'), by contrast with the more mechanistic naturalism associated especially with Epicurus.

However, in some respects, the Stoic theory fits uneasily in Galen's schema. This is a point on which it is useful to refer to the broad conceptual differences between Galen and Stoicism highlighted in Chapter 1.[206] The difference derives from the combination of revisionism and holism that is highly characteristic of Stoicism. By 'revisionism' I mean their willingness to revise and replace familiar or received categories and distinctions, including those established in previous philosophical frameworks. The idea of holism is, of course, a broad one, centring on the tendency to analyse entities in terms of

[202] LS 47, esp. 47 A–B (four elements), G, H–I (also section 48) (total blending), C, N–O (innate vitality and other functions).

[203] See LS 47 I–J and 48, also Moraux 1984: 740–1. The issue (as presented in *Nat. Fac.* II.5, cited in text to n. 200 above) is whether blending takes place at a fundamental level (the Stoic view) or affects only the properties of substances (the Peripatetic view, reflecting the Aristotelian idea that elements are properties of substances, which constitute the primary units of reality).

[204] *Hipp. Elem.* 9.35–9 De Lacy; see also Kupreeva 2004: 81–2.

[205] *Nat. Fac.* II.5 (1.2), II.92 (2.4), also *Prop. Plac.* 15.1 Nutton.

[206] See Ch. 1 above, text to nn. 40–51.

whole states rather than component parts. I have tried to give more precision to this idea by referring to the distinction, deployed by Harte in connection with Plato, between competing ways of analysing the part–whole distinction, namely, in terms of competing 'structure' or 'composition' (or holistic and atomistic) conceptions of the part–whole relationship. There are several issues on which the Stoic combination of revisionism and holism generates a significant difference of view from Galen's thinking. As stressed in Chapter 1, this is not because these features are wholly absent from Galen's thought; on the contrary, there are a number of ways in which we can find similar tendencies in his thinking. But on several points the Stoics go significantly further in this direction than Galen does. These points may give rise to explicit conflict between the theories, as we find in certain parts of *PHP*. But they may also give rise to a lack of conceptual fit or dislocation between the two theories, though one that may not be recognized by Galen himself. This is the case here, I think. This lack of conceptual fit coexists with some important shared features, notably those I am associating with 'high naturalism'.

The aspects of Stoic theory which Galen cites (the idea of elements and total blending), form part of an over-arching analysis of principles and causes, the scope of which goes beyond defining the material basis of *living* entities, which is Galen's concern here.[207] The two fundamental principles are presented as being an active cause (sometimes identified with *pneuma*) and a passive one (*hulē*), both of which are conceived as material or bodily in nature. These principles are the core features of an explanatory framework, centred on the type or degree of 'tension' (*tonos*) in the blending of active and passive causes. This framework provides the basis for analysing unity or structure in different kinds of entity: the spectrum of tension runs from *hexis* in lifeless objects to *phusis* in plants, psyche in animals, and rationality in adult humans and gods.[208] This summary by Philo of Alexandria encapsulates some of the radical implications of this idea:

> Intelligence (or mind, *nous*) has many powers, the tenor kind, the physical, the psychic, the rational, the calculative... Tenor (*hexis*) is also shared by

[207] The following two paragraphs constitute a modified version of Gill 2007*a*: 100–1.

[208] See LS 44 B, 45 G–H, 47 *passim*; also LS vol. 1: pp. 270–1, 286–9.

lifeless things, stones and logs, and our bones, which resemble stones, also participate in it. *Phusis* also extends to plants, and in us too there are things like plants—nails and hair. *Phusis* is *hexis* in actual motion. Psyche is *phusis* which has also acquired impression and impulse. This is also shared by irrational animals.[209]

One of the implications of the Stoic theory is that *all* entities, both natural and non-natural, can be understood as manifestations of the 'complete blending' of god (or the active principle, or fire) with matter (or the passive principle, or the other elements).[210] This difference comes out if we juxtapose a passage from Galen's *MM*, cited earlier, to a summary of a related aspect of Stoic theory.

For it was Hippocrates who first of all introduced the doctrine of the Hot, the Cold, the Dry, and the Wet; later Aristotle gave a demonstration of it. Chrysippus and his followers took it over ready-made, and did not indulge in futile strife, but say that everything is blended (*kekrasthai*) from these things, and that they act and react upon each other, and that nature is constructive (*technikēn phusin*); and they accept all the other Hippocratic doctrines, except in one small matter in which they differ from Aristotle.[211]

The Stoics made god out to be intelligent, a designing fire (*pur technikon*), which methodically proceeds towards creation of the world, and encompasses all the seminal principles according to which everything comes about according to fate, and a breath pervading the whole world, which takes on different names owing to the alterations of the matter through which it passes.[212]

The contrast between the two conceptions can be exemplified by the difference between two seemingly similar phrases: Galen's 'constructive (or craft-like) nature' (*technikēn phusin*) and the Stoic 'designing fire' (*pur technikon*). Galen's concern is with showing how the blending of the four elements provides the basis for understanding the nature of living things, especially their inbuilt teleological ('craft-like') functions. The Stoic theory is intended to show how the blending of god or designing fire with matter provides a unified

[209] Philo, *Allegories of the Laws* 2.22–3, trans. LS 47 P, slightly modified.
[210] See further Long 1996: 227–9 and LS vol. 1: pp. 270–2, 286–9, 292–4.
[211] *MM* X.16, 1.2.10, trans. Hankinson 1991*c*.
[212] Aëtius 1.7.33, trans. LS 46 A.

explanatory framework for *all* entities, including those that are structured by *hexis* rather than *phusis*. This point of difference exemplifies the conceptual contrast outlined earlier. Although both these Galenic and Stoic theories aim at a unified or holistic account, the Stoic analysis is more—or more systematically—holistic, for instance, in cutting across the standard distinction between natural and non-natural entities, which remains important in Galen's framework.

A similar tendency can be seen in another passage, Galen's characterization of the Stoic theory of psyche in *QAM*, which is relevant in several ways for understanding the relationship between Stoic and Galenic ways of thinking. This passage brings out the linkage in Galen's mind between his philosophy of nature and his thinking about psychology. It also exhibits the shared naturalism in Galenic and Stoic thinking about psychology. The comment also illustrates the contrast between Galenic or Stoic body-based thinking about psychology and (Platonic-style) psyche–body dualism, which is explicitly rejected in this treatise. It also shows the shared adoption by Galen and Stoicism of 'high naturalism', at least in the linkage made between psychology and the theory of the elements and blending or mixture. However, the passage also brings out certain subtle but important differences in the way in which this naturalistic conception of psychology is understood. For one thing, it shows how Galen's description assimilates the Stoic account of the psyche to the Aristotelian one, which Galen himself seems inclined to accept. For another, Galen's comments on this aspect of Stoic thought, like those on the Stoic theory of elements, fail to bring out its more radically revisionist and holistic features.

The relevant passage comes in a treatise (*QAM*) in which Galen maintains that the physiological make-up and state of humans and other animals, understood in terms of the 'mixtures' of elements, has a determining effect on their psychological capacities and individual character. In support of this thesis, he cites quotations and ideas from a whole series of earlier thinkers, including Hippocrates, Aristotle, and the Stoics, as well as selected aspects of Plato's writings. The precise nature of Galen's thesis in *QAM* and its relationship to other aspects of his thought, are considered later (3.5). Here, my concern is simply with Galen's characterization of the Stoic theory of psyche, taken as illustrating a shared naturalism, but one conceived in significantly different ways.

Before citing Galen's comments on Stoicism, it is useful to consider his characterization of Aristotle's idea of psyche, which provides some of the conceptual language in which Galen analyses Stoic thinking on this subject.[213] This passage is one of the places in *QAM* where Galen articulates the physicalist conception of psyche that he comes close to adopting in this work, despite his normal reluctance to take up a position on the substance of the psyche. He does so by commenting on what, in his view, Aristotle's account of psyche implies. He begins from Aristotle's standard definition of the psyche as the 'form' (*eidos*) of the body,[214] and then argues that 'form', in effect, means the basis of material composition, that is, the specific mixture of the elements. The rationale for Galen's move is the claim that only this factor (mixture of elements) is common to both levels of bodily composition: that of uniform (homoeomerous) parts such as flesh or sinew and also that of bodily organs. Therefore, 'form' must refer to this factor, rather than to 'shape' (*morphē*) or arrangement, which could only apply to organs such as the heart or brain.[215] He formulates the implications of Aristotle's view in this way:

Now, given that all such bodies are composed of matter and form, and, as Aristotle himself thinks, when the four qualities are generated in the matter of physical things, bodily mixture is generated out of them, he must posit this latter as the form. So the substance of the psyche must be some sort of mixture of the four: of wet and dry, cold and hot, if you want to call them qualities, or, if you prefer, of the wet, hot, cold and dry bodies; and hence we will show that the powers of the psyche are consequent upon [or 'follow', *hepomenas*] its substance.[216]

[213] The remainder of this section is close in content to Gill 2007*a*: 102–4.

[214] See Arist. *De An.* 2.1, esp. 412^{a}19–21, 27–8.

[215] *QAM* IV.773–4, *SM* 2.37.5–15; see also Lloyd 1988: 24, Hankinson 2006: 246. On Galen's thinking about bodily composition, see text to nn. 163–9 above.

[216] *QAM* IV.774, *SM* 2.37.16–26 (the last clause is bracketed as dubious by the editors of *SM* but seems to be in line with Galen's argument here), trans. Hankinson 2006: 246; see also the translation of Singer 1997*a*: 153 (which omits the last clause).

Galen thus interprets Aristotle's theory of psyche as the form of the body in the light of Aristotle's own theory of elemental transformation in *GC* 2.2–4,[217] and on this basis he attributes to him the core thesis of *QAM* about the dependence of psychological on physiological character. This type of conceptual recasting of other theories to assimilate them to Galen's main claim is typical of *QAM* and is even more strongly marked in the case of Stoic theory.

Galen characterizes the Stoic theory in these terms:

> [The Stoics] hold that the psyche, like nature [*phusis*] is a kind of breath (*pneuma*) but that of nature is more humid and colder, whereas that of psyche is drier and hotter. That is why this *pneuma* too is a kind of matter (*hulē*) appropriate to the psyche and the form (*eidos*) of the matter is such-and-such a mixture (*krasis*), consisting in a proportion of the airy and fiery substance (*ousia*)... It has, then, become clear to you now that in the view of the Stoics the substance of the psyche comes to be according to a particular mixture of air and fire. And Chrysippus has been made intelligent because of the well-tempered mixture of these two [elements], while the sons of Hippocrates... [have been made] swinish because of the boundless heat.[218]

The general character of Galen's analysis is similar to that applied to Aristotle, and Galen uses Aristotelian language to analyse the Stoic theory. We find again the idea that the 'form' is a certain mixture or proportion of the elements, or at least two of them (fire and air). This form is said to be the 'substance' of the psyche; at least, the psyche 'comes to be' (*gignetai*) according to this mixture. On this basis, Galen presents the Stoic conception of psyche as being (in effect at least) a mixture of elements, and he illustrates the principle of the impact of physical factors on psychology by the contrasting intellectual abilities of Chrysippus (the Stoic) and the sons of Hippocrates (who are not related to the great medical writer).

How credible is Galen's attribution of this idea to the Stoics? From what one might call a 'middle-distance' perspective, the ideas look similar to those found in modern scholarly accounts of Stoic psychology. The linkage between fire and air (or *pneuma*) and animating functions including *phusis* and psyche is a central part of Stoic

[217] On Aristotle's theory, and its relationship to Galen's, see Kupreeva 2004: 81.

[218] *QAM* IV.783–4, *SM* 2.45.5–11, 21–4 (part of *SVF* 2.787), trans. Tieleman 2003*a*: 149–50, slightly modified; see also the translation of Singer 1997*a*: 157–8.

thinking, as is the idea of the four elements and of (total) blending or mixture (*krasis*).[219] Galen also alludes to the important Stoic idea that nature can be seen as a spectrum of types of 'tension' (or modalities of *pneuma*), of which *phusis* and psyche are two of the types or levels.[220] There are also Stoic parallels, highlighted by Tieleman, for the idea that individual long-term characteristics have a physical basis and that transient psychological states manifest themselves as exceptional degrees of hot and cold.[221] However, Galen's treatment also involves a good deal of recasting to make the Stoic theory fit the required pattern. For instance, the idea that psyche constitutes the 'form' of a material body is an Aristotelian, rather than Stoic, idea. Also, in so far as the 'form–matter' distinction is relevant to this aspect of Stoic thought, *pneuma* (or fiery air) is normally conceived as the 'formal' or 'active' cause, by contrast with the passive material cause (*hulē*). Here, however, *pneuma* is presented as the 'matter', while 'mixture' (or air and fire) appears as the 'form'.[222] This difference is an index of a larger contrast between the two theories. Galen presents these Stoic ideas as constituting their version of answers to a relatively familiar set of questions, which are cast in Platonic–Aristotelian terms, such as 'what is the psyche?', and 'how do we define the psyche–body relationship?'[223] I think that the Stoic framework is more revisionist than Galen's presentation suggests; in particular, the Stoic theory of tension, outlined earlier, is intended to offer a radically holistic framework, in which notions such as *hexis* and psyche function as levels or grades of a unified framework.[224] The psyche–body distinction,

[219] See LS 47A–J; also text to nn. 202–3 above. See e.g. Long 1996: 227–39 and von Staden 2000: 100–4. [220] LS 47 K–R.

[221] In addition to the passage cited above, see also the lines omitted (*QAM* IV.783–4, *SM* 2.45.11–21, translation in Singer 1997*a*: 158). See Tieleman 2003*a*: ch. 4, esp. 194, referring to Cic. *Fat.* 7–9 (environmental influences on character-formation), and 157–8, referring to *SVF* 2.886 (*PHP* VI.291, 3.1.25 De Lacy) on anger as transient heat.

[222] See *QAM* IV.783–4, *SM* 2.45.8–11 (also 5–8). Contrast LS 47 F, I, L, and LS, vol. 1: pp. 287–9.

[223] On the role of doxography, drawing predominantly on Platonic–Aristotelian ideas, in shaping Galen's conceptual framework in psychology and the questions he poses, see Tieleman 2003*a*: chs. 1–2, esp. 34–5, 2003*b*: 141–51.

[224] In other words, the framework expresses a 'structure', rather than 'composition', conception; for this contrast (as applied to Stoic and Galenic thinking), see Ch. 1 above, text to nn. 40–51.

which, in a more familiar Platonic–Aristotelian framework, constitutes a fundamental distinction between categories of being, does not have the same significance in Stoicism. In fact, the notion of 'body' (*sōma*) disappears from the Stoic schema, being replaced, in effect, by *hexis*. Though the idea of 'psyche' remains, it now constitutes a further stage or degree of 'tension', calibrated, alongside *hexis* and *phusis*, on a single spectrum of states.[225] Galen's approach, which treats the Stoic framework as directly comparable with the Aristotelian one, thus understates its radically revisionist and holistic character.

In spite of these indications of difference in conceptual framework, Galen's presentation of the Stoics as sharing common ground as regards the effect of physiological factors on psychology is striking. It complements the similarities between his thought and Stoic theory regarding the basic constituents of matter which Galen himself underlines and those highlighted earlier regarding teleology, both of which are seen here as making up an outlook of 'high naturalism'. This makes all the more surprising Galen's uniformly negative and critical response to Stoic psychology in *PHP* 2–5. It is this response to which I turn in the next two chapters, which illustrates most graphically how far Galen is from Stoic ideas on psychology and yet how close he could have come.

[225] For some related points about the distinctive character of the Stoic theory, see Gill 2006: 30–2.

3

Psychology and the Body

3.1 PRELIMINARIES

I continue this exploration of the relationship between Galen and Stoicism by considering their respective ideas about the relationship between psychology and the body. I focus on three Galenic texts: *On the Doctrines of Hippocrates and Plato* (*PHP*), particularly Books 1–3, *The Construction of the Embryo* (*Foet. Form.*), and *Psychological Faculties Depend on Bodily Mixtures* (*QAM*). These texts, especially *PHP*, are ones in which Galen engages explicitly and sometimes at length with Stoic thinking. This subject, in particular as treated in *PHP* 1–3, brings out vividly the central paradox highlighted in Chapter 1. This is that, although Galen shares with the Stoics a naturalistic approach to psychology, his main explicit response to Stoic ideas, in *PHP* 2–5, is a consistently negative or critical one. The discussion of Chapter 2 has deepened this paradox by examining in more detail what this shared naturalism of approach consists in. In broad terms, it consists in a shared form of 'high naturalism', combining a 'biological' and a teleological conception of natural entities. This shared naturalistic approach is reflected in their ideas about embodied psychology, in ways partly indicated in the preceding chapter.[1] Also, as regards the methodology of natural inquiry, despite some obvious differences of approach and focus, there are several partly shared strands. Galen's distinctive logico-empirical method draws on Stoic thinking on logic and causation, and both Galenic and Stoic theories have in common a non-sceptical and largely empirical

[1] See Ch. 2 above, text to nn. 102–5, 137–51, 213–25.

approach to knowledge (2.2 above). These shared or converging features render more surprising Galen's generally negative attitude to Stoic psychology (especially in *PHP*) and his decision to frame his main study of psychology (*PHP*) as a synthesis of medical ('Hippocratic') and Platonic ideas, despite the fact, sometimes acknowledged by Galen himself, that Plato often adopts a non-naturalistic or idealist conception of the psyche, which is developed by many subsequent Platonists.

There are various ways of explaining this paradox and of accounting for Galen's strongly critical response to Stoic psychology. A crucial factor is Galen's disagreement with the Stoics, as well as Aristotle, regarding the location in the body of the ruling part of the psyche. A related factor is his low evaluation of the methodology of natural inquiry that leads the Stoics to adopt the heart, rather than the brain, as this location. Another, more general influence, I think, is the (partial) contrast between 'structure' and 'composition' approaches to the part–whole relationship.[2] However, the similarities between the two theories remain striking. I focus especially on the idea that the two theories are, in important ways, conceptually compatible and complementary. For instance, I suggest that the Stoics might have done well not only to adopt the Galenic logico-empirical method of natural inquiry, but also its main outcome, Galen's account of the function of the brain and the central nervous system. Apart from the fact that the Galenic account is more effectively supported by empirically based inquiry, it can also be argued that the Galenic account of the brain fits the role of the Stoic 'control-centre' (*hēgemonikon*) better than the Stoic account of the heart does. By the same token, it can also be argued that the Stoic model of embodied psychology, with its single, inclusive centre, provides a better framework for Galen's account of the function of the brain than does Galen's own account, based on a three-centre model adopted from Plato.

I begin this discussion by making these two suggestions, as a way of exploring the relationship between the Galenic and Stoic theories of embodied psychology, especially as presented in *PHP* 1–3 (3.2–3). Subsequently, I examine Galen's critique of Stoic (and Aristotelian)

[2] On the first two factors, see 2.2 above; on the third, see Ch. 1 above, text to nn. 40–51. See further on this question below 4.1 and 5.4, text to nn. 331–46.

ideas about the development of the embryo in *Foet. Form.* I ask whether the critique reflects fundamental conceptual differences or, rather, localized disagreements within a largely shared approach to this question (3.4). Finally, I discuss Galen's thinking about the psyche–body relationship, as expressed in *QAM* and *Prop. Plac.* (3.5). In *QAM* in particular, Galen comes close to an explicit adoption of psychological physicalism, though in a form that has a number of important ambiguities and is also at least potentially in conflict with views about rational agency he holds elsewhere. Here too, I suggest that Galen might usefully have adopted a Stoic (or at least Stoic-style) approach, combining an explicitly physicalist approach to psychology with a clear distinction between the causal role of rational and non-rational agency. This suggestion brings out in another way the conceptual compatibility between these two ancient versions of naturalist psychology. Needless to say, all these suggestions are highly controversial, as well as hypothetical in character, and need to be developed in some depth if they are to be at all credible. But they are suggestions that follow logically from the overall conclusion of Chapter 2, that the Galenic and Stoic theories exhibit in different ways a shared naturalism of approach to psychology.

3.2 STOIC PSYCHOLOGY AND GALEN'S BRAIN

Before examining what Galen and the Stoics might usefully have adopted from each other, I consider Galen's overall project in *PHP* and the kind of evidence that this treatise provides for my inquiry. In *PHP* Galen's main explicit engagement with Stoicism comes in Books 2–3, where he criticizes Stoic arguments for locating the ruling part of the psyche in the heart, and in Books 4–5, where he challenges the Stoic unified account of psychological functions. However, these two critiques need to be placed within the larger context of the structure of *PHP* as a whole and of its underlying objectives.

PHP is, even by Galen's standards, a big and complex treatise with an ambitious intellectual programme. There were, it seems, two phases of composition; Books 1–6 were completed during Galen's first stay in Rome in 162–6 and Books 7–9 in his second period in Rome in 169–75.[3] Within these two phases of work, Galen signals several changes of plan in the course of composition. These include the extension of the two critiques of Stoic ideas from one to two books each, and the decision to defer a planned discussion of the virtues, a topic linked with that of psychological functions. Books 7–9 are explicitly presented as a sequel to Books 1–6 and make several backward references to them.[4] Even so, a relatively clear structure emerges, at least in Books 1–6. Book 1, which survives only in part,[5] and Books 2–3 deal with the question of the location in the body of the *hēgemonikon*, the ruling part of the psyche or 'control-centre'. The main focus is on presenting Galen's own account, centred on the brain and the nervous system, and disputing the heart-centred account offered by Aristotle (criticized mainly in Book 1) and the Stoics, especially Chrysippus in his work *On the Psyche.* This account is rounded off in Book 6 with an analysis of Galen's three-centre picture of embodied psychology, though the focus here is on the role of the third part, the liver.[6] The topic of Books 4–5, that of psychological functions, centred on a critique of Stoic unified psychology, is presented as, in one sense, a digression from the main theme of the treatise, the bodily location of psychological functions.[7] However, the theme of *PHP* 4–5 is related in several clear and important ways with the question of location of functions; and the type of discussion, ethical psychology, is one in which Galen has an independent interest.[8] This explains the scale of the digression, two whole books, and also the return to the related question of the virtues at the start

[3] Both parts also contain references to Galenic works written after these dates and so were probably revised subsequently: De Lacy 2005: 46–8.

[4] De Lacy 2005: 48–50. The treatment of the virtues is finally offered in V.589–600, 7.1.9–3.1 De Lacy; but this is presented as only provisional (V.600, 7.3.1 De Lacy).

[5] De Lacy 2005: 12–13 estimates that the surviving part of Book 1 is about a third of the whole book; this is V.181–210, 1.5.1–10.20 De Lacy, preceded by various other pieces of Galenic evidence that seem to cover the missing material (pp. 66–71 De Lacy).

[6] The other two key parts, brain and heart, were discussed extensively in Books 1–3. Book 6 begins by discussing several important categories and concepts for the topic, including activity (*energeia*) and affection or passion (*pathos*) and form (*eidos*) or part (*meros*): V.505–19, 6.1.1–2.17 De Lacy.

[7] *PHP* V.428–9, 5.1.1–3 De Lacy, V.505–6, 6.1.1–2 De Lacy.

[8] See further Ch. 4 below.

of Book 7.[9] In Books 7–9 Galen returns to questions of embodied psychology and associated medical or philosophical topics. Book 7 examines the roles of brain, nerves, and sense organs, with special attention to sight. Books 8–9 discuss other points of contact between Hippocrates and Plato. Galen considers in Book 8 their ideas on elements and humours as a factor bearing on health, and in Book 9, their methods of classification, which is finally linked with the main theme of the treatise by reference to the subdivision of the psyche.[10]

What is the intellectual programme underlying this complex structure? Tieleman, building on work by other scholars, especially Mansfeld, underlines the significance of an evolving Greek tradition of inquiry into the nature and properties of the psyche since, at least, Aristotle. This tradition is found in its most systematic and elaborate form in certain late (fourth- or fifth-century AD) handbooks or doxographies. But the process presented there of defining key issues and setting out the main positions taken on these issues goes back much earlier. Mansfeld has suggested that the influence of this doxographical tradition is already visible in evidence for Chrysippus' *On the Psyche* provided by Galen, and Tieleman points to much more extensive indications of such influence on Galen's approach in *PHP*.[11] However, Tieleman also highlights respects in which Galen's treatment does not match what seems to be the standard pattern either in earlier philosophical discussions or in doxographical accounts. In particular, Galen largely omits discussion of the essence or substance of the psyche, for instance, whether it is bodily or non-bodily by nature. He also discusses the question of the location of the ruling part of the psyche (in *PHP* 1–3) before considering whether the psyche has parts, a question which is tackled in *PHP* 4–5, although the former question was usually taken first and is logically prior to that of location.[12] These divergences from standard doxographical

[9] See n. 4 above.

[10] For the latter topic, see V.793–827, 9.9.7–46 De Lacy. See also De Lacy 2005: 50.

[11] Galen's report of Chrysippus: *PHP* V.287–8, 3.1.9–14 De Lacy. See Mansfeld 1989 on Chrysippus and doxography, and Mansfeld 1990 on doxography on the psyche in general. On Galen and doxography, see Tieleman 2003*a*: 61–88, esp. 80–8.

[12] Tieleman 2003*a*: 20–9, contrasting Galen's approach with, e.g., Arist. *De An.* 1.1, 402ᵃ23–ᵇ3 and sections IV.2–6 of the (reconstructed) handbook of Aëtius. On Galen's reticence about the question of the substance of the psyche, see Ch. 2 above, text to n. 4.

or philosophical patterns suggest that Galen's project needs to be explained, primarily at least, by reference to other factors.

Galen himself presents as his fundamental objective investigating the shared views of Hippocrates and Plato about 'the capacities (or faculties, *dunameis*) that govern us, their number, the nature of each, and the place that each occupies in the body'.[13] But what does this programme actually mean, when we relate it to the specific form of Galen's treatise? As indicated already, much of Books 1–5 take the form of an extended critique of Stoic (and sometimes Aristotelian) ideas on psychology, with Plato or, less commonly, Hippocrates cited in support of Galen's independent view.[14] It is not until Book 6 that Galen attempts, in a detailed way, to correlate Platonic and Hippocratic ideas about embodied psychology with each other and with Galen's own account. His treatment of the ideas of both thinkers in Book 6 is highly selective and is strongly shaped by the concern to find support for his own picture. For instance, Galen conflates the Platonic accounts of the tripartite psyche in the *Republic* (435–41) and the *Timaeus* (69–72), eliding salient differences of emphasis and theme. As regards the *Timaeus* version, Galen ignores Plato's lack of specificity about the location of the third part of the psyche and the fact that Plato's account of the function of the liver is quite different from his own.[15] Galen also does not go very far towards supporting the claim that Hippocrates shares Platonic thinking about the tripartite psyche. He finds brief Hippocratic comments relating to the heart and liver that he takes as offering some support, but cites no material to show the role of the brain in this connection, although this would have been possible.[16] These points indicate that Galen's programme in *PHP* is not the relatively straightforward matter of

[13] p. 68.3–7 De Lacy, Testimony 2 to Book 1 (cf. V.211, 2.1.1 De Lacy), trans. De Lacy slightly modified.

[14] The most detailed discussion of Plato in Books 1–6 is of *R.* 435e–441c in V.479–501, 5.7.1–82 De Lacy.

[15] See further Tieleman 1996: xxix–xxxi, Gill 2006: 297–8. On his selective treatment of Plato, see also text to nn. 121–39 below.

[16] Texts cited include Hipp. *Epid.* II, 5.16, V.130 Littré (*PHP* V.574–5, 6.8.46 De Lacy) and *Alim.* 31 (*PHP* V.577, 6.8.56 De Lacy), supporting the Galenic view of the heart and the liver. Galen does not cite other Hippocratic texts that might have supported his view of the role of the brain, including *Morb. Sacr.* 14 and *Epid.* II, 4.4, V.124.9 ff. Littré. See further Tieleman 1996: xxxi–xxxv.

summarizing and integrating the ideas of Hippocrates and Plato that his comment cited earlier might seem to suggest. The project has other, and broader, objectives, even if these can in some sense be characterized as the synthesis of Hippocratic and Platonic approaches to psychology.

In fact, I think it is fairly clear what his main aim is. At the core of the treatise is the attempt by Galen to draw on the results of his anatomical work in order to resolve the longstanding question of the location of the ruling part of the psyche. Books 1–6 of *PHP* were written during the same period (162–6) when Galen, as he tells us himself, was establishing his medical standing at the highest level in Rome by public displays of anatomical skill.[17] Central to these displays was Galen's demonstration of the respective roles of brain and heart in controlling speech functions and sensation.[18] These demonstrations drew on his expertise in anatomy, developed during his lengthy education (conducted partly in Alexandria, where Herophilus and Erasistratus had done their pioneering studies on the brain and nerves) and through his surgical work as doctor of the gladiators in his home city of Pergamon.[19] Thus, by the time of his arrival in Rome, Galen had a well-developed, research-based, theory about the respective roles of brain and heart. Galen seems to have seen *PHP* 1–6 and *UP* (*On the Utility of the Parts*), of which Book 1 was written in this period, as vehicles by which he could contribute decisively to major philosophical debates such as that on the location of the ruling part of the psyche or between teleological and non-teleological views of the human body.[20]

Hence, when Galen talks about combining the thinking of Hippocrates and Plato on psychology, it seems clear he has in view a grander and more innovative programme than one might expect. This is none other than the combination of (what Galen sees as) the results of the best work on psychology from both medical and philosophical standpoints. Central to this project is the conviction

[17] See Rocca 2003: 6–11, 2008: 244–5, referring to Galen's own reports in *Praen.*

[18] See Ch. 2 above, text to nn. 102–5, 137–40.

[19] See *AA* II.651–706, XI.4, 11. Galen's education took place in 146–57 (153–7 was spent in Alexandria) and his role as doctor of the gladiators lasted from 157 to 162. See also Ch. 2 above, text to nn. 11–14.

[20] See further Rocca 2003: 17–21, 46–7.

that Galen's anatomical findings, building on earlier medical research, lend decisive confirmation to the brain-based account of the ruling part of the psyche. Also crucial is the belief that these findings are consistent with, and support, Plato's three-centre picture of the psyche, as presented in the *Republic* and the *Timaeus*. A further dimension, which may have emerged only in the course of composing the work, is the conviction that he was able—and perhaps needed—to become involved in another well-established issue of debate. This is that between part-based (Platonic–Aristotelian) or unified (Stoic) accounts of psychological functions, an issue that was interlocked in various ways with the question of the location of the ruling part of the psyche. Although Galen's anatomical work was not directly relevant to the latter debate, he saw the reassertion of the Platonic (part-based) side of the argument as crucial for his larger objectives.[21] Thus, the detailed account of the three-centre psychophysiological model in Book 6 is, comprehensibly, presented as the culmination of the main part of Galen's medico-philosophical analysis of psychology in *PHP*.

An implication of this view of Galen's project is that, when he talks about combining Hippocratic and Platonic ideas about psychology, 'Hippocratic' signifies, in effect, 'medical', and more specifically 'Galenic', especially regarding the role of brain and nerves. To say this is not to understate Galen's view of Hippocrates as the supreme medical authority and a crucial inspiration for Galen's work and for some of his central ideas, especially regarding the elements and the humours. In *PHP* 8–9 at least, Galen does engage in something much closer to detailed exegesis or commentary on Hippocratic material, as he does extensively elsewhere.[22] But in *PHP* 1–6, Hippocrates mostly plays a more marginal or symbolic role, although Galen does attempt to show in Book 6 that his three-centre psychology can claim Hippocratic as well as Platonic support. Galen's deployment of Hippocrates, and to a lesser degree Plato, needs to be understood against the larger background of the use of earlier authorities in first- and second-century Greco-Roman intellectual life. From the first

[21] On the nature of the linkage, see Ch. 4 below, text to nn. 8–14.

[22] See the comprehensive treatment of Galen as a commentator on Hippocrates in Manetti and Roselli 1994; also Flemming 2008, von Staden 2009.

century BC onwards, the emergence of commentaries as a standard feature of intellectual life enabled a spectrum of possible modes, ranging from faithful and detailed exegesis to creative interpretation or virtually independent thought.[23] Galen's use of Hippocrates, and to some extent Plato, in *PHP* falls in the more creative end of the spectrum. There, as often elsewhere, the appeal to the authority of 'the ancients' is used to challenge more recent (but still earlier) thinkers and also contemporary—though usually unnamed—opponents.[24] The appeal is seriously meant, but it also serves as the vehicle of an independent, often strongly innovative, conceptual project, as in *PHP* or *Nat. Fac.*[25]

In Galen's programme in *PHP* a key assumption is that the brain-centred account of psychology that emerges from his anatomical research is consistent with the Platonic three-centre picture rather than the Stoic unified one. But is this assumption justified? I think that, on the contrary, there is a strong case for claiming the consistency of the brain-centred account with the Stoic picture rather than the Platonic one. I explore this view, first by suggesting that the Stoics might have done well to adopt the brain-centred account[26] and then, in the next section, by arguing that Galen would have benefited by adopting important features of the Stoic picture.[27]

There are various grounds for claiming that the Stoics could consistently have adopted the brain-centred account and would, indeed, have improved their theory by doing so. Earlier, I outlined Galen's critique of Stoic methods of argument on the location of the ruling part of the psyche question and the underlying rationale of the Stoic approach. As Tieleman has argued, the Stoic arguments are much better conceived than Galen claims and reflect a credible type of methodology, centred on the 'articulation' of concepts embodied in a range of types of beliefs.[28] None the less, I think it is hard not to conclude that, on the question of the location of the ruling part of the

[23] On the emergence of an intellectual culture in this period in which commentary (with a variety of modes) has a central role, see Sedley 1997, M. Frede 1999*a*.

[24] See further Vegetti 1986, Lloyd 1993; also Hankinson 1991*c*: 86.

[25] On *Nat. Fac.*, see Vegetti 1999, and Ch. 2 above, text to nn. 163–72.

[26] For a similar suggestion, see Long 1999: 568–9.

[27] For a preliminary account of the main claims of these two sections, see Gill 2009.

[28] See Ch. 2 above, text to nn. 147–8.

psyche, Galen has the better of the argument. Galen's position on this question reflects a carefully considered combination of logical inference and empirical observation. It is widely seen by modern scholars as one of the most impressive outcomes of ancient natural inquiry, and one that can seriously be considered as a precursor of modern experimental method.[29] The strongest argument on the Stoic side, linking the heart and speech-functions, is not of comparable cogency, at least as far as the question of location is concerned.[30] Also, I can see no obvious philosophical reason why the Stoics should not have accepted the force of Galen's argument. Their epistemological approach is, broadly speaking at least, an empirical one.[31] More specifically, there is no evidence that they regarded the question of the role and location of the heart as one to be determined on purely theoretical grounds. Although Chrysippus, like other Stoics, did not claim to have done independent work on anatomy, the school seems to have taken note of the findings of those who did undertake such work.[32] Their approach to psychology is 'naturalistic' in the sense that it reflects key features of their philosophy of nature, which converge with salient aspects of Galen's thinking (2.3 above). So, in methodological terms, it seems reasonable to suggest that they could consistently have accepted Galen's arguments for the brain-centred account of animal psychology.

Did the Stoics at least take note of such arguments, even if they did not accept them? Chrysippus, the most systematic and influential Stoic theorist, lived after the pioneering work on the brain and nerves by the Ptolemaic doctors, Herophilus and Erasistratus.[33] There is one passage, cited by Galen, which indicates that he may have responded to their views, though he may be responding more generally to those who place the ruling part in the head. Chrysippus' reported words include this comment: 'Surely the same sort of statement that they

[29] See e.g. Tieleman 2002: 256, Rocca 2003: 51.

[30] On this debate, see Ch. 2 above, text to nn. 102–10, 137–40.

[31] The main (seemingly) 'idealist' dimension is the belief that human beings have an innate disposition to form 'preconceptions'; but this is combined with an empirical conception of the acquisition of knowledge; see Scott 1995: 190–210, M. Frede 1999*c*: 321–2.

[32] See Ch. 2 above, text to nn. 150–2.

[33] Their respective dates are: Herophilus (*c.*330–250), Erasistratus (*c.*320–240), Chrysippus (*c.*280–*c.*206) (all BC).

[advocates of the head] might make about speech, that it is carried out of the chest through the windpipe with an initiation of some kind coming from the head, can be made if the governing part is in the heart but the beginning of movements is from the head.'[34] What Chrysippus seems to be saying is (as Tieleman suggests), 'even if it is granted that the brain is the source of the nervous system, this still leaves open the possibility that the intellect resides in the heart and the brain functions as some sort of auxiliary centre which receives stimuli from the heart and passes them on to all parts of the body'.[35] The fact that, as Galen reports, Chrysippus opposed those who placed the source of the nerves in the head by referring to Praxagoras, who located them in the heart, also indicates an acknowledgement of the arguments for the brain-centred approach.[36] Mansfeld, in his review of doxographical evidence on this debate, also cites some sources for Stoic thought in the first centuries BC and AD in which rational functions were seen as located in the head rather than the heart. The context of debate seems in these cases to be that of mythical interpretation (for instance, that relating to the birth of Athena from the head of Zeus), rather than of arguments based on medical or anatomical inquiry.[37] However, the fact that certain Stoics were prepared to entertain this idea at all indicates that the question of location, by itself, may have been less important for them than Galen suggests, a point pursued further shortly.

However, my suggestion is not that the Stoics actually did adopt the brain-centred picture but that it would have been theoretically consistent for them to do so. The main distinctive feature of the Stoic account, considered in relation to other ancient theories, is a highly unified psychological centre, which serves as the focus and director of

[34] *PHP* V.255, 2.5.70, p. 140.28–31 De Lacy, trans. De Lacy.

[35] Tieleman 1996: 51–2, cf. also Solmsen 1961: 192, 195. As Tieleman notes, Chrysippus seems to model this line of reasoning on an analogous hypothesis made by his opponents (which Galen also adopts), that speech comes from the chest but is directed by the brain.

[36] Gal. *PHP* V.189, 1.7.1 De Lacy. Praxagoras (flourished *c*.300 BC) preceded and may have taught Herophilus. On his influence on Chrysippus and Diogenes of Babylon, a later head of the Stoic school, see Tieleman 1996: 83–6.

[37] Mansfeld 1990: 3095, n. 145, referring to Philodemus, *De Pietate* IX.9 ff. (=*SVF* 2.910), [ps.] Heraclitus, *Homeric Problems*, ch. 19, 1–2, and Cornutus, 35.9–15.

a unified communication system running throughout the body.[38] The notion of the psychological 'ruling part' or 'control-centre' (*hēgemonikon*) linked with this conception is one that seems to have originated in Stoicism, though the term became widely used in ancient psychology more generally, with meanings that vary according to the theory. This distinctive Stoic feature emerges clearly in a passage of Chrysippus' *On the Psyche* cited by Galen:

The psyche is *pneuma* integral to our nature [or 'connate', *sumphuton*], extending continuously throughout the body as long as the regular breath of life is present in the body. Of the parts of the psyche which are assigned to each segment of the body, the one that extends to the throat is voice; that to the eyes, sight; that to the ears, hearing; that to the nostrils, smell; that to the tongue, taste; that to the entire flesh, touch; and that which extends to the genital organs, since it has a different principle (*logos*), is seminal. The heart is the location of the part where these all meet, which is the governing part (*hēgemonikon*) of the psyche.[39]

This passage brings out two aspects reflected in other sources too. There is a single centre operating both as the receiving agent and assessor of the evidence of the senses,[40] and as the locus of cognitive functions and source of motivation to movement and action.[41] The control-centre operates (by means of *pneuma*) throughout the body, and the body interpenetrated by pneumatic agency constitutes a single integrated system.[42] The unified character of this view of embodied psychology is brought out, here or elsewhere, by a series of images: a tree-trunk and its branches, an octopus and its tentacles, a spider in the centre of

[38] The closest parallel is the Epicurean account, including a unified centre of psychological agency (in Lucretius' terms, *animus*) with a network of communication for sensation and motivation of action running through the body (*anima*); both Epicurean and Stoic accounts are physicalist in conception. See LS 14, esp. B (Lucr. 3.136–76); also Annas 1992: 144–51, Everson 1999: 543–6.

[39] Gal. *PHP* V.287–8, 3.10–11, p. 170.9–16 De Lacy, trans. Long 1999: 567, slightly modified.

[40] 'The psyche as a whole despatches the senses (which are its proper functions) like branches from the trunk-like control-centre to be reporters of what they sense, while itself like a monarch passing judgement on their reports', LS 53 G(8) (Calcidius *in Timaeum* 220), trans. LS, slightly modified.

[41] 'The Stoics say the control-centre is the highest part of the psyche, which produces impressions, assents, perception and impulses', LS 53 H(1) (Aëtius 4.21.1), trans. LS, slightly modified. Cf. LS 53 K, and, on impulse and action, J, L, Q–S.

[42] See esp. Hierocles' account (LS 53 B); and below.

its web.[43] The control-centre is not, in most sources, responsible for all bodily functions, notably not for digestion and growth, which fall under *phusis* (nature), rather than psyche.[44] But it is consistently presented as the central or coordinating agency for sensation, the seat of cognitive processes (impression and assent), and the source of motivation ('impulse', *hormē*) and movement or action.

The Stoics located this unified centre in the heart. Various factors influenced this decision, including the widespread belief that anger and other emotions occurred in the region of the heart and the supposed linkage between heart, chest, throat, and speech-functions, the latter being taken as rational ones.[45] A further possible factor is the evident role of the heart as the centre of a physical network running throughout the body (that of blood vessels). However, the Stoics saw the vehicle of psychological communication not as blood but (psychic) *pneuma*, which they did not identify with any single material entity, such as blood or air.[46] How important for the Stoics was the question of the location of the control-centre? We know, of course, that, having settled on the heart as the base for the control-centre, they offered quite extensive arguments for this view, with which Galen engages vigorously and at length. But this does not mean that the question of location had the same importance for them as for Galen. A crucial difference is that Galen's view is based on a well-established programme of independent anatomical research and a theory of the body as a system of embodied functions (set out in *UP* especially). Although the Stoics based their choice on a variety of factors, their thinking about anatomy and psychological functions relied on the investigations of other thinkers, notably Praxagoras.[47] What seems to have been most important for their theory was the

[43] LS 53 G(7), H.

[44] Calcidius, exceptionally, presents the control-centre as responsible for nutrition and growth, as well as locomotion, sensation, and impulse (LS 53 G(6)); but this is not reflected in other sources. See further Long 1996: 238, Tieleman 1996: 95–9, and text to nn. 59–65 below.

[45] On the argument from anger and other passions, see e.g. Gal. *PHP* V.268, 2.7.8 De Lacy, V.321, 3.5.2 De Lacy; the corollary (on their assumptions) is that reasoning and deliberation also occurs there. On the arguments relating to speech, see text to nn. 49–51 below.

[46] See further Annas 1992: 25–6, 35–8, 45–6, Tieleman 1996: 87–95, Long 1999: 568–9.

[47] See text to nn. 32, 36 above.

idea of a unified centre that operated as the locus of an integrated communication system. Where, precisely, this centre was located seems likely to have been a secondary consideration.

That this is the case is indicated, for instance, by the passage Galen cites from Chrysippus' *On Psyche*, quoted in part earlier (text to n. 39 above). The first and main point stressed is the existence of a unified control-centre, acting as the focus of the embodied network of psychic *pneuma*. Although this control-centre is located in the heart, Chrysippus goes on to acknowledge the variety of views held on this point and the difficulty in determining its location definitively.[48] A similar conclusion can be drawn from the arguments for the heart by successive Stoic thinkers that Galen also records. Although there is a clear commitment to the heart-centred view and evidence of increasing elaboration of this claim in terms of bodily organization, the fundamental thesis seems to be that a complex of psychological functions converge in a single centre. This point emerges, for instance, from Chrysippus' arguments for the heart by reference to speech-functions.

It is reasonable that the destination of meanings and the source of discourse (*logos*) is the governing part of the psyche. The source of discourse is not different from the source of thought, nor again is the source of voice different from that of discourse, nor (to state the whole point simply) is the source of voice different from the governing part of the psyche... In general, the source from which discourse issues must be where reasoning occurs and thinking and the preparation of language, as I said. But these latter plainly occur in the region of the heart since both voice and discourse issue from the heart through the windpipe. It is plausible in addition that the place to which language conveys meaning should be the place where is acquires meaning and that words should come from there in the way described.[49]

The claim that is made repeatedly here is the linkage between the functions of voice, language, and reasoning, taken as implying that

[48] As Tieleman stresses (1996: 158–60), this passage, which is preliminary to Chrysippus' positive arguments, need not be taken as indicating lack of conviction in the heart-based location; but it suggests, none the less, that the question of location is less fundamental for the Stoics than that of the unification of psychological functions.

[49] Gal. *PHP* V.242–3, 2.5.15–20, pp. 130.24–132.2 De Lacy, trans. Long 1999: 570, slightly modified.

they derive from the same source. Although this is used to support the idea that these functions are to be located in the heart, the emphasis falls on the idea of convergence within a single centre.[50] A similar emphasis is found in the arguments of Diogenes of Babylon, which Galen also cites. Although Diogenes, in this respect and in others, links the argument more closely with bodily organization, the theme of the convergence of psychological functions is still the dominant one.[51] The fact that, as noted earlier, some later Stoics were prepared to locate reasoning (that is, presumably, the control-centre as a whole) in the head, rather than the heart, indicates that the question of location was secondary to the unitary character of psychological functions.[52]

A corollary of the points just made about the Stoic theory is that the Stoics could have adopted the brain-centred anatomy advocated by Galen and still have advanced their main claims about animal (especially human) psychology. The combination of brain and nervous system could have provided the anatomical basis for the two features that were of most importance to Stoic theory. These are the idea of a unified psychological centre and a communication system radiating from the control-centre and running through the body. The core functions of the Stoic control-centre, those of coordinating perception and acting as a source for movement and motivation, are precisely those of the brain, acting through the nervous system, as Galen shows by his demonstrations, building on the earlier work of the Ptolemaic doctors. The logical conclusion is that, as Long points out, 'Chrysippus' most interesting contributions could fit a brain-centred model of mind just as well as a cardiovascular one'.[53] Indeed, I want to suggest that, in some respects, the brain-centred model would fit the Stoic account *better* than the heart-centred one. One reason, already indicated, is that the arguments for the brain-centred account, based on Galen's highly developed logico-empirical method, are stronger than those offered by Stoic thinkers for the heart. I can see no philosophical reason, as regards the Stoic theory of

[50] For a similar view, see Long 1999: 570–1.

[51] Gal. *PHP* V.241–2, 2.5.9–13 De Lacy. On Diogenes' contribution, see Tieleman 1996: 79–105.

[52] See text to n. 37 above.

[53] Long 1999: 569.

knowledge or methodology of inquiry, why the Stoics should not have accepted the force of Galen's argument, as he formulates it. So I think their theory would have been strengthened by combining the main features of their psychological account with a more credible picture of the workings of the animal body.[54]

This claim can be reinforced by a further suggestion. A striking feature of the Stoic theory, noted in Chapter 2, is the analysis of the spectrum of natural kinds (or *scala naturae*) in terms of varying modalities of 'tension' (*tonos*). A corollary of this theory is that some functions allocated by earlier thinkers to psyche, notably growth and nutrition, were allocated to a lower level of 'tension', namely nature (*phusis*).[55] Thus, in animals, including human beings, it would seem, the operation of growth and nutrition falls under 'nature' in this sense, while psyche is the agency for the operation of more advanced functions including perception, movement, and motivation. The brain-centred account could accommodate this distinction more easily than the heart-centred one. The distinctively psychic functions could be allocated to the combination of brain and nervous system, whereas the 'natural' functions of growth and nutrition could be allocated to the workings of other organs, such as the heart, stomach, or liver. The resulting picture would be that of a single overall system, which accommodates different types or levels of process, also understood as different modalities of tension, in various subsystems of the body. An advantage of this revised version of the Stoic theory is that it resolves the problem which arises otherwise of knowing quite how different levels of psychic *pneuma* ('nature' and psyche) operate in the same organ, namely the heart seen as the seat of the control-centre.[56]

Heinrich von Staden provides supporting evidence for this suggestion. He points out that we can find analogues for the Stoic psyche–nature distinction in the thinking about embodied psychology of the

[54] Galen claims, in fact, at the start of Book 7 of *PHP* (written some time after Books 1–6) that 'No Stoic or Peripatetic philosopher and no physician is as bold as before, and some, at least, have publicly changed over to the true account' (V.588, 7.1.4, p. 428.17–19 De Lacy, trans. De Lacy).

[55] See Ch. 2, text to nn. 207–12, also discussion below.

[56] Tieleman (1996: 99) raises this question about the Stoic theory: did it 'involve an actual [physical] separation' between the two types of function?

Ptolemaic doctors who discovered the roles of brain and nervous system, Herophilus and Erasistratus, and in Galen, at least in certain strands in his thought. More specifically, he suggests that the version of this distinction offered by Herophilus and Erasistratus, linked with their pioneering work on the brain, might have actually influenced the thinking of Chrysippus at least, and could certainly have shaped that of Galen.[57] The relevant distinctions are, in the case of Herophilus, between the activation of sensation, movement, and voluntary action (*prohairesis*) through the nerves, and involuntary movements, such as pulse and respiration, which he calls 'natural activities'. Erasistratus sees the body as interpenetrated by 'triple webs' (*triplokiai*) of arteries, veins, and nerves. Psychic *pneuma*, conveyed from the brain through the nerves, acts as the vehicle of sensation, cognition, and movement, while 'natural activities', such as pulse, respiration, digestion, and reproduction, are administered by blood or 'natural' *pneuma*. The similarity between these distinctions and that found in Stoic theory, apparently as systematized by Chrysippus, make it plausible to see either direct influence or at least strong affinity between these theories.[58] Von Staden identifies a similar set of distinctions in certain aspects of Galen's thinking, though these are in tension with other features of his psychology, which are based on Plato's tripartite model, as I bring out later (3.3 below). This line of thought reinforces the idea that the Stoics could consistently have adopted the brain-centred account in conjunction with central features of their analysis of animal psychology.

It has to be acknowledged, however, that the evidence for this aspect of Stoic thought is not wholly straightforward. At least one source (Calcidius) allocates the functions of growth and nutrition to the control-centre and to the operation of psychic *pneuma* rather than to 'nature'.[59] Diogenes of Babylon, head of the Stoic school in the mid-second century BC, also presents the source of nourishment and of voluntary movements (the heart as the seat of the control-centre)

[57] Chrysippus lived in *c.*280–*c.*206, i.e. well after Herophilus (*c.*330–250) and Erasistratus (*c.*320–240).

[58] See von Staden 2000: 88–90, 95–6, 101–4.

[59] Calcidius, *In Timaeum* 220 (*SVF* 2.879), LS 53 G(6); the functions of psychic *pneuma* (*uitali spiritu*) are listed as including 'nutrition, growth, locomotion, sensation, impulse to action' (trans. LS).

as one and the same.[60] On the other hand, most of our evidence points to a clear-cut distinction between psychic functions and natural ones including those of growth and nutrition.[61] Scholars have responded in different ways to this diversity in our evidence. Some have supposed that, although we are told by Stoic sources that, at birth, the animal develops psyche in addition to *phusis*, growth and nutrition may be in some way subsumed within psychic ones.[62] Tieleman posits a change of Stoic thinking on this topic in the course of the second century BC, leading towards a sharper contrast between the roles of psyche and nature.[63] However, A. A. Long and, more recently, Anna Ju have argued strongly that the 'psyche–nature' distinction formed a consistent part of Stoic thought from Zeno and Chrysippus onwards, and that the evidence of Calcidius, in particular, is misleading and unrepresentative.[64] Ju supplements this argument by pointing out that there is some reason to think that there are two conceptions of psyche in Stoic thought, a broader one (as 'natural *pneuma*') and a narrower one (linked with the eightfold psychic functions that belong to animals). The broader sense can be seen as the source of all animal functions, including growth and nutrition, whereas the narrower one is consistently contrasted with 'nature'. Hence, Ju suggests, Calcidius' attribution of growth and nutrition to psyche reflects confusion between the broader and narrower account of psyche in Stoicism.[65] Although

[60] Gal. *PHP* V.282, 2.8.44 De Lacy; see further Tieleman 1996: 87–95.

[61] See e.g. [Galen], *Int.* 3 (XIV.726 K = *SVF* 2.716), Gal. *Adv. Jul.* 5 (XVIIIA.266 K = *SVF* 2.718), S.E. *M.* 9.83–4 (part of *SVF* 2.1013); see further Ju 2007: 98–9.

[62] For the transition from *phusis* to psyche, see esp. LS 53 B(2–3), Hierocles' account of birth. For the suggestion that natural processes are somehow subsumed under psychic ones, see Philo, *Quaest. et solut. in Genesin* 2.4 (*SVF* 2.802). Bonhöffer 1890: 69 (also 105–6) and Pohlenz 1959, vol. 1, 87, conclude that psyche subsumes natural functions.

[63] Tieleman 1996: 95–9. As he notes, Diogenes' pupil Panaetius (*c.* 185–109 BC) presents reproduction as a function of 'nature' (Panaetius fr. 86 van Straaten, LS 53 I), which implies that nutrition and growth were already attributed to 'nature' by then.

[64] Long 1996: 237–9 (a slightly more nuanced view is given in LS, vol. 1: 320), Ju 2007: 97–9.

[65] Ju 2007: 99–108. Both Calcidius (ref. in n. 59 above) and Galen (*PHP* V.287–8, 3.1.10–11) begin by citing the broader meaning of psyche (connate *pneuma*) and then isolate the narrower meaning (linked with the eight psychic functions, those of the five senses, the control-centre, voice, and sexuality); but Calcidius also includes growth and nutrition along with the latter functions.

there is, clearly, room for continuing debate on this topic, I follow Long and Ju here in assuming that the distinction between psyche and *phusis* is a well-attested feature of Stoic thought. Certainly, much of our evidence is consistent with a clear subdivision of functions between the control-centre and more basic natural processes such as automatic growth and digestion. To this extent, the suggestion that the Stoic theory could profitably have adopted the brain-centred model, and the associated contrast between brain-based and 'natural' processes, holds good.

3.3 GALENIC PSYCHOPHYSIOLOGY: TRIPARTITE AND UNIFIED STRANDS

A corollary of the point made in the previous section, that the brain-centred model is compatible with key features of Stoic psychology, is that those features of Stoic thought are also compatible with a central strand in Galen's thinking about psychology. If it is right to suggest that the Stoic ideas of a unitary psychological centre and associated communication system go well with the combination of a directing brain and a central nervous system, it follows that they are compatible with the core feature of Galen's account. But, if this is right, it is highly paradoxical that Galen devotes so much energy to arguing against the Stoic picture in *PHP* 2–3, and, regarding psychological functions, in *PHP* 4–5. Of course, in Books 2–3, Galen's chief target is Stoic thinking about the location of the ruling part of the psyche, a subject on which, I have suggested, Galen has the better of the argument. But Galen himself makes no attempt to distinguish, in the way done in 3.2 above, between the core distinctive features of the Stoic theory and their choice of location. Had he done so, it is at least conceivable that he would have seen the links highlighted here between Stoic thinking about the control-centre and the account of the brain and nerves that Galen advocates. However, another important aspect of Galen's thinking might have prevented him from recognizing this linkage. This is his conviction that the brain-centred account is compatible with the Platonic tripartite picture of the psyche. More precisely, he is convinced that the brain-centred model is compatible with *his version* of the Platonic tripartite psyche.[66] Since there are major differences between the Galenic–Platonic tripartite account and Stoic psychology, it is unsurprising that Galen does not accentuate, or perhaps even recognize, the linkage between the brain-centred model and Stoic psychology highlighted here.

But is Galen justified in his conviction about the compatibility of the brain-centred model and the tripartite psyche? In recent years, different scholars have pointed to a number of serious problems, including inconsistencies, in Galen's account of the embodied psyche in *PHP* 1–3, 6. These problems do not derive from Galen's arguments about the directive role of the brain, as exercised through the nervous system, which are generally seen as highly cogent. What is more problematic is the account Galen offers of the relationship between the functions of the brain and the other two organs (heart and liver) that he presents as seats of distinct psychological parts or agencies. More precisely, the difficulties arise from Galen's attempt to reconcile the results of his anatomical work, focused on the brain and nerves, with a psychological model derived from Plato that subdivides motivation and agency between three separate parts or sources. I begin by summarizing the problems that scholars have identified and considering whether the difficulties can be resolved. I then highlight the presence in Galen's thought outside *PHP*, and possibly also within it, of a more unified psychological model that is more consistent with his brain-centred anatomy and also with aspects of Stoic thinking. I conclude by considering whether Plato's picture of embodied psychology in *Timaeus* 69–72 is more compatible with the tripartite strand in Galen's thinking or with the more unified strand in his psychology.

What, exactly, is the psychological account that Galen defends in *PHP* 1–6? Two quotations illustrate his main thesis well and also indicate some of the complexities in the theory.

My purpose is to show that it is not in a single part (*morion*) of the psyche nor by virtue of a single faculty (*dunamis*) of it that both judgements and affections (or 'emotions', *pathē*) occur, as Chrysippus claimed, but that the psyche has a plurality of faculties of different kinds, and a plurality of parts. Posidonius and Aristotle grant that the faculties of the psyche are three in number, and that by them we desire, feel anger, and reason: but that they are

[66] On the significance of this point, see text to nn. 120–39 below.

also spatially separate from each other, and that our psyche not only contains many faculties but is composed of parts that are different in kind (*heterogeneis*) and in substance (*ousia*), this is the doctrine of Hippocrates and Plato.[67]

I have proved that an animal after birth is governed by three sources (*archai*), one located in the head, whose work is by itself to provide imagination and memory and recollection, knowledge and thought and reasoning, and in its relation to the other parts of the animal to guide the sensation of the sensory parts and the motion of the parts that move voluntarily. A second source is located in the heart; its work is by itself to provide the 'tone' (*tonos*) of the psyche, to be constant and unyielding in the things that reason commands, and in states of passion (*pathos*) to provide the boiling, as it were, of the innate heat, as the psyche at such times desires to avenge itself on the supposed wrongdoer, and this kind of thing is called anger; in its relation to other things its work is to be a source of warmth for the several parts and of pulsing motion for the arteries. The remaining faculty, seated in the liver, has as its work all the things that have to do with nutrition in the animal, the most important of which in us and in all sanguineous animals is the production of blood. To this same faculty belongs also the enjoyment of pleasures, and when it is moved by this enjoyment more than it should be, it produces intemperance and licentiousness.[68]

The first passage illustrates the intellectual options from which Galen chooses his approach to psychology and his conceptual vocabulary in this area.[69] The second, in which Galen sums up his thesis in Books 1–6, brings out clearly certain points indicated in the first passage, notably the linkage between spatially separate parts or organs of the body (*moria*) and determinate and quasi-independent psychological faculties or capacities (*dunameis*), which are also characterized as 'sources' (*archai*) of certain types of bodily and psychological process. The physical parts are brain, heart, and liver, seen as sources of distinct bodily networks, namely those of nerves, arteries, and veins, respectively.[70] The corresponding psychological functions,

[67] Gal. V.454–5, *PHP* 5.4.2–3, p. 312.25–34 De Lacy, trans. De Lacy, slightly modified.

[68] *PHP* V.600–1, 7.3.2–3, pp. 438.28–440.8 De Lacy, trans. De Lacy, slightly modified.

[69] See further Tieleman 2003*b*: 142–4, discussing this passage and *PHP* V.515–16, 6.2.5–6 De Lacy.

[70] See esp. *PHP* Book 6, e.g. V.519–22, 6.3.1–9 De Lacy.

clearly based on Plato's tripartite psyche, are, roughly, those of reasoning and voluntary action, anger and other emotions, and sensual desires. The passage distinguishes between the functions, both physical and psychological, that each part or organ has by itself and those that it has in conjunction with other parts of the body. Also, as will become clear, the passage indicates two, rather divergent ways in which Galen's psychological theory can be understood.[71]

What are the problems that scholars have identified in this tripartite theory? Some problems at least centre on the question whether the psychological functions allocated to specific parts are consistent with their physiological character, as Galen conceives this. Mansfeld, for instance, suggests that Galen's anatomical demonstrations of the role of the brain and nerves, while convincing in their own right, also invalidate Galen's presentation of the other two parts as seats of psychological agency and motivation.

> Because there are no motor nerves issuing from either the heart (the seat of anger, according to Galen) or the liver (the seat of desire, according to Galen), the two non-rational parts are in fact precluded from moving any muscle; there is, in the literal sense of the word, no way in which they can determine our actions, because it is reason, and reason alone, which makes the muscles move by means of the connecting nerves.[72]

Hence, when Galen, as he often does, speaks of the other parts as being stronger than reason, Mansfeld argues that he must mean that reason somehow intervenes on behalf of the other part (against itself) and moves the nerves in a relevant way. But Galen does not explain how this process would work, which is left puzzling at both the psychological and physiological level.[73] Tieleman reinforces this criticism: '[Galen in *PHP*] fails to account for the anatomical and physiological basis for the necessary interaction between the three parts . . . This problem seems to subvert his whole enterprise.'[74]

[71] See further von Staden 2000: 109–110, summarizing the passage and outlining the competing strands in Galen's thought; see also his 106–11, discussed below.

[72] Mansfeld 1991: 141.

[73] Mansfeld 1991: 141–2; on the idea of other parts being stronger than reason in Galen (and in Posidonius, as presented by Galen), see Mansfeld 1991: 133–5. Galen's depiction of Medea's state of mind is a clear example, *PHP* V.306–7, 3.3.14–16 De Lacy (see further Gill 2006: 255–6).

[74] Tieleman 2003*b*: 155. See further his 155–60 and discussion below.

Related problems emerge in trying to define the relationship between psychological and physiological functions in connection with the heart and liver. Galen argues that the independence of the heart from the brain, at the physiological level, is demonstrated, for instance, by the fact that the hearts of sacrificed animals sometimes continue to beat for a while even when cut out of the body and separated from the brain. The automatism of the heartbeat is taken by Galen to show that the heart is an independent source or principle of motion, like the brain.[75] Analogously, heightened palpitation of the heart is frequently noted in the case of strong emotions such as anger or fear, which Galen sometimes takes to be self-evidently non-rational responses and hence not dependent on the orders of the brain. This is held to show that the heart, as the seat of emotions such as anger, is a source of motivational response at the psychological level.[76] The second claim, though crucial for Galen's argument against Stoic unified psychology,[77] is more questionable, and is not supported by observational evidence in the same way as the point about the automatism of the heartbeat.[78] But a more immediate problem, which I underline here, is how we should understand the relationship between the physiological process and the psychological faculty. Simply highlighting the linkage between palpitation and emotion, combined with the assertion of the independence of both of these from the function of reason, does not, by itself, explain how this linkage is to be analysed.

This problem arises also in connection with the idea of the liver as the source of sensual desires. Galen's presentation of the liver gives rise, in fact, to a whole cluster of difficulties. Galen himself highlights one of these. In Galen's view, the functions of brain and heart as the starting-points of physiological networks and sources of motivation

[75] *PHP* V.239, 2.4.48–9 De Lacy, V.277–8, 2.8.23–5 De Lacy; see also Tieleman 1996: 44, 2002: 265. On Galen's experiments with cutting access to arteries and thus showing the role of the heart and pulse (as he supposes), see *On Whether Blood is Contained in the Arteries* (*Art. Sang.*), IV.702–36.

[76] *PHP* V.655, 8.1.22–4 De Lacy.

[77] See e.g. *PHP* V.270–2, 2.7.17–21 De Lacy, V.291–3, 3.1.25–33 De Lacy.

[78] Cf. Tieleman 2002: 265: 'It is one thing to show experimentally that the heart is the source of the pulse; it is another to prove that the heart is the dwelling place of emotions like fear and anger.'

can be shown by observational investigation, especially by the use of ligature (cutting access to nerves or arteries).

> But in the case of the liver we are unable to make any such demonstration, whether by exposing it and applying pressure, or by ligating the veins. For it is not the source of obvious motion, as the heart is of pulsation and the brain of sensation and volition. Nor is it the cause of rapid injury, as each of the others is, but time is required for the weakness of the liver to harm the animal's nutrition and colouring.[79]

Similarly, and by contrast with the other cases, the premises of the argument 'are not taken from the very nature of the thing under investigation, but are from properties peculiar to it'.[80] That is, the premises fall short of those taken by Galen to support the kind of demonstration that provides secure knowledge.[81] Hence, as Hankinson brings out, Galen has to fall back on arguments from analogy and strong teleological assumptions to support his claims about the function of the liver. He argues from structural similarities between liver and heart that the liver, like the heart, is a source (*archē*) of a physiological network and a specific function. He also maintains that the liver does not merely contribute to the body's nutrition, in various senses, but is the (unique) starting-point for this process, exercised through the network of veins of which it is taken to be the (sole) source. For the liver to act as (sole) source and starting-point in this way is to fulfil its distinctive teleological role, which constitutes fulfilling 'properties peculiar to' the liver.[82] Although the line of argument is not inconsistent with Galen's method of natural inquiry, the absence of proof by controlled observation leads him to place great weight on some very strong, and questionable, assumptions about the teleological function of the liver and its relationship to other parts, especially the heart.

The problem of correlating the physiological and psychological roles of the liver is still more acute. How does Galen bridge the

[79] *PHP* V.520, 6.2.5, pp. 372.32–374.4 De Lacy, trans. De Lacy.

[80] *PHP* V.519, 6.2.2, p. 372.21–2 De Lacy, trans. De Lacy.

[81] For the methodology presupposed here, see Ch. 2 above, text to nn. 92–110.

[82] Hankinson 1991*a*: 223–7, referring esp. to *PHP* V.526–7, 6.3.20–4 De Lacy, V.533–4, 6.4.1–7 De Lacy, V.546, 6.5.30–1 De Lacy. On Galen's teleological assumptions, see Ch. 2 above, text to nn. 157–62. See also text to n. 70 above.

gap—it would seem, a large one—between the roles of producing blood and so nourishing the body and acting as a source of sensual appetites and desires in general? The difficulty is still more acute because Galen elsewhere says that hunger and thirst arise in the stomach and are transmitted by a nerve to the brain, not the liver.[83] In another context, he presents the genital organs as a fourth source (*archē*) of functioning and motivation, comparable with brain and heart.[84] This indicates a rather different, and on the face of it, more plausible picture, in which different types of desire are distributed to different centres or arise out of the coordinated functioning of a number of parts.[85] Phillip De Lacy highlights the apparent conflict between the picture of the liver offered in *PHP*, as a centralized locus for certain types of basic faculties (attraction, retention, alternation, and expulsion), and the picture offered elsewhere in Galen. In other contexts, 'the four natural powers [faculties] peculiar to this part of the soul [the liver] are decentralized, each part of the body possessing and using them autonomously'. In other words, elsewhere, 'in the nutritive chain the liver is simply one link out of many', rather than being the sole physiological and psychological source of these functions that is depicted in *PHP*. [86]

What justifies the move made in *PHP* of identifying a single organ which functions both as the source of the vein-system and sensual appetites? Galen, while not addressing this question in analytic terms, brings together Hippocratic and Platonic material in a way that seems designed to suggest an answer. The Hippocratic material presents the liver as the 'root' (*rhizōsis*) of a nexus of veins that, like a root system, links digestive organs such as the stomach and spleen with each other and with the heart.[87] The Platonic material (from the *Timaeus*) presents the same region of the body as the location of the appetitive (*epithumētikon*) part of the psyche.[88] These are presented as

[83] *UP* 1.201–2 Helmreich (III.275.8–15), *On Hippocrates 'Epidemics'* (*Hipp. Epid.*) XVIIA.664–5; see also De Lacy 1988: 62, Tieleman 2003*b*: 158.

[84] *Art of Medicine (Ars Med.)* I.319, *Therapeutics to Glaucon (MMG)* XI.97, *On Semen* (*Sem.*) IV.585; see further De Lacy 1988: 62–3, Tieleman 2003*a*: 160, 164–5.

[85] See further on this point discussion below.

[86] De Lacy 1988: 61 (also 56–7), referring to, e.g., *Nat. Fac.* II. 29–30, 1.12, *SM* 3.122.9–16, *On Affected Parts* (*Loc. Aff.*), VII.66.9–15, 1.7.

[87] *PHP* V.578–9, 6.8.59–66 De Lacy, based on Hipp. *Epid.* 2.4.1, *De Nat. Oss.* 10.

[88] *PHP* V.580, 6.8.67–70, citing Pl. *Ti.* 70d7–e5.

complementary (medical and philosophical) types of description.[89] The implication of the passage seems to be that the vein-system, centred in the liver, acts as the seat for the complex of sensual appetites associated with the processes that take place in this whole region (those of stomach, genitals, and so on). The reason for seeing these desires as focused in this area, specifically, the liver, and as not involving the brain is not stated explicitly here. But Hankinson offers some suggestions on Galen's behalf. He suggests that Galen is seeking to define a primitive type of appetite or desire, without a cognitive component, and that it makes teleological sense to localize this type of desire in one organ or at least region.[90] Viewed in this way, Galen has at least some kind of justification for his presentation of the liver in *PHP*; but it is open to question whether this is the best account he can offer of the relationship between physiological function and psychological faculty or motive in connection with the workings of this part of the body.[91]

I think that most of these problems or puzzles stem from a single cause, which is Galen's attempt in *PHP* to combine his anatomically based account of the brain and nervous system with a Platonically inspired picture of three independent psychological sources with separate bodily locations. The anatomical account implies a unitary source of psychological agency and motivation, exercised through the body as a whole, by contrast with the three-centre psychophysiological model presented in *PHP*. The difficulties that arise in linking physiological features and psychological role in the case of the heart and liver are an index of the mismatch between the findings of anatomy and Galen's Platonic-style paradigm. As a way of pursuing this suggestion, I take note of various features of Galen's psychological thinking outside *PHP* that seem to avoid the

[89] See esp. 'in the case of the liver, (Plato) and (Hippocrates) proceeded as if they had parcelled out the arguments, the one speaking of the organs, the other of the faculty that governs them'; in the case of the heart (but not the liver) both thinkers are also said to 'combine both accounts' in certain respects, *PHP* V.580–1, 6.8.71, 73, esp. p. 422.9–11, 20–2, De Lacy, trans. De Lacy slightly modified.

[90] Hankinson 1991*a*: 229–31: a further suggestion is that Galen's account implies what is in modern terms a behaviourist or functionalist view that trying to get something implies wanting it; in this sense, the fact that the liver absorbs materials signifies 'desire'.

[91] For an alternative account, in terms of the contrast between 'psychic' and 'natural' functions used by Galen elsewhere, see text to n. 114 below.

problems I have outlined. These features are ones that have been discussed by scholars who also highlight the problematic aspects of the psychology of *PHP*. These points can be seen as adding up to a rather different picture of embodied psychology, one that is more consistent with Galen's anatomical account of brain and nerves—and also with key aspects of Stoic psychology.

One of the problems highlighted by scholars including Mansfeld and Tieleman is that Galen does not provide in *PHP* an account of the interaction between psychological parts in a form that is consistent with Galen's anatomically based view of the role of the brain and nervous system.[92] Both these scholars also cite passages in other Galenic works that indicate how this interaction might be understood. Mansfeld refers to a passage from *Character Traits* (*Mor.*), in which Galen refers to the tripartite psychology of *PHP*. Galen then goes on to say: 'It makes no difference how I refer to these things in this book, whether as separate souls, as part of the one human soul or as three different faculties of the same essence.' Mansfeld notes another passage from the same context in which Galen analyses action by reference to a sequence in which a decision following reflection produces desire which activates bodily movement: 'This deliberate movement... sets in motion the hands, feet, tongue, larynx, chest, eyes, mouth or other similar members'.[93] The first passage shows a notable lack of commitment to the distinctive theory of *PHP*, in which the three distinct and independent faculties, with different essences, have three separate locations.[94] The second passage suggests an account of action that implies a unitary locus of decision-making and desire, which activates the body as a coordinated system. I think that the approach taken and the kind of terminology used reflect the type of treatise involved, namely ethical psychology, rather than signalling a substantive change of theory.[95] But the

[92] See text to nn. 72–4 above.

[93] Mansfeld 1991: 143–4, referring to *Mor.* XXVI Kraus, trans. Mattock 1972.

[94] See e.g. the passages cited in text to nn. 67–8 above, illustrating the distinctive character of the theory.

[95] The treatise is an Arabic abstract of a Greek original, but it is not difficult to reconstruct the kind of terminology Galen would have used. Mansfeld is inclined to see an unacknowledged change of doctrine, but this may be too strong an inference. For Galen's psychological language and approach in *Mor.*, and other works of this kind, see 5.2 below.

fact that Galen is prepared to characterize psychological structure and action in this way is none the less significant, especially when coupled with other indications of a unified conception of psychological structure and workings in other, more technical, treatises.

Tieleman underlines further passages from works other than *PHP* that point in a similar direction. One is a fragment from Galen's commentary on Plato's *Timaeus*: 'that all the nerves in the animal evidently have their origin in the brain, from which small offshoots (*paraphuseis*) reach the heart. This [the heart] needs to take part in this higher principle (or 'source', *archē*), in view of the fact that it [the heart] serves it [the principle].'[96] Galen is commenting on a Platonic passage in which the spirited part in the chest is said to respond to reason in the brain, when this reports wrongdoing and calls for revenge (*Ti.* 70a7–b8). As Tieleman points out, the psychology implied in the passage, involving a coordinated psychophysiological response by brain and heart, is very different from the view stressed in *PHP* of brain and heart as centres of two distinct physiological and psychological networks.[97]

Tieleman also cites in the same connection a passage from Galen's *On the Preservation of Health* (*San. Tu.*): 'Anger is not simply an increase, but a kind of boiling, so to speak, of the heat in the heart; this is why the most distinguished philosophers say that its substance is of such a kind. For the craving for revenge is an inessential property (*sumbebēkos*) rather than the substance (*ousia*) of anger.'[98] Galen's comment alludes to Aristotle's statement that the dialectical definition of anger (as the desire for revenge) refers to the 'form and definition' (that is, essence) of anger whereas that of the philosopher of nature (as the boiling of blood around the heart) refers to its 'matter' (*hulē*). However, Galen—writing from the standpoint of the philosophy of nature—revises Aristotle's view, presenting the physical side of anger as its 'essence' and the motivational side (desire for anger) as an incidental attribute.[99] What this implies, Tieleman suggests, is a view of anger similar to that of Plato, in *Timaeus*

[96] *Plat. Tim.* fr. 14, lines 1–4 Larrain, my trans.

[97] Tieleman 2003*b*: 153–4, referring to, e.g., *PHP* V.262–7, 2.6.1–6.

[98] VI.138.7–12, 2.9.5–6, p. 61.24–8 Koch, trans. Tieleman 2003*b*: 156.

[99] See Arist. *De An.* 1.1, 403^{a}29–32; for related ancient definitions of anger, see Tieleman 2003*b*: 156 n. 62.

70a7–b9, as, essentially, a physiological reaction, but one correlated with (and, by implication, triggered by) the judgement of the rational part. This idea matches the passage just cited from Galen's commentary on the *Timaeus*, in which the heart responds to a message sent through the nervous system to the heart, which is prepared to respond to this message. Tieleman also cites the point noted earlier that hunger and thirst are presented in *UP* as arising in the stomach and as transmitted by a nerve to the brain, not to the liver or to the brain via the liver.[100] One might expect that this line of communication would be extended to the liver, which is, indeed, presented as forming part of the nervous system in *UP*. But Galen says that the connecting nerve is a small one which only penetrates the surface (or 'tunic') of the liver; he also adds: 'Insofar as this organ is the source of the nutritive psyche, the kind that is also in plants, it appears to have no need for a nerve. I pass over the question whether it should be called nature (*phusis*) or nutritive psyche.'[101] The significance of the final comment (about 'nature') is considered shortly.

The passages cited by Mansfeld and Tieleman imply a significantly different picture of embodied psychology from the one that is dominant in *PHP*. In place of the focus on the operation of three distinct centres or sources, we see indications of a more unified psychological and physiological structure. Motivation radiates through the nervous system from the brain and activates the body as an interconnected whole. In the case of anger, the heart provides the reactive component (boiling of the blood), in response to the messages sent from the brain through the nerves. The liver, or liver-based, system operates in a more independent way, but also at a more basic (plant-like) level, carrying forward low-level processes of nutrition. Von Staden has suggested that the picture just outlined is prevalent in Galen's works outside *PHP*. He points, in particular, to Galen's frequent use of the psyche–nature contrast in a way that is closely parallel with that found in the theories of Herophilus and Erasistratus and also the Stoics. For instance, in *Differences of Symptoms* (*Symp. Diff.*), the natural activities of a living being are said to include 'appetite or "striving",

100 Tieleman 2003*b*; 158; cf. n. 83 above.

101 *UP* 1.226.18–22 Helmreich (May 1968: 228), trans. Tieleman 2003*b*: 158, slightly modified.

digestion, the distribution of nutriment, the generation of blood, the pulse, and the excretion of residues . . . whereas the "psychic" activities are restricted . . . to cognitive and voluntary motor activity'.[102] 'Natural' activities are explained by reference to four 'natural faculties' or capacities, namely those for attraction, retention, alternation, and secretion; these are, usually, seen as operative in each part of the body—by contrast with *PHP* where the stress falls on the idea of the liver as the primary source of these capacities.[103] Again, outside *PHP*, psychic activities are not presented as inbuilt in all parts of the body but 'flow to the instruments of the psyche from its source [*archē*, that is, the brain], similar to the light of the sun [radiating out]'.[104] As in Herophilus, Erasistratus, and Stoicism, psychic activities tend, outside *PHP*, to be grouped under the headings of perception (*aisthēsis*) and movement (*kinēsis*), sometimes with the addition of 'activities that belong to the ruling part (*hēgemonikon*) of the psyche'.[105]

Von Staden suggests that these features of Galen's thought form a pattern that is consistent with, and probably influenced by, the brain-centred account of animal (including human) psychology developed by Herophilus and Erasistratus, and consolidated by Galen's own studies. The psyche–nature contrast is also prominent in Stoic thought and is combined there with the idea of a unified control-centre (though one located in the heart).[106] However, von Staden sees in *PHP* explanatory models which are 'to some extent . . . on a collision course' with the features of Galenic thought just outlined.[107] In particular, 'Galen's Platonic view that the lower functions too—not only heat and pulse, but also the vegetative, nutritive, reproductive, desiderative functions (especially desires for food, drink, and sexual

[102] See von Staden 2000: 107, referring to *Symp. Diff.* VII.55 (see other refs. in his n. 72).

[103] Von Staden 2000: 107, referring e.g. to *On My Own Opinions* (*Prop. Plac.*), IV.759 (13.7 Nutton, Boudon–Millot and Pietrobelli 2005: 187.2–6), *Symp. Diff.* VII.63. For the contrast with the account of the liver in *PHP* see also De Lacy 1988: 61–2 (also 56–7).

[104] *Loc. Aff.* VIII.66–8, trans. von Staden 2000: 108, slightly modified.

[105] Von Staden 2000: 108–9, referring e.g. to *Symp. Diff.* VII.55, and outlining the rich variety of cognitive, sensory, and voluntary motor functions allocated to the ruling part of the psyche (and categorized as 'psychic'). On Galen's use of the psyche–nature distinction, see also De Lacy 1988: 53–6.

[106] See 3.2 above, text to nn. 56–65.

[107] Von Staden 2000: 109.

pleasure) are activities of the *soul*, and that human beings share this desiderative kind of soul with plants, is hardly compatible with the Galenic views traced above, and especially not with his distinction between *physis* and *psyche*'.[108] As is often noted, Galen often expresses indifference about whether one should use the terminology of 'nutritive psyche' (or sometimes desiderative psyche) or 'nature'; he often presents this variation as unimportant in terms of doctrine. However, von Staden suggests that this indifference is best taken as marking an ambivalence or tension between two psychological models operating in his thought, which comes out especially in the contrast between patterns dominant in *PHP* and elsewhere.[109]

However, as von Staden also implies (2000: 110), not all aspects of the psychology of *PHP* are in conflict with the more unified psychological picture, associated with the psyche–nature contrast, found elsewhere in Galenic thought. It is worth re-examining in this connection the passage in *PHP* 7.3.2 (V.600–1) cited earlier, which summarizes the tripartite theory.[110] The description of the ruling part of the psyche is made in terms of the combination of cognitive functions and (in conjunction with other parts of the body) perceptive and voluntary motor functions that are, elsewhere in Galen, characterized as psychic rather than natural.[111] It is not difficult to see how this description could form part of a unified account of psychology and physiology of the type found elsewhere in Galen. The characterization of the heart-based part is also particularly suggestive in this connection:

> its work is by itself to provide the 'tone' (*tonos*) of the psyche, to be constant and unyielding in the things that reason commands, and in states of passion (*pathos*) to provide the boiling, as it were, of the innate heat, as the psyche at such times desires to avenge itself on the supposed wrongdoer, and this kind of thing is called anger; in its relation to other things its work is to be a source of warmth for the several parts and of pulsing motion for the arteries.[112]

[108] Von Staden 2000: 110, his italics.

[109] Von Staden 2000: 110–11, esp. n. 83: 'a lacunose, vacillating (even though richly detailed) theory lurks behind his shimmering nomenclature'. For expressions of this indifference, see e.g. *MM* X.635.14–15, *UP* 1.226.18–25 Helmreich, *Nat. Fac.* II.1–2, 1.1; also n. 101 above.

[110] See text to n. 68 above.

[111] *PHP* V.600, 7.3.2, p. 438.29–33 De Lacy; cf. von Staden 2000: 108–9.

[112] *PHP* V.601, 7.3.2, p. 438.33–440.3.

Some aspects of the role are purely physiological, for instance, being a source of warmth. Others, however, fulfil the function of providing the physiological response to a cognitive message sent from the brain (the 'boiling' in response to reason's command) that also figures in the passage cited earlier from Galen's commentary on the *Timaeus*. In both cases, the role of the heart-based part is that of reacting in a physiological way appropriate to its character by 'pulsing' activity in response to a rational command, presented in the *Timaeus* commentary as sent from the brain via the nerves.[113] The characterization of the third part juxtaposes physiological and psychological functions in a way that is less easy to assimilate to a unified picture and that is, in any case, rather problematic, as suggested earlier. A view more consistent with this unified picture would be either (1) that the functions of the liver are purely 'natural' and not psychic or (2) that the liver acts in a basic, 'natural', way, but also responds (via the nervous system) to commands from the brain.[114] However, the passage, taken as a whole, indicates that the psychology of *PHP* could have been worked out in a way that would be more fully compatible with the brain-based anatomy adopted by Galen. The psychological pattern could have been presented as one in which motivation (voluntary movement) derives entirely from the brain-based *hēgemonikon*, communicated through the nervous system. The functions of the other two parts would be characterized either as 'natural' or as physiological reactions activated by the messages of the control-centre. This is, of course, *not*, for the most part, how Galen formulates his psychological theory in *PHP*; the stress is, rather, on the independence of the three psychic-physiological parts. But it is possible to see how this kind of account could have been offered, if Galen's objectives had been rather different.

What I have suggested so far is that much of Galen's psychological thinking, especially outside *PHP*, is consistent with the brain-centred psychophysiology to which he attaches such importance. In fact, there are some aspects of *PHP* that are consistent with this picture, though there are other features (notably the idea of three autonomous

[113] Cf. n. 96 above. This kind of division could be characterized in terms of the contrast between psychic and natural, though that is not used here.

[114] See text to nn. 100–1 above. See also Tieleman 2003*b*: 158–9.

psychological centres) that are much harder to match with this picture. The aspects of his psychological thinking that are compatible with a unified, brain-centred view are, as von Staden stresses, also largely consistent with the theories of Herophilus and Erasistratus, as far as we can recover these, and also with the Stoic unified theory. An important common strand is the distinction between psychological functions located in, or deriving from, the control-centre and natural functions operating in the rest of the body.[115] It follows then, as suggested at the start of this section, that much Galenic psychological thinking, as well as the brain-centred anatomy on which he places so much emphasis, is compatible with the Stoic idea of a unified psychological control-centre. This renders paradoxical the fact that in *PHP* so much of the argument takes the form of a sustained critique of Stoic psychology. The paradox is somewhat lessened by the fact that in Books 1–3, the argument is mainly directed at Stoic (and Aristotelian) thinking about the location of the ruling part of the psyche, particularly the alleged defects of Stoic methodology in maintaining the heart-centred view.[116] However, in Book 6, Galen also strongly asserts the validity of a tripartite psychological and physiological picture, in contrast to the unified Stoic one. If I am right to suggest that there are, in fact, significant common features between the Galen and Stoic models (alongside obvious differences), why does Galen show so little sign of recognizing this point, at least in *PHP*?[117]

As already suggested (in 3.1), it is a rather complex matter to explain Galen's consistently negative or critical approach to Stoic psychology in *PHP* and his failure to explore possible common ground between the two theories; and different aspects of this question are examined in the course of this study. The disagreement about the location of the ruling part of the psyche, stemming from the methodological differences considered in 2.2 above, is one very important factor. Another, discussed in Chapter 4, is Galen's conviction, maintained at length in *PHP* 4–5, that the Stoic analysis of

115 Von Staden 2000: 105–9, outlined above.

116 See Ch. 2 above, text to nn. 137–40.

117 In 2.3 above, text to nn. 197–201, I highlighted contexts, outside *PHP*, in which Galen does acknowledge points of similarity with Stoic thinking, especially regarding the philosophy of nature.

psychological functions, especially the relationship between reason and emotion or desire, is radically misguided. Although this issue is not directly linked with the question of the relationship between psychology and bodily functions, it clearly has a substantial impact on Galen's overall evaluation of Stoic psychology. A broader question, outlined in Chapter 1, and explored further in Chapter 4, is whether Galen's attitude to Stoicism reflects underlying conceptual differences, bearing especially on their respective thinking about the part–whole relationship.[118] However, a further important factor is Galen's objective, fundamental to the project of *PHP*, of bringing out common ground between Platonic and 'Hippocratic' psychology, the latter signifying, in part at least, the results of Galen's own medical, especially anatomical, investigation.[119] Galen's general view is that, on several key questions, especially that of the location of the ruling part of the psyche and the relationship between reason and emotions, the Platonic picture is both correct and is sharply different from the Stoic one. This is, no doubt, a further reason why Galen does not give serious thought in *PHP* to the question whether his own theory has more in common with Stoic psychology than he often allows.

But is Galen right to think that Platonic psychology supports his side of the argument? Elsewhere, I have argued that the Stoics, as well as Galen, could have found support and inspiration in Plato's accounts of psychology in the *Timaeus* 69–72 and the *Republic*—and that perhaps the Stoics (as well as Galen) *did* find inspiration there.[120] Here, I focus on the more limited, though related, question of which strand of Galen's thinking about embodied psychology is best supported by Plato's description of the embodied tripartite psyche in *Timaeus* 69–72. The two strands I have in mind are those outlined earlier: one is the more unified, brain-centred psychology that is closer to Stoicism and which includes the psyche–nature distinction and the other is the tripartite psychology (and physiology) that is the dominant strand in *PHP*. Galen himself, obviously,

[118] See Ch. 1 above, text to nn. 40–51, and Ch. 4 below, esp. text to nn. 36–55, 257–68. [119] See text to nn. 13–21 above.

[120] See Gill 2006: 291–322, where I juxtapose Galenic and Stoic 'readings' of Platonic psychology in the *Timaeus* and *Republic*, the Stoic ones being constructed (speculatively) on the basis of similarities between Stoic and Platonic theory.

believes that *Timaeus* 69–72 supports the tripartite pattern (with three separate and independent psychophysiological sources), and cites the passage extensively in Book 6 as well as sometimes elsewhere in that connection. But there are reasons for thinking that Plato's passage lends some support to the other, more Stoic, strand; and that Galen's own comments indicate this point, though without drawing larger conclusions from it.

In *PHP* in general, Galen underpins his psychological theory by combining aspects of these two Platonic dialogues that reinforce the separateness and autonomy of the three parts. In particular, he stresses in the *Republic* the argument in book 4 (435–41) for the idea of the three parts as independent and potentially competing sources of motivation and in *Timaeus* 69–72 the fact that the three psychic parts are given a distinct bodily location and function. Both points are referred to near the start of *PHP* and they are used to support the key claim of the treatise, noted earlier, that the three psychic sources are 'forms' (*eidē*) and 'parts' (*moria*) which differ in their 'essence' or 'substance' (*ousia*).[121]As well as referring to these two Platonic accounts, Galen tends to conflate them. For instance, in this context, he uses the terms 'dog' and 'many-headed beast', which occur in the *Republic*'s characterization of the conflicting parts of the psyche, to describe the (rather differently conceived) parts of *Timaeus* 69–72.[122] It is not difficult to see how this kind of conflation supports the Galenic tripartite (psychophysiological) account, for instance, by linking the third (liver-based) part with the broad range of appetites, including sexual one, associated with this part in the *Republic*, rather than the rather different set of functions described in *Ti.* 70e–72d.[123] Also, in his references to *Ti.* 69–72,

[121] *PHP* V.514–18, 6.2.1–12 De Lacy brings together these Platonic passages and others to support the Galenic thesis about the separateness of the three psychic parts, contrasted with other views, including Chrysippus' (V.515, 6.2.5 De Lacy). See also text to n. 67 above. *R.* 435–41 is also referred to in *PHP* V.512–13, 6.2.25–7 De Lacy, and discussed extensively in V.480–502, 5.7.1–82 De Lacy.

[122] *PHP* V.518, 6.2.14, p. 372.4–5 De Lacy, which uses the terms of *R.* 440c–d and 588c–589b to characterize the relation between parts in *Ti.* 70a–b. On the differences between the two accounts, see further below.

[123] For the sexual connotations of the third part, see *R.* 439d6, 439e–440a (Leontius example), 580e4; this connotation is absent from *Ti.* 70e–72d and is ruled out by the location specified in 77b4. On Galen's ambiguity (or variation) about the scope of the liver, see text to nn. 79–91 above.

Galen cites repeatedly the Platonic phrases, 'fountain-head of blood that moves violently (*sphodrōs*) through all the limbs' (linked with the heart) and 'appetitive (*epithumētikon*) of food and drink'. Although Galen uses these phrases to make various points, including purely physiological ones, they tend to reinforce the core Galenic thesis that the three organ-parts are sources of distinct and autonomous psychological agency.[124]

However, there are important aspects of the presentation of the embodied tripartite psyche in *Ti.* 69–72 that are different in their implications from the features of the *Republic* stressed by Galen. In the *Timaeus*, the emphasis is less on the idea of the psyche as a collection of independent and potentially conflicting sources of motivation and more on the idea of the psyche (and body) as an integrated set of functions.[125] This emphasis involves themes that are more congenial to Stoic psychology, and to the strand of Galenic psychology that resembles this. One such theme is that reason or the mind, situated in the head, communicates directly with the heart-based spirited part, in a way that triggers a physiological response, and more indirectly with the liver-based appetitive part. The spirited part responds to grounds for anger, 'when reason gives the message that some unjust action is occurring'. Especially striking is the linkage between the reason-sent message and the physiological response. It is when 'reason gives the message' that 'the excitement (*menos*) of spirit boils', which in turn, stimulates 'the blood that moves violently through all the limbs' (one of the phrases accentuated by Galen).[126] The third (appetitive) part, though presented as incapable of responding to reason in the same way as the second part (spirit-heart) is adapted to be guided by images (*psuchagōgein*). Although these images are, on the face of it, merely physiological reactions (such as bilious contractions produced in the liver), they are also, in some sense, the product of 'thoughts sent down from the mind'. This linkage is reinforced by reference to the traditional idea of the liver as the seat of divination. Prophetic dreams are located here; in this way,

[124] For these phrases, see *Ti.* 70b1–3, d7–8. See e.g. (for the first phrase), *PHP* V.566, 576, 581, 6.8.40, 49, 72 De Lacy (also V.292, 3.1.31 De Lacy); for the second, see V.576, 580, 6.8.51–2, 69–70 De Lacy.

[125] For this point, cf. Gill 2006: 294, also Johansen 2004: 153–9.

[126] *Ti.* 70a7–b4; for the Galenic passages, see n. 124 above.

a part of us that 'has no share in reason and understanding' has 'some grasp of the truth'.[127]

These features of *Ti.* 69–72 can be seen as prefiguring salient aspects of Stoic psychology. The description of the heart's responses in anger evokes the idea of an intense physiological response to a rational judgement that is the characteristic mark of a Stoic emotion or passion (*pathos*).[128] The Platonic characterization of the reactions of the third part maps less straightforwardly onto Stoic patterns. But it can be seen partly as expressing the kind of automatic, non-cognitive process that is associated with the work of 'nature', rather than psyche. At the same time, it prefigures other Stoic ideas, such as that even seemingly non-rational processes such as sexual desire express the operation of the control-centre and that the natural functions of a human being contribute to the teleological or providential structure that is proper to human beings.[129] I have suggested that we can find in Galenic thought a comparable strand to that of Stoicism, alongside the programmatic tripartite psychology that is the dominant strand in *PHP.* To what extent do Galen's comments on *Ti.* 69–72 in *PHP* or elsewhere provide evidence that he read Plato's description in a way that reflects this strand in his thought?

I noted earlier a fragment from Galen's commentary on the *Timaeus,* analysing the Platonic picture of spirit-heart responding to reason with anger (70a–b) in terms of Galenic anatomy, namely as communication from the brain through the nervous system.[130] A second passage noted by Tieleman refers to an Aristotelian account of anger, but it may also reflect Galen's reading of the same Platonic passage. This Galenic passage implies a conception of anger as a physiological response ('boiling of blood') which is non-rational in itself but which is correlated with (and presumably triggered by) the judgement of reason that an act calls for revenge.[131] I suggested

[127] *Ti.* 71a–e, esp. a3–7, b3–4, d4, e1; for a fuller analysis, see Gill 2006: 300–2.

[128] In Stoic passions, assent to a rational impression e.g. that 'it is appropriate to react with anger' triggers (automatically) an intense reaction, such as swelling of the (bodily) control-centre. See e.g. LS 65 A (Andronicus, *On Passions* 1) and LS 65 D (*PHP* V.336–7, 4.2.1–6 De Lacy); see further Brennan 1998, 2003, Graver 2007: 24–34.

[129] On psyche and nature in Stoicism, see text to nn. 38–44, 59–65 above, on the control-centre and the genitals, see LS 53 H(4); on Stoic thinking on the stomach as expressing a teleological (providential) role, see Cic. *N.D.* 2.156–7.

[130] See text to n. 96 above. [131] See text to nn. 98–9 above.

earlier that a similar pattern might be seen as implied in the summary of the function of the heart-based, spirited part at the start of *PHP* Book 7.[132] The description of anger in *Ti.* 70a–b is cited explicitly by Galen in a passage in *PHP* Book 6 that suggests parallels between the Platonic characterization of psychic functions and the Hippocratic characterization of physical organs. The Galenic passage also states, in the case of anger at least, that both Plato and Hippocrates also highlight some links between physiological and psychic responses.[133] The main explicit function of this passage seems to be, in the case of both heart and liver, to promote the correlation of organ and psychic function or motivational source in line with the main thesis of *PHP*, that there are three psychophysiological centres.[134] However, the passage is not very explicit about the nature of the correlation involved; and it *might* be possible to take the comment as expressing a view of anger more in line with the other passages just noted, namely as a physiological response to a rational command. If so, the passage runs counter to the presentation of the heart as the seat of an independent source of emotions such as anger that is the dominant view in *PHP*.[135] If this reading is possible, this passage suggests that the unified (Stoic-style) conception of anger may make an appearance in *PHP* too, at least in Book 6.

Galen also cites in the same passage part of Plato's description of the third part of the psyche, based in the region including the liver. Galen couples it with Hippocrates' account of the vein-system in this part of the body, and comments: 'in the case of the liver (Plato) and (Hippocrates) proceeded as if they had parcelled out the arguments, the one speaking of the organs, the other of the faculty that governs them'.[136] This subdivision of the topic, perhaps tactically, enables Galen to avoid spelling out the considerable differences between his conception of the liver as a physiological organ and that of Plato. Non-Platonic features in Galen's account include a different understanding of its role in digestion and growth.[137]

[132] See text to n. 112 above.

[133] *PHP* V.575–82, 6.8.48–76 De Lacy, esp. V.581–2, 6.8.72–5 De Lacy.

[134] See text to nn. 68–70 above.

[135] For this type of presentation of anger in *PHP*, see e.g. V.655, 8.1.22–4 De Lacy.

[136] *PHP* V.580, 6.8.71, p. 422.9–11 De Lacy, trans. De Lacy, slightly modified.

[137] See Tieleman 2003*b*: 153–4, referring to Arist. *PA* 3.7, 670^{a}27 as the first expression of the post-Platonic view of the liver.

They also include the elimination of the rather complex or elusive type of communication with the rational centre described in *Ti.* 71a–e. As noted earlier, although Galen envisages in *UP* a small nerve reaching the liver, he analyses its functions in purely organic or automatic (not cognitive) terms.[138] The more positive implications of Galen's juxtaposition in *PHP* 6 of Hippocrates' physiological description and Plato's psychological one are more difficult to spell out. Hankinson takes the passage as implying that, in the case of a relatively basic organ such as the liver, 'desire' *means* fulfilling the appropriate digestive or nourishing function.[139] This could be taken as Galen's way of linking the role of the liver as psychological agent and physiological organ; and this is what the passage explicitly suggests. But, given how little content the idea of 'psychological' has, in this interpretation, the implication could be that the liver's role is simply a 'natural' one—a form of description that Galen, like the Stoics, uses elsewhere for this kind of function. In this passage, as in the one on the heart just discussed, firm interpretation is difficult in the absence of analytic commentary by Galen himself. What is clear is that, regarding the third part, Galen's view diverges in most respects from Plato's in a way that calls into question his claim to be combining Platonic and Hippocratic elements. But the divergence *might be* taken as bringing Galen's account closer to a more Stoic-style conception, of the kind found elsewhere in Galen, in which the role of the liver is analysed as 'natural' rather than psychic.

In this section, I have argued that, in Galen's thought as a whole, there are two psychological patterns, which are, sometimes uneasily, combined. The first is the tripartite psychophysiological pattern that is the dominant strand in *PHP*. The second, which predominates outside *PHP*, presents the body as a unified psychophysical system, in which cognitive motivation derives from the control-centre and other, more basic ('natural'), processes are carried forward by other organs, working as a connected system. The second pattern is more clearly consistent with the outcome of Galen's research, building on the work of Herophilus and Erasistratus, on the brain and nervous system. It also exhibits some striking similarities with Stoic thought (especially in the contrast sometimes drawn between psychic and natural functions) despite Galen's intense critique of Stoic embodied

[138] See text to n. 101 above. [139] See text to n. 90 above.

psychology in *PHP* 1–3, 6. Galen's tripartite psychology gives rise to a number of problems and obscurities,[140] which do not arise in the same way in the more unified aspects of his psychophysiology. There are some indications even in *PHP* of ideas that could fit in with a more unified psychology, or that could, at least, be modified to do so. A key objective of the project of *PHP* is the desire to bring out the consistency between the picture of brain and nervous system shown by Galen's anatomical research and the tripartite psychology found in Plato's *Republic* and *Timaeus*.[141] This objective seems to generate a number of the problems in Galen's tripartite model noted earlier. However, there are reasons for thinking that some aspects of Plato's picture of the embodied psyche in *Ti.* 69–72 might actually fit better with the more unified (Stoic-style) psychophysiology found in Galen outside *PHP*. Although the account of Galenic thought offered here is a rather complex one, the overall impression, as in the previous section, is to accentuate actual or potential points of contact between Galenic and Stoic thinking about embodied psychology, in spite of Galen's resolute criticism of this in *PHP* 2–3.

3.4 THE CONSTRUCTION OF THE EMBRYO

The Construction of the Embryo (*Foet. Form.*), is another work bearing on psychology and the body in which Galen engages directly with Stoic ideas. It is a relatively short essay, written much later in Galen's life.[142] The comments on Stoic thought are briefer and more restricted in scope, focusing on their ideas about the development of the embryo. Discussion of this Galenic essay complements the preceding treatment of *PHP* (in 3.2–3) in a number of ways. Although similar issues reappear here, for instance, about the roles of the three main organs, brain, heart, and liver, and about the methodology of natural inquiry, there are certain salient differences of approach from the earlier work. Despite the retention of the

[140] See text to nn. 71–90 above. [141] See text to nn. 17–21 above.

[142] It falls within the works in the last period of Galen's life, between 193 and *c.*210; see Nickel 2001: 44.

tripartite psychology and physiology, Galen's work also presents the body and its psychological functions as constituting a relatively unified structure. For related reasons, there is less evidence of tension between different strands within Galenic psychological thought. Also, although Galen has serious criticisms of the Stoic and Aristotelian approach on this question, the gap between his standpoint and theirs emerges as less great than in *PHP*. On one key aspect of the discussion, that of teleology, Galen is on the same side as Aristotle and the Stoics, even if he draws somewhat different conclusions from this shared standpoint. To put the point differently, this is a work in which we are conscious that all three theories, to a large extent, share the world-view that I characterized in 2.3 as 'high naturalism', even if they have localized disagreements regarding the development of the embryo. Platonic thinking plays a more marginal role in this treatise—markedly so by comparison with *PHP*—and the Aristotelian and Stoic theories emerge as the philosophical theories that Galen feels he needs to take seriously on this question.

What are Galen's overall objectives in *Foet. Form.*, and how does Stoic thought, usually taken together with Aristotelian thought in this essay, relate to these objectives? At the start of the work, and at some subsequent points, Galen highlights certain methodological defects, regarding the topic of the construction of the embryo, which he wants to address here. One is the failure to base one's conclusions on properly conducted anatomical work. Another is that of using inappropriate premises (or 'non-evident' assumptions), a defect linked with that of failing to begin one's inquiry from the nature of the specific subject under investigation.[143] These criticisms recall those made of the Stoics in *PHP* regarding the location of the ruling part of the psyche;[144] and the criticisms are directed primarily at the Stoics here, though they are coupled with Aristotle and his followers. The main inappropriate premise seems to be that the heart serves as the organizing centre of physiological and psychological activity, which underlies the claim that the heart is constructed

[143] *Foet. Form.* IV.652, 1.1 Nickel, IV.675–6, 4.4–5, p. 80.2–5 Nickel. (Singer 1997*a* contains a translation of *Foet. Form.*, which cites Kühn page refs.) On Galen's objectives in the work, see also Nickel 2001: 46, 48.

[144] See Ch. 2 above, text to nn. 136–40.

first in the embryo and that the heart, once formed, manages the formation of the other parts. The premise is said to be 'non-evident', and not appropriate to the essence of the subject in question, because it is not based on anatomical research on the animal embryo (or, in the case of the Stoics, not based on anatomical research at all).[145] Despite the fact that criticism of the Stoic (and Aristotelian) position is presented as the main objective of the work, another passage suggests that the treatise is directed primarily at thinkers from those schools. Towards the end of the essay, Galen makes it clear that the work is chiefly addressed to those who share the teleological approach to the subject adopted here.[146] This could include Platonists as well as followers of Aristotle and the Stoics, but, given the relatively minor role of Platonic ideas in the work,[147] the other two groups seem to be meant, along with medical readers who share Galen's teleological standpoint.

The work may also have another key objective, though this is not emphasized in the same way. Before he makes his criticisms of the Stoic and Aristotelian approach, Galen comments that he has, in fact, changed his mind on the question of the order in which organs are formed in the embryo, a topic that is central for this essay. In an earlier work, *On Semen*, he maintained that the heart was formed, along with the liver, in the first few days after conception. He says that he based this view on the exceptional importance of the heart in the fully developed animal. However, Galen says here that he has changed his mind in light of the consensus among philosophers and doctors that the embryo's operation is initially plant-like, which Galen takes as implying that its functions are managed by the nutritive work of the liver rather than the heart. Hence, in this work, Galen strongly maintains the thesis that the liver develops earlier than the heart and has the prime role in shaping the early stages, by contrast with the Stoic and Aristotelian view that this role is played by the heart.[148] So it seems likely that another important

[145] *Foet. Form.* IV.674–8, 4.1–9, esp. pp. 78.12–16, 89.14–25 Nickel.

[146] *Foet. Form.* IV.688, 6.5, p. 92.22–3 Nickel.

[147] See further on this point, text to nn. 182–9 below.

[148] *Foet. Form.* IV.663–6, 3.9–14, esp. p. 66.19–28 Nickel. See also *On Semen* (*Sem.*), 1.8.8–9.7, pp. 92.4–94.6 De Lacy. For his criticisms of Stoic–Aristotelian views, see below.

aim in the work is to explore and present this revised Galenic position. The disagreement with the Stoics and Aristotelians, who take a view closer to Galen's earlier thinking, thus emerges, in part at least, as a consequence of Galen's own shift in thinking.

Galen's acknowledgement of a change of opinion is interesting, and rather unusual. In *On My Own Opinions* (*Prop. Plac.*), written slightly later than *Foet. Form.* (but also during 193–210), he says that he was originally drawn to the view that the heart developed first, though he then realized that the formation of the heart depends on the pre-existence of the liver.[149] In *UP* 15, written in the same general period as *On Semen* (169–75), but probably rather later than that work, he also suggests that the greater size of the liver in the embryo implies that it develops first.[150] So, if Galen's report of his own earlier view is correct in *Prop. Plac.*, we seem to have three stages in Galen's thinking: (1) the heart is formed first; (2) both organs are formed about the same time (*On Semen*); (3) the liver is formed first.[151] As Diethard Nickel points out, these variations of view on Galen's part are not entirely surprising, since he did not actually have the technical resources to make accurate measurements of the relative size of organs in the early stages of embryonic development. Galen himself reports in *Foet. Form.* that in foetuses aborted after thirty days, all three organs are formed, though the liver is much bigger; and this seems to be more or less all the evidence he is able to draw on. Galen acknowledges that he cannot determine the exact time of the emergence of the heart. According to a modern medical handbook cited by Nickel, by the end of a month's growth of the embryo, the liver has been formed and the embryonic heart has begun to beat.[152] Galen's admissions of these variations in his own view, taken with the limitations, partly acknowledged, in his observations, might lead us to be rather sceptical about the validity of Galen's objectives

[149] *Prop. Plac.* 11.1–5, pp. 90.18–94.16 Nutton, Boudon-Millot and Pietrobelli 2005: 182.16–183.15.

[150] *UP* 2.359–60 Helmreich, 15.6.

[151] See further Nickel 1989: 80–2, 2001: 121–3, Nutton 1999: 177–8.

[152] *Foet. Form.* IV.662–3, 3.5–8, p. 676.5–18 Nickel, also referring to Hippocrates' report of a six-day foetus, cited in IV. 654–5, 1.5–7 Nickel. See further Nickel 1989: 82–3. See also Blakemore and Jennett 2001: 36 (article on 'Antenatal development'); 'Between the fourth and eighth week after conception, most of the major organ systems start to form in the embryo, although it is much later before these start to function properly.'

in this essay. If Galen's position is so provisional and rests on such limited observational evidence, what is it that justifies his methodological critique of the Stoic and Aristotelian position, which is central for his project in this work?[153] Certainly, on this topic, Galen is not able to draw on observation-based demonstrations that have the cogency of his work on the brain and nerves.[154] However, as brought out shortly, Galen may be justified in some of the critical points he makes about the heart-centred view, even though his own account remains largely conjectural and is only indirectly supported by anatomical observation of fully formed animals.

To form a clearer view of Galen's response to Stoic and Aristotelian ideas, and to correlate these with his approach in *PHP* and elsewhere, we need to locate his comments within the structure of his whole argument.[155] Roughly speaking, in the first three chapters, Galen sets out his own account of the development of the embryo; chapters 4–5 are centred on correction of the Stoic–Aristotelian views, and chapter 6 includes criticisms of their views as part of a tentative overall conclusion. In more detail, the work begins (ch. 1) with a Hippocratic account of a six-day old foetus, of which Galen then offers an anatomical analysis in ch. 2. This then serves as the basis for an account (ch. 3) of the development of the embryo. This chapter includes Galen's acknowledgement of his change of view and the rationale for his revised position.[156] This account includes a certain amount of anatomical detail, though it is not claimed that this is based on detailed first-hand examination of the human (or animal) foetus. Galen seems to be drawing on his work on the anatomy of fully formed animals to support his current position on the sequence of development of organs in the embryo.[157] Chapters 4–5 are centred on the criticisms of the Stoic and Aristotelian view that the heart developed first and that it manages the subsequent development of the embryo. Chapter 4 focuses on weaknesses in methodology, especially the failure (by the Stoics) to make use of anatomical

[153] On his objectives in *Foet. Form.*, see text to nn. 143–5 above.

[154] On his work on the brain and nerves, see Ch. 2 above, text to nn. 11–18, 102–10. This work is referred to in *Foet. Form.* V.679, 5.2–3 Nickel.

[155] See also the outline of contents in Nickel 2001: 46–8, and, on the work as a response to Stoic ideas, Nickel 1993.

[156] See text to n. 148 above.

[157] Cf. Nickel 1989: 82.

observation. Chapter 5 amplifies this criticism with arguments based on (Galen's view of) the functions of the organs involved, also supported by reference to anatomical evidence. The final chapter (6) attempts to give a teleological analysis of the development of the embryo. Again, the Stoic–Aristotelian view on the function of the heart is criticized, though Galen admits that his own alternative account is sketchy and incomplete in certain ways.

How does Galen's response to Stoic thought in this work compare with that in *PHP*, discussed earlier in this chapter? What does Galen's response indicate about his own position on embodied psychology and about the nature and internal coherence of this position? Clearly, from what has been said so far, much of the argumentation recalls the arguments of *PHP* 1–3, 6, also directed against Stoic (and to some extent Aristotelian) heart-centred psychology.[158] The position Galen adopts here on the development of the embryo is based on the three-centre physiology for which he argues in *PHP* and involves rejection of the (more unified) heart-centred picture that underlies the Stoic–Aristotelian position.[159] As in *PHP*, Galen stigmatizes the Stoics for their defective methodology of natural inquiry, especially their failure to make proper use of systematic anatomical observation.[160] As in *PHP*, Galen's competing picture of animal physiology is presented as depending on controlled observation, including the use of ligature (blocking access to organs).[161] The links with the earlier debate come out most plainly towards the end of the work where Galen argues that their view that the heart develops first reflects, and is coupled with, their general picture of the heart as the psychological centre. 'In the first place... they [Peripatetics and Stoics] assume that the heart is generated before anything else. Secondly, that the heart generates the other parts... Thirdly, as a consequence, they claim that even the

158 In *PHP*, the critique of Aristotle is mainly concentrated in what remains of Book 1, though he is often coupled with the Stoics for his maintenance of heart–centred psychology.

159 See esp. *Foet. Form.* IV.667, 672–3, 676–7, 685–6, 698, 3.17–18, 27–9, 4.5–8, 5.12.17–19, 6.27 Nickel.

160 *Foet. Form.* IV.676–7, 4.6–8 Nickel, IV.686, 5.20–1 (by implication directed against the Stoics), 698–9, 6.27–8 Nickel. See also text to n. 144 above, and Ch. 2 above, text to nn. 136–40.

161 *Foet. Form.* IV.679–81, 4.2–4 Nickel; as noted in the text to nn. 152–4 above, Galen is (obviously) not able to apply this method in the case of embryos.

deliberative part of our psyche is situated in the heart.'[162] In these respects, *Foet. Form.* presents itself as a sequel to the argument of *PHP*[163] and seems to reflect the same approach to Stoic thinking. Perhaps it therefore raises similar questions about the nature and coherence of Galenic psychophysiology to those discussed in *PHP* (3.3 above).

In fact, I think *Foet. Form.* does give rise to one inconsistency or at least ambivalence, which arises in part out of his retention of the tripartite model.[164] But, in general, Galen's thinking in this essay is markedly less problematic than that of *PHP* and the question of consistency of approach is less acute. There are several reasons for this. One is that the issue of the relationship between psychological faculties and physiological organs is much less prominent than in *PHP.* Advanced or complex psychological faculties, such as being the seat of appetite or anger and other emotions, are not relevant to the undeveloped state of the embryo. Hence, the problems that figure in *PHP,* about how to understand the relationship between psychological and physiological characteristics (especially in the case of heart and liver) and about whether Galen's brain-centred anatomy is consistent with tripartite psychology, do not arise in the same way in this essay.[165] A second significant factor is that Galen stresses here the idea of the body as a coherent system of organs with interlocking functions as much as, or more than, the tripartite model.[166] The former idea is fully consistent with Galen's brain-centred anatomy, and with the more unified psychology sometimes associated with this anatomy (including the psyche–nature distinction) discussed earlier.[167] This is a further reason why Galen's thinking about physiology and psychology in *Foet. Form.* raises fewer issues regarding consistency.

Returning to the question of the relationship between physiological and psychological character, in so far as this does give rise to problems, it is in connection with the Stoic–Aristotelian position

[162] *Foet. Form.* IV.698, 6.27, p. 102.12–17 Nickel, trans. LS 53 D, slightly modified.

[163] Galen refers explicitly to *PHP* in *Foet. Form.* IV.679, 5.2 Nickel, and ends the work by reaffirming the three-centre physiology and psychology (IV.701, 6.33–4, p. 106.5–10 Nickel). See also Nickel 1989: 79–80.

[164] See text to nn. 174–7 below.

[165] On these problems in *PHP,* see 3.3 above, text to nn. 72–91.

[166] See e.g. *Foet. Form.* IV.685–6, 689–91, 693–5, 5.17–19, 6.7–11, 16–19 Nickel; see further text to nn. 175–9 below.

[167] See text to nn. 101–15 above.

criticized by Galen. This position, Galen maintains, attributes to the heart a formative and directive role that is both inappropriate for its physiological character and is inconsistent with the Stoic–Aristotelian view that the embryonic condition is primitive and plant-like. The Stoic–Aristotelian position, as presented by Galen, is 'that the heart is constructed first; and then . . . that the other parts are formed by the heart, and that it is in charge (*hēgemōn*) not only of their formation (*genesis*) but of their management too (*dioikēsis*)'.[168] Against this position, Galen makes a number of criticisms. One is that this view conflates two distinct concepts, that of the source of formation and the source of management.[169] Another is that the allocation of both roles (formation and management) to the heart runs counter to the findings of anatomy about the functional roles of the organs in the case of fully formed animals, which provide the only available basis for inquiry into the roles of the organs in the development of the embryo.[170] Linked with both these criticisms is the point that—as is widely accepted, by thinkers including Stoics and Aristotelians—the state of the embryo is primitive or plant-like. It follows from this that the liver, the main organ involved in the formation of the body, must develop first, followed by the heart, the source of the pulse, while the brain, which is the locus of management in the fully formed animal, develops last.[171] The Stoic–Aristotelian view, attributing both a formative and a managing role to the heart of the embryo, runs counter to a plausible picture of embryonic development, as well as resting on a false picture of the role of the heart as the seat of the ruling part of the psyche in the adult animal.[172] So, on Galen's account, it is the Stoics and Aristotelians who make inappropriate or unjustified

[168] *Foet. Form.* IV.677, 4.7, p. 80.20–5, trans. Singer 1997*a*: 189. Cf. the account of their position in IV.698, 6.27 Nickel, cited above.

[169] *Foet. Form.* IV.674–5, 677–8, 4.1–3, 7–8 Nickel.

[170] This is the main theme of ch. 5 of *Foet. Form.*; see also (in ch. 4), IV.676–7, 4.5–8 Nickel.

[171] See *Foet. Form.* ch. 3, esp. IV.663–4, 665, 672–3, 3.9–10, 13–14, 27–8 Nickel.

[172] See esp. 'The belief . . . (1) that the part first constructed by Nature goes on to construct the others, and (2) that this part is the heart, is false on both counts [i.e. the heart has neither role]; but even if both these points were conceded, it would not necessarily follow that the activities of the fully developed animal are the responsibility of that organ.' *Foet. Form.* IV.686–7, 5.21, p. 90.20–5 Nickel, trans. Singer 1997*a*: 193–4, slightly modified. This sums up the argument of chs. 4–5. On Galen's critique of the Stoic–Aristotelian view, see also Nickel 1989: 77–9, 1993: 81–3.

connections between the physiological nature and the psychological functions of the embryo.

Galen's critique of the Stoic–Aristotelian position is quite powerful, at least if we accept his—largely credible—assumptions.[173] But what, exactly, is his alternative account and how far is it consistent and well supported? As explained earlier, in ch. 3, Galen argues that the organs develop in a step-by-step sequence (liver, heart, brain) that reflects the needs and relative complexity of the embryo at the relevant time. The main basis for this claim is what he presents as the consensus that the embryo's condition is plant-like or, in Galen's version, that it moves from plant-like to animal status during embryonic development.[174] However, in the fuller account of development in ch. 5, Galen seems to nuance or vary this rather straightforward three-stage picture. We are told that 'neither the liver nor the heart is the first item to be formed; for their formation clearly requires bloodlike substance, which comes to them from the womb along the vessels'.[175] Galen adds that this process is likely to be contemporaneous with that of other parts, in the same region of the embryo and in other regions: 'For the power that constructs plants and animals will never stand still; all the power will attach itself to all parts simultaneously, and augment them.'[176] This point is supported by an account of the embryonic body as an emergent system of organs, each of which have their own distinct function but which are also mutually supporting. The main explicit aim of this account is to suggest that the embryo develops gradually as a whole system, rather than that the later organs develop as offshoots of the earlier ones (that is, liver or heart).[177] Although Galen does not

[173] The main assumptions are (1) his view of the functions of the main organs, and (2) the idea that the embryo functions in a primitive, initially plant-like, way. On the question whether his report of Stoic and Aristotelian theory is accurate, see text to nn. 190–6 below.

[174] *Foet. Form.* IV.663–4, 670–1, 672–3, 3.9–10, 24, 27–8 Nickel.

[175] See also: 'the formation of the [blood vessels] must be the first thing to come into being, followed by liver and heart—in the same way as the foundations of a house or the keel of a ship'. *Foet. Form.* IV.682, 5.10–11, p. 86.14–17, 19–20 Nickel, trans Singer 1997*a*: 191.

[176] *Foet. Form.* IV.683, 5.12, p. 86.25–6 Nickel, trans. Singer 1997*a*: 191.

[177] *Foet. Form.* IV.683–6, 5.13–19 Nickel, esp. 'the same force which is responsible for the formation of arteries and veins also subdivides them and brings them on into

explicitly acknowledge any tension between these accounts, we may sense here two competing ideas about what it means to say that the embryo is in a primitive state. One is that *certain parts* (especially those associated with primitive processes, such as nutrition, especially the liver) develop before others and play a key role in enabling the production of the other parts. The other is that the embryo develops *as a whole interconnected system*, but in a primitive form, in which (all) the organs only gradually play their full function. These two ideas are not necessarily in direct conflict; even in the second version, some parts, for instance, the liver, may develop rather faster than others and thus contribute towards the systemic process of growth out of which other organs are formed.[178] But these ideas imply rather different views of what it means for the embryo to be in a primitive state, and also rather different conceptions of the part–whole relationship, as I bring out later.[179] It is important to bear these competing ideas in mind when seeking to correlate Galen's picture with that of other theories.

In considering Galen's positive account of embryonic development, we need to take note of a further issue, signalled in ch. 5, which becomes the main subject of ch. 6. This is how to provide an account of the development of the embryo that matches the teleological world-view to which Galen is strongly committed, which is linked with his understanding of the body as a system of organs with interlocking functions.[180] Galen dismisses without argument the Epicurean view that the development of the embryo, like other processes, can be explained without reference to natural design.[181] However, he acknowledges real difficulty in explaining how the

every part of the embryo, and constructs the parts around them in their proper places' (IV.684, p. 88.13–15, trans Singer 1997*a*: 192). This section strongly evokes the analysis of the body as an interconnected system in *UP*, a work referred to in IV.685, p. 90.7 Nickel. This point is coupled with an outright rejection of the Stoic–Aristotelian view that the heart is formed first and constructs the other parts (IV.683, 685, 5.13, 25, p. 88.3–4, 25 Nickel); but this rejection also has implications for Galen's view that the liver develops first.

178 See e.g. the comparison of liver and heart to foundation or keel (n. 175 above).

179 See Ch. 4 below, text to nn. 41–55, 258–69.

180 See *Foet. Form.* IV.689–90, 693–5, 6.6–8, 17–19 Nickel; see also n. 146 above.

181 *Foet. Form.* IV.688–9, 6.3–5 Nickel. The Epicurean view of generation is, in fact, much less random than Galen suggests: see e.g. Epicur. *Ep. Hdt.* 39, Lucr. 1.159–73, S.E. *PH* 3.17–18.

embryo realizes this design. Does some element within the emerging animal serve as the vehicle of the design or is the design somehow fulfilled from outside? Galen's approach to this question is an interesting indicator of his general world-view and of its relationship to other ideas of his day. Although Galen does consider, without adopting, the idea that the psyche might be the vehicle of the body's design, he shows no inclination to adopt a Platonic-style dualist version of this idea, in which the embryo is the product of a non-material psyche and matter.[182] Galen notes an idea offered by one of his Platonist teachers that the teleological construction of the embryo should be attributed to the world-psyche, an idea based on the *Timaeus*, presumably. But he dismisses this idea on the ground that it is inconceivable that a cosmic force would be responsible for the construction of such minor and destructive creatures as scorpions, venomous spiders, and mosquitoes.[183] The idea to which he seems most attracted is that the seed or semen contains 'the scheme (*logos*) of the craftsman'; and that the gradual emergence of the embryo as a coordinated system of organs with interlocking functions expresses this scheme.[184] He proposes this idea as preferable to the Stoic–Aristotelian idea that one part of the body (specifically the heart) serves as the source and manager of the emerging system.[185] He is less sure about whether this means that the psyche in the seed acts as the key agent in fulfilling the design, in part because he disclaims, here and elsewhere, a definite view about the nature of the psyche.[186] To this extent, his inquiry ends inconclusively, although he is confident

[182] *Foet. Form.* IV.692–3, 6.12–16 Nickel (considering the idea that the existence of innate or instinctive capacities implies that the psyche is the agent of the system); it is unclear exactly whose theory Galen has in view (cf. Nickel 2001: 156–7). See also *Foet. Form.* IV.699–70, 6.29–30, esp. p. 104.3–7, 11–12 Nickel. Despite the seemingly Platonic dualism, it seems that Galen has some kind of Aristotelian position in mind. See further Nickel 2001: 163–7, referring e.g. to Arist. *GA* 2.3, 737^{a}7–9.

[183] *Foet. Form.* IV.700–1, 6.32, pp. 104.25–106.32 Nickel; cf. Pl. *Ti.* 34b–37c. For Galen's reasons for rejecting this idea, see Nickel 2001: 168–9, M. Frede 2003: 76–7, 122–3.

[184] *Foet. Form.* IV.682–3, 5.11–12, esp. p. 86.18 Nickel, trans. Singer 1997*a*: 191.

[185] *Foet. Form.* IV.683, 685, 5.13, 17 Nickel, IV.698–9, 6.27–8 Nickel. See also IV.699, 6.29–30, p. 104.7–11 Nickel, referring to the Stoic idea that the seed, or the *pneuma* it conveys, is the (demiurgic) craftsman, i.e. the Stoic god, an idea Galen says he has discussed elsewhere.

[186] *Foet. Form.* IV.700, 6.31 Nickel; a particular difficulty is that of understanding how a primitive level of psyche can act as the agent of a complex design.

that some kind of teleological explanation for the embryo's development is correct. Galen's preferred model anticipates in some respects the modern idea that the embryo's development is genetically programmed (the programme being carried in what for Galen would be the seed), though Galen lacks the conceptual or methodological resources to evolve this idea.[187]

Taking this essay as a whole, how should we characterize Galen's relationship to Stoic (and Aristotelian) thought on embodied psychology, taken in comparison with *PHP*? The last chapter discussed (ch. 6) brings out a feature that underlies his response to Stoicism throughout the essay. Despite disagreement on specific points, Galen's approach to embryonic development exhibits the kind of naturalism, more precisely, 'high naturalism', that, I suggested earlier, Galen shares with Stoicism, and Aristotelianism in many respects.[188] Neither in discussing teleology in ch. 6 nor elsewhere in the work does Galen show any serious inclination to analyse the issues in terms of Platonic psyche–body dualism. For Galen, as for the Stoics and Aristotle, the functions of the embryo, including psychological ones (in so far as these are present in the embryo) are those of a fundamentally embodied organism that forms an integral part of the natural world. For all three theories, also, living entities are viewed as bearers of inbuilt animation, and as coherent organic structures, which serve as the base for an interlocking set of natural faculties. The fact that Galen repeatedly refers to specific points of difference with Stoic–Aristotelian thought, which centre on the role of the heart, reflects the point that, in other respects, his approach to the embryo is similar to theirs. Hence, as regards anatomy, or natural faculties, or teleology (the main themes of chs. 4, 5, and 6, respectively), engaging with the Stoic–Aristotelian position on embryonic development enables him to think through the distinctive features of his view. Put differently, critical reflection on their view enables him to define his distinctive version of a 'high naturalistic' approach to embryology in a way that could not be done, for instance, by reference to a dualistic version of Platonism. Although Platonic influence persists in the essay in the form of the tripartite model,

[187] For a modern parallel to Galen's picture, see text to nn. 206–7 below.
[188] See 2.3 above.

centred on brain, heart, and liver, the problematic dimensions of this idea are much less evident than in *PHP* and the idea of the body as a unified nexus of organs and functions is much more prominent.[189]

One further question remains to be considered here about Galen's attitude to Stoic and Aristotelian thought about embryonic development. Is Galen accurate in his report of their views and in coupling these together? This question is easier to answer as regards Aristotle. The two main points that Galen ascribes to the two theories can be securely identified in Aristotle's *Generation of Animals* (*GA*). These are that the heart is the first organ to be formed in the embryo and plays the major role in the formation of the other organs, and that the state of the embryo is a plant-like one.[190] But what about Stoicism? Galen confidently asserts that both theories hold that the heart develops first in the embryo and forms the other parts.[191] Perhaps he is right to do so; but, as far as I am aware, there is no other evidence for the claim that this idea formed part of Stoic thought.[192] As regards the second point, that the embryo is plant-like, Galen seems to be referring to what certainly *was* an important and distinctive Stoic theory.[193] This is that the life of an embryo is shaped entirely by 'nature' (*phusis*), and only at birth does it develop psyche. The fullest evidence for this idea is from the second-century AD Stoic Hierocles; but the idea itself is attested as an orthodox Stoic one.[194]

[189] See text to nn. 166–7 and 175–9 above.

[190] See, respectively, *GA* 2.4, 740^{a}3–23; 2.3, 736^{b}12, 3.2, 753^{b}27, 5.1, 779^{a}1; see further Nickel 1993: 84. Also relevant, of course, is Aristotle's heart-centred psychology and physiology, though Aristotle's thinking on this subject is less systematic and unequivocal than that of Stoicism; see van der Eijk 2000: 68–9.

[191] *Foet. Form.* IV.674, 677, 698, 4.1, 7, 6.27 Nickel.

[192] *SVF* 2.761 consists of the three Galenic passages listed in the preceding note; no other supporting evidence for this thesis is cited here or elsewhere, as far as I know. On the relationship between Galen's evidence and Stoic thinking, see also Nickel 1993: 79 n. 5, and 84, Long 1996: 237. If Galen is supplying this Stoic idea, he might feel justified in doing so on the basis that, if the Stoics share the Aristotelian heart-centred view of the fully formed animal, they must share his view of embryonic development as originating with the heart.

[193] See *Foet. Form.* IV.663–4, 3.9, p. 66.25–6 Nickel, where Galen ascribes this belief to 'all other doctors and philosophers' (other than Galen, at this stage in his thinking), taken together with the equation of 'nature' (as conceived by Stoics) with 'nutritive psyche' (as conceived by Plato and Aristotle), IV.665, 3.15 Nickel.

[194] See LS 53 B(2–3), cf. Plu. *Mor.* 1052 F (=*SVF* 2.806); see further Long 1996: 237, also (on parallels with Diogenes of Babylon) Tieleman 1991. On Hierocles'

Galen, here as elsewhere, presents the Stoic idea of 'nature', which, as we have seen, he also sometimes adopts, as interchangeable with the Platonic–Aristotelian one of nutritive psyche, a faculty seen as shared with plants by Plato and Aristotle.[195] On this basis, Galen claims that there is a consensus about the idea that the life of the embryo is plant-like. This is, initially at least, taken to support the claim that the liver, not the heart, is the first of the organs to be formed in the embryo, though he later explores the idea of a plant-like state as one consisting in the simultaneous but incomplete development of the whole system of organs.[196]

On the face of it, Galen's use of the Stoic idea of 'nature' seems reasonable. But it involves at least some distortion, and it also helps to prevent Galen from using Stoic thought to develop another, and perhaps more promising, aspect of his thinking. Both these points bear on the question of the part–whole relationship and the related contrast between holistic and part-based (or 'composition') approaches to this relationship.[197] The Stoic use of the idea of 'nature' reflects their holistic approach in at least two ways. As pointed out earlier, this idea forms part of a radically innovative *scala naturae* (spectrum of natural kinds) that applies to *all* entities, not just living things. It also provides a framework that replaces—or at least substantially modifies—the received contrast between body and psyche.[198] Hence, for Galen to identify the Stoic idea of 'nature' with the Platonic–Aristotelian 'nutritive psyche', that is, the most basic type of psyche possessed by living things, is to blunt the innovative holism of the Stoic move, even if there is a clear analogy between the two ideas.

A related point arises out of the Stoic use of the idea of 'nature' in connection with the embryo. A distinctive feature of Stoic thinking about the embryo is that its functions are wholly governed by 'nature' until birth. At birth there is an instantaneous and total shift, as the embryo, now independent of the mother, becomes for the first time

account of birth, see further Bastianini and Long 1992: 296–300 (text), 373–8 (commentary), also 368–73 (introduction), including 372–3 on Galenic evidence for Stoic thinking in *Foet. Form.* and in the pseudo-Galenic, *Is the Embryo an Animal?* (*An. Ut.*). On later ancient treatments of the latter question, see Mansfeld 1990: 3186–90.

[195] *Foet. Form.* IV.665, 3.15 Nickel.

[196] See text to nn. 175–9 above.

[197] On these larger questions, see Ch. 4 below, esp. 4.4.

[198] See Ch. 2 above, text to nn. 206–12.

an animal, most of whose functions are now shaped, in a unified or coordinated way, by psyche, though growth and nutrition continue to be directed by 'nature'.[199] This picture differs from the Galenic one in several ways.[200] But one potentially fruitful link is the idea that the embryo functions in a primitive way *as a whole.* I noted earlier that Galen's account of the embryo's primitive (plant-like) state accommodates two, partly competing, lines of thought. One is that the organ that houses the most primitive functions develops first (the liver) followed by those that house more complex or advanced functions (heart, brain). The other is that the embryo develops *as a whole* but in an incomplete, primitive way.[201] The second line of thought brings Galen close to the Stoic view of the embryo (namely, that it functions as a whole, but shaped by 'nature'). It is also a line of thought that fits well with other Galenic ideas, notably the idea of the embryo, like the fully developed animal, as a teleologically designed system of organs with interlocking functions.[202] The Stoic view that the heart develops first in the embryo might seem to introduce another dimension, which brings their view closer to the first strand in Galenic thought, stressing the temporal priority of one part rather than others. But, as pointed out earlier, Galen provides our only evidence for this idea, which might represent a conflation of Stoic and Aristotelian ideas.[203] If the idea is actually part of Stoic thought, it surely reflects in another way their unified or holistic view of the animal organism (including the animal embryo), since the heart is for them the source of unification and agency in the developed

[199] This transition comes out very clearly in Hierocles' account, LS 53 B(2–3), esp.: 'Yet throughout this time—I mean the time from conception to birth—it remains [in the form of] *phusis*, i.e breath, having changed from seed and moving methodically from beginning to end... For just as the breath in stones is immediately kindled by a blow... so the *phusis* of a ripe embryo, once it is born, does not hesitate to change into psyche...', trans. LS, slightly modified. The idea that the animal, once born, also functions in a highly unified way (now involving psyche) is very clear in LS 53 B(5–9). See further Inwood 1984: 173–7, Long 1996: 257–61, and refs. in n. 194 above. For the interpretation assumed here of the relationship between psyche and 'nature' in the animal, see text to nn. 59–65 above.

[200] These include the fact that, in Galen's account, the embryo changes from plant–like to animal status during embryonic development, when the heart begins to function, *Foet. Form.* IV 670–1, 3.24–5 Nickel.

[201] See text to nn. 175–9 above.

[202] For this idea, see text to nn. 166, 188–9 above.

[203] See n. 192 above.

animal.[204] Hence, in various ways, the Stoic picture might offer support for a potentially fruitful approach to the embryo, stressing its primitive character in a way that also recognizes its status as a whole, connected entity.

We can also see links between the suggestion just made and aspects of modern thought about the embryo. It is, of course, misleading to present modern thought as, in itself, confirming or disconfirming the validity of ancient ideas, since ancient and modern lines of thought are, often, supported by different lines of reasoning or methods of verification. However, points of connection and contrast with modern thought can be, at least, interesting and, at most, strikingly parallel in ideas or methodology.[205] I noted earlier one point of comparison between modern and Galenic thought, namely between the idea of genetic programming and Galen's idea of the seed as the vehicle of a teleological scheme.[206] It is noteworthy that an outline of antenatal development in a modern handbook brings together the idea of genetic programming and the idea of systemic, but incomplete, development, an idea just noted in both Galen and Stoicism.

> Between the fourth and eighth week after conception, most of the major organ systems start to form in the embryo, although it is very much later before these start to function properly. The process of embryogenesis is very complex. Major advances are now taking place in our understanding of the genetic control of the cell migrations, cell proliferation and programmed cell death . . . that need to happen in a highly coordinated fashion over a short time-scale for the successful development of an individual. [207]

As in the second line of thought noted in Galen's thinking on embryonic development and in the Stoic idea of the embryo as uniformly shaped by 'nature', this account stresses the idea of organs developing at the same time in a coordinated, but incomplete, way. The first Galenic line of thought, found also in Aristotle (and ascribed to Stoicism by Galen), that some organs develop before others and

[204] On this view, see further text to nn. 45–52 above.

[205] See e.g. the parallel between Galen's thought on the role of the brain and in his (quasi-) experimental method and modern thought on both these points: see further Rocca 2003: ch. 2, and Ch. 2 above, text to nn. 104–10. On parallels between ancient and modern thought on psychology and types of therapy, see Ch. 6 below.

[206] See text to n. 187 above.

[207] Blakemore and Jennett 2001: 36, italics deleted.

play a key role in carrying forward the developmental process, does not appear in this modern survey. Hence, this is another point on which we can see fruitful potential lines of connection between (some) Galenic and (some) Stoic thought, which, in this instance, intersect at least with a modern approach to the topic.

3.5 GALEN AND STOICS ON THE PSYCHE–BODY RELATIONSHIP

So far, in this discussion of Galen's relationship to Stoic thought on psychology and the body, I have set aside one, rather fundamental, question. How does Galen understand the relationship, in general terms, between psyche and body? A related question is this: what, exactly, is Galen's thesis in *QAM* (*Psychological Faculties Depend on Bodily Mixtures*), the Galenic work that comes closest to being a theoretical study of the relationship between psyche and body? As I explain, both of these questions are, in fact, very hard to answer. This is partly because of Galen's attitude towards these questions and partly because of certain ambiguous or apparently inconsistent features in the kind of answers he gives. In addressing these complex questions, I make two main suggestions. One is that Galen's general position on the psyche–body relationship, although it sometimes seems needlessly elusive and ill-defined, has a distinct rationale. Broadly speaking, this is that any views he offers on this question should reflect what are, in modern terms, the findings of his research programme and should not consist in ungrounded statements about areas of inquiry where he has not done independent work. This point also illuminates the project of *QAM*, which is designed, I think, to draw out the implications of one important strand in his philosophy of nature for the question of the psyche–body relationship.

My second suggestion relates to the relation between Galenic and Stoic thought. I think that, on both the questions considered here, Galen's position could be improved by closer engagement with Stoic ideas. On the psyche–body question in general, Galen seems to be drawn towards a certain kind of physicalist account, which reflects a key strand in his philosophy of nature. Stoicism offers a more fully articulated physicalist position, of a kind that is also compatible with this strand of thinking about the philosophy of nature. Hence, Galen might either have adopted the Stoic physicalist account or at least used it to define more precisely his own version. Secondly, the Stoic version of physicalism is fully compatible with the idea that human beings are rational agents who are properly held responsible for their actions and in some ways responsible for the formation of their characters. In *QAM*, Galen seems to think that the position he adopts on the psyche–body relationship entails that human character and actions are wholly determined by inborn, physically based, psychological characteristics. One can argue that this is not a necessary corollary of his position on the psyche–body relationship and also that it is inconsistent with the assumption he makes elsewhere, that human beings are properly held responsible for their actions and are to some degree able to shape their own character. Fuller engagement with the Stoic position might have helped Galen to formulate his ideas about responsibility in *QAM* in a way that is more consistent with his thinking about the psyche–body relationship there and with his thinking about responsibility elsewhere. Hence, overall, this is another area where Galenic thought is closer to Stoic thinking on psychology and the body than he acknowledges and where fuller engagement might have worked for the improvement and greater consistency of his ideas.

Galen's thinking about the relationship between psyche and body has been quite intensively discussed in recent years;[208] and discussion has focused on certain puzzling and seemingly inconsistent features of his thinking on this topic. On the one hand, he repeatedly refuses to take a position on the question of the 'substance' or 'essence' (*ousia*) of the psyche.[209] By this stage in ancient thought, this was generally taken to mean whether the psyche (in whole or in part) was mortal or immortal, and material or non-material.[210] His refusal is often linked with the

[208] Two recent, acute treatments are Hankinson 2006 and Donini 2008.

[209] See e.g. *PHP* V.793, 9.9.7, p. 598.27–9 De Lacy, *Prop. Plac.* 3.1–2, pp. 58.22–60.11 Nutton, Boudon-Millot and Pietrobelli 2005: 173.13–18.

[210] Other standard questions include whether or not the psyche exists, how many faculties it has and of what kind and where these are located in the body. This set of questions reflects both earlier philosophical discussions (esp. Arist. *De An.*) and the systematization of key questions and positions in handbooks; see further Tieleman 2003*b*: 137–9, Hankinson 2008*a*: 178–80.

claim that this question, unlike other questions about the psyche, belongs to purely speculative philosophical inquiry and is not relevant for medicine or practical ethics.[211] On the other hand, Galen makes a number of comments that come close to being a statement on this question, particularly in *QAM* (a late work) and in what seems to be his last work, *On My Own Opinions* (*Prop. Plac.*).[212] In these works especially, he comes very close to adopting a physicalist or materialist position on the nature of the psyche.[213] His attitude is puzzling because he officially declines to adopt a formal position while seeming to embrace a materialist approach. Scholars have wondered whether he is reluctant to make a formal break with Platonism by adopting a full-hearted materialist view. They have also sometimes tried to trace a development in his position over time away from a more Platonic and towards a more materialist view. But there are several difficulties with a developmental approach to this question, including the apparent equivocation in his thinking even in the final period of his work.[214]

Despite these problems, I think we can see an underlying rationale in Galen's comments on this topic, which comes out most clearly in his own résumé of the outcomes of his medical work in *Prop. Plac.*[215] The core point is that what matters regarding the substance of the psyche, as

[211] See e.g. *Prop. Plac.* 14.4–5, esp. p. 114.22–3 Nutton, 15.5 Nutton, Boudon-Millot and Pietrobelli 2005: 188. 6–20, 189.11–16. *PHP* V.780–2, 9.7.9–19 De Lacy gives a list of questions that belong to purely speculative philosophy (among which, by implication, the question of the substance of the psyche belongs), by contrast with questions that are useful for medicine or practical ethics (p. 588.7–9 De Lacy).

[212] On this duality in Galen's approach to this question, see Hankinson 2006: 236–9, Donini 2008: 185–6.

[213] Physicalism is sometimes distinguished from materialism, but I am using them here as synonyms, meaning that the psyche is a physical or material, by contrast with non-material, object; on these terms, as applied to ancient theories, see Annas 1992: 3, Everson 1999: 546–50.

[214] A further problem with a developmental approach is that, even in *PHP*, when Galen is adopting an approach to psychology that is 'Platonic' in some sense, he does not adopt Platonic-style psyche–body dualism. See further Singer 1991: 47–9, 1997*b*: 540–1, dissenting from the more developmental approach of Moraux 1984: 778–80; also, reviewing the debate, Nutton 1999: 143–4.

[215] We now have a full Greek text of this work, from a newly rediscovered manuscript, edited with French translation (Boudon-Millot and Pietrobelli 2005). Previously, our knowledge of this work depended on a medieval Latin translation of an Arabic version, with only the three final chapters given completely in Greek, though there were Greek extracts of some earlier sections: see Nutton 1999: 14–49.

on other subjects, is not what a specific person happens to believe but what claims can be justified by properly conducted inquiry. One relevant kind of inquiry is speculative philosophical analysis of the nature of the psyche, including the question whether it is immortal or material, as conducted by, for instance, Plato in the *Phaedo*, or Aristotle and Chrysippus in their works *On the Psyche*.[216] Galen does not engage in this type of speculative analysis, and sometimes distinguishes it from the more practically oriented medical or ethical activity in which he does engage.[217] However, he does not therefore regard this kind of speculative inquiry as intrinsically invalid or incapable of reaching well-grounded conclusions. His frequent statements of agnosticism on the nature of the substance of the psyche mark his recognition that he has not engaged in philosophical analysis of the kind that would enable him to reach independent, securely grounded conclusions. However, he is confident that his natural inquiry, though practically oriented (towards medicine), has enabled him to reach sound conclusions about some aspects of the nature and workings of the psyche. He is most confident about the implications of his work for the question of the location of psychological functions in the body, a topic that he sees as important for medical practice as well as philosophical inquiry.[218] He also seems sure that other key features of his philosophy of nature, notably that relating to elements and natural faculties, have implications for the understanding of the nature of the embodied psyche. Thus, while not engaging in separate philosophical analysis or argument about the nature of the psyche (in particular about its substance), he does suppose that his medically oriented natural inquiries have crucially informed this type of analysis—though the epistemological implications of this belief are not wholly easy to pin down.

This line of thought seems to underlie Galen's comments in *Prop. Plac.* on the outcome of *PHP* for inquiry into the nature of the psyche:

Like everyone, I am convinced that we have a psyche. I see that what everyone calls a psyche is what is responsible for deliberate movement and

[216] On this genre of philosophical discussion (from Plato to Iamblichus), see Tieleman 2003*b*: 137.

[217] On the (lost) Galenic work with this title, see Ch. 2 above, n. 3.

[218] See e.g. *PHP* V.793–4, 9.9.7–9 De Lacy.

sensation by means of sense-organs. But I confess that I do not know what the substance (*ousia*) of the psyche is—still less if it is immortal or mortal. So, when I wrote some books *On the Doctrines of Hippocrates and Plato*... I made no statement about whether the psyche is mortal or immortal or whether it is non-corporeal or corporeal. But... I did set down the arguments (or 'proofs', *apodeixeis*) which convinced me, to the effect that there are three different sources of movement, in the brain, the heart, and the liver. Indeed, I am prepared to say that from the brain our memories and thoughts derive... To go much further, I am prepared to say that each of the parts of the body is equipped from these sources with motivational or deliberate movement... and the same goes for the recognition by means of the sense-organs of external perceptible objects. I also stated that the heart is the source of the movement of the pulse... and that the boiling of the innate heat comes from this source... [and that] there is so much heat in the heart that its boiling occurs along with anger.[219]

This passage clearly highlights the linkage between the outcome and the method of Galen's inquiries. Here, as in comparable passages in *PHP* itself, agnosticism on (what Galen sees as) purely speculative questions about the psyche is coupled with confidence about matters where he has been able to provide 'proofs' (*apodeixeis*).[220] He gives emphasis to the most important outcome of the application of his distinctive logico-empirical method, the demonstration that the source of volition and sensation is located in the brain and not the heart.[221] He also refers, though less emphatically, to his alleged findings on the psychological roles of the heart and liver.[222] It seems likely that Galen's proof of the role of the brain to which he, understandably, attaches such significance has shaped his whole view of what he can and cannot contribute to psychological inquiry. The location of the ruling part of the psyche, like the question of the corporeality and mortality of the psyche, fell squarely within the questions about the psyche debated by philosophers, as well as

[219] *Prop. Plac.*, ch. 3, Boudon-Millot and Pietrobelli 2005: 173.13–174.3, my translation of relevant passages from this chapter. For the equivalent chapter in the Latin version, see Nutton 1999: 58–63.

[220] See esp. *PHP* V.793–5, 9.9.7–14 De Lacy.

[221] See Ch. 2 above, text to nn. 11–18, 101–10.

[222] Cf. the statement of his findings on this in *PHP* V.600–1, 7.3.2–3, cited in 3.3 above, text to n. 68; there are gaps in the relevant part of *Prop. Plac.*, ch. 3 in both Greek and Latin versions.

medical writers, which are in any case overlapping groups.[223] But this is a question that, as Galen sees the matter, admits of definite proof one way or the other, which he has helped to provide. This conviction probably underlies his view, apparent in his comments on this topic, that he can make substantive contributions to some topics of debate about the psyche, even while he explicitly withdraws from others.

I think it is relatively clear why Galen thinks that his findings about the respective psychophysiological roles of brain and heart are well grounded and also how he thinks they can inform debate about the bodily location of functions. More elusive, or problematic, are the conclusions that Galen seems to draw from his approach to the philosophy of nature for the understanding of the psyche as an embodied entity in both *QAM* and *Prop. Plac.* Earlier (2.3 above), I outlined key features of Galenic (and Stoic) thinking that I associated with the idea of 'high naturalism'. Most relevant for the present topic is his belief that matter can be analysed, ultimately, in terms of a complete fusion or mixture of elements and that this mixture provides the basis for the inbuilt vitality of natural entities. This postulate of inbuilt vitality underlies, in turn, Galen's conception of living things as coherent complexes of natural faculties or capacities. The contrasting view, which Galen rejects, is that matter consists in atomic units, and that all natural processes, including what we call 'life', represent a product of the mechanical combination and separation of these atoms.[224] In *QAM* and *Prop. Plac.* (chs. 7, 14–15), we can see Galen exploring the implications of this understanding of nature for philosophical debate about the psyche. This exploration takes a rather different form in the two works. In *QAM* Galen argues for what is—up to a point at least—a relatively determinate claim and draws out what he sees as being the implications of this claim for philosophical analysis of psyche–body relations. In *Prop. Plac.* Galen applies a similar approach, and one that presupposes the argument of *QAM*, but does so in a more methodologically self-aware form, and with greater theoretical caution. In both cases, it is more difficult to specify the theoretical outcome of Galen's arguments than it is with regard to his experimental work on the brain. This is partly because, as suggested earlier, the methodological and

[223] On the agenda of these debates, see n. 210 above.

[224] See Ch. 2 above, text to nn. 163–73.

epistemological basis for his approach to the philosophy of nature is less well defined, and perhaps less cogent, than for his anatomical work on the brain.[225] Also, Galen seeks in this connection to draw out the implications of this approach for questions that are more theoretically challenging than that of the location of psychological functions. He raises the broader question of the relationship between the psyche, in part or as a whole, and the body and thus—virtually or by implication—tackles one part of the question of the essence or substance of the psyche, its corporeal or incorporeal nature. But Galen does so in a way that acknowledges that he is not engaging in the kind of purely philosophical argument in which those issues were normally discussed. This is a delicate balancing act that, in *Prop. Plac.* especially, comes close to breaking point on several occasions.

In *QAM*, the thesis and underlying project is explicit in the title, which is the same as the first words of the essay: 'That the faculties (*dunameis*) of the psyche follow (or 'depend on', *hepesthai*) the mixtures (*kraseis*) of the body'. As Jacques Jouanna has recently argued, the traditional Latin title (*quod animi mores corporis temperamenta sequantur*) misrepresents the topic by omitting the idea of 'faculties.'[226] These opening words signal clearly the linkage with two ideas central for Galen's approach to the philosophy of nature, namely those of (natural) faculties and mixtures. The core project of the essay is that of thinking through the implications for psychology of these features of Galen's thought. Galen summarizes these features in the opening chapters, as well as explaining his understanding of key terms such as 'faculty' and 'substance'.[227] A notable feature of *QAM* is that Galen carries forward his argument by summary and quotations (sometimes lengthy) of previous

[225] See Ch. 2 above, text to nn. 194–6.

[226] Hence, (Jouanna 2009: 192), we should abbreviate the work as *QAF*, a view I accept, though, here as elsewhere, I use the standard Latin titles and abbreviations for Galen's works. Jouanna also stresses that Galen's thesis applies to the faculties of the rational part of the psyche and not just the non-rational part(s), as might be implied by the use of *mores* (=*ēthē*).

[227] See *QAM* IV.768–70, ch. 2, *SM* 2.33.4–34.16 (on 'faculties'), IV.772–3, ch. 3, *SM* 2.36.9–37.2 (on 'substance', 'forms' or 'parts' of the psyche, and 'matter'), IV.785, ch. 5, *SM* 2.46.8–47.2 (on the contrast between 'biological' and 'atomic' views of living entities, cf. *Nat. Fac.* 1.12 and Ch. 2 above, text to nn. 163–73). On Galen's concepts and assumptions in *QAM* see Hankinson 2006: 240–5, and on his psychological categories more broadly, Tieleman 2003*b*: 141–51.

medical and philosophical writers, who are presented—more or less plausibly—as stating one or other aspect of Galen's central thesis.[228] The intellectual idiom is rather curious. Galen comments, positively or negatively on psychological theories, such as those of Plato, Aristotle, and the Stoics, on the basis of certain highly determinate assumptions, those of his own approach to the philosophy of nature. But he does not present a formal analytic argument either for this approach or for the conclusions he draws about psychology. His conclusions emerge obliquely, through the comments he makes on the theories of earlier medical and philosophical thinkers. In this way, Galen engages with (what he elsewhere calls) purely speculative philosophy on the psyche, without claiming to practise this type of theorizing himself.

This approach underlies, for instance, Galen's (re-)interpretation of Aristotle's idea of the psyche as the 'form' (*eidos*) of the body, cited in an earlier chapter. On the face of it, Galen is—rather arbitrarily—replacing Aristotle's idea of psyche as 'form' with that of 'matter' (specifically, mixture of qualities):

> Now, given that all such bodies are composed of matter and form, and, as Aristotle himself thinks, when the four qualities are generated in the matter of physical things, bodily mixture is generated out of them, he must posit this latter as the form. So the substance of the psyche must be some sort of mixture of the four: of wet and dry, cold and hot, if you want to call them qualities, or, if you prefer, of the wet, hot, cold and dry bodies; and hence we will show that the powers of the psyche are consequent upon [or 'follow', *hepomenas*] its substance.[229]

The basis for Galen's move is that the mixture of elements can be conceived as the 'form' of matter at every level of bodily composition, including 'homoeomerous' parts such as sinew and bone as well as organs or living entities.[230] Hence, when Aristotle says that psyche is the 'form' of the body, Galen is saying that he means, in effect, 'mixture of elements'. Although this comment has some basis in

[228] See further Lloyd 1988: 15–33, highlighting Galen's highly selective and sometimes tendentious use of quotation in *QAM*.

[229] *QAM* IV.774, *SM* 2.37.16–26, trans. Hankinson 2006: 246; see also the translation of Singer 1997*a*: 153, which omits the last clause. For citation and discussion of this passage, see also p. 81 above.

[230] *QAM* IV.773–4, *SM* 2.37.5–15.

Aristotelian thought, it is, essentially, a recasting of Aristotelian ideas in the light of Galen's own theory of elements as the core constituents of all natural entities.[231] The effect, of course, is to produce a more physicalist version of Aristotle's theory, but without Galen formally arguing for this type of theory or engaging explicitly in theory about the nature and substance of the psyche.

In the same style of exposition, Galen offers what comes closest in his works to an assertion of a physicalist account of the substance of psyche:

> And Andronicus the Peripatetic actually dared to state that it [the mixture of elements in the body] was the substance (*ousia*) of the psyche, without any shilly-shallying, and I praise and welcome the man's position (*prohairesis*)... But when he says 'either a mixture or a faculty dependent on the mixture', I take issue with his addition of 'a faculty', since, while the psyche *has* many faculties it *is* a substance, as Aristotle rightly said... while 'substance' can mean either matter, form, or a composite of the two, Aristotle held it was substance in the sense of form [taken to mean 'mixture' of elements].[232]

The basis for Galen's revision of Andronicus' formulation is his (Aristotelian-style) view that the psyche is a substance which possesses faculties,[233] and his earlier interpretation of Aristotelian form as mixture of elements. Hence, in effect, Galen adopts explicitly a physicalist account of psyche, though still couched in the form of exegesis of an earlier thinker, in this case Andronicus' version of Aristotle.

It is useful to contrast Galen's approach here with that of Alexander of Aphrodisias, head of the Aristotelian school in the generation after Galen. We know that Alexander sometimes wrote explicitly contesting Galen's views.[234] Even when the allusion is only implicit, it is sometimes

[231] The comment reformulates Aristotle's theory of psyche in *De An.* 2.1, esp. 412ᵃ19–21, 27–8, in the light of his theory of elemental transformation in *GC* 2.2–4; see Kupreeva 2004: 81, also Lloyd 1988: 24, Hankinson 2006: 246.

[232] *QAM* IV.782–4, *SM* 2.44.12–45.2, my trans. after Singer 1997*a*: 157 and Hankinson 2006: 250. For Aristotle's thinking on substance, see *Metaph.* 7.3. Andronicus of Rhodes (1st cent. BC) was credited with producing the first critical edition of Aristotle's school texts.

[233] See Hankinson 2006: 241–4.

[234] Alexander probably held the chair of Peripatetic philosophy in Athens at some point between 198 and 209; he is therefore not to be identified with the earlier (Peripatetic) Alexander whom Galen encountered (*AA* II.218, 1.1, and *Praen.* 96.5–98.9 Nutton). Alexander wrote a refutation of Galen's theory of motion. See further Donini 1974: 148–50, Tieleman 1996: 75–6, esp. n. 34.

highly plausible to see an attempt to challenge or revise Galen's claims. Alexander's views on the psyche–body relationship seem also to represent a nuanced response to those of Galen. He accepts, on the one hand, the idea that occurrent emotions can be understood, in part at least, as the product of bodily states.[235] On the other hand, he dissents from Galen's view, just illustrated, that the psyche (or most of it) is a 'mixture' of bodily elements. Alexander maintains that the psyche is a 'form' (*eidos*) or 'faculty' (*dunamis*), which in some sense 'supervenes' on the blend or 'harmony' of bodily elements.[236] This represents a divergence from the position of the earlier Aristotelian Andronicus, cited approvingly by Galen in *QAM*, who presented the psyche as 'following' the blend of bodily elements. Alexander's position gives the psyche a rather more independent status than is suggested by Andronicus' formulation, and thus implicitly rejects Galen's presentation in *QAM* of the psyche as a blend of bodily elements.[237]

In the passage just cited from *QAM*, Galen is referring specifically to the non-rational part (or parts) of the psyche, which can more readily be regarded as bodily and mortal in a Platonic–Aristotelian framework of thinking.[238] But he is also inclined to challenge Plato's view, as he presents this, that the rational part of the psyche is immortal. Following his reinterpretation of Aristotle's idea of psyche as form, cited earlier, he continues: 'So if the reasoning faculty is a form of the psyche, it will be mortal, since it too will be a certain mixture [of elements] in the brain. But if it is immortal, as Plato wants, he would have done well to tell us why it is separated [from the body] when the brain is excessively cooled or heated or dried or moistened.'[239] Galen presses the point in unusually sardonic terms

[235] Alex. Aphr. *De An.* 13.1–8 (also 12.16–17), cf. Arist. *De An.* 1.1, 403^{a}19–24. See also Sorabji 2000: 261 and 2004: 193–4, which cite the main relevant passage.

[236] See Alex. Aphr. *De An.* 24.1–5, 24.18–25.9, 26.7–30; a related point is that health is better characterized as 'harmony' than psyche is (*De An.* 24.18–23). He also thinks that the idea of psyche as 'harmony' fits the Stoic or Epicurean (materialist) accounts better than his own (Aristotelian) one, *De An.* 26.20–2. See further Sorabji 2000: 261–2, also the passages cited in Sorabji 2004: 193–5.

[237] *QAM* IV.782–3, *SM* 2.44.12–45.3, trans. Singer 1997*a*: 157, also cited in Sorabji 2004: 187. See also Sorabji 2000: 261–2, and Donini 1974: 151–6, who discusses in some detail how far Alexander's view can be considered a response (implicit or explicit) to Galen's views in *QAM*.

[238] *QAM* IV.782, *SM* 2.44.4–8.

[239] *QAM* IV.774–5, *SM* 2.37.26–38.4, my trans.

(his treatment of Plato is usually respectful), wanting to know from Plato himself, 'if he were alive' why such things as a drink of hemlock should separate psyche from body, on the Platonic view of psyche. The underlying thought is that, if the rational psyche is susceptible to physical alterations, it is unclear why we should not suppose that it is itself a physical object.[240] Thus, Galen advances in this indirect way a virtually physicalist conception of psyche (as a whole), while still maintaining that 'I am unable to make a confident assertion one way or the other'.[241]

In *Prop. Plac.*, Galen expresses similar ideas but in a more theoretically self-aware way. Chapters 7 and 14–15 present the same line of thought but the second discussion does so in a more fully articulated way.[242] Galen sets out in ch. 14 a range of theoretical positions on the psyche–body relationship;[243] he also specifies with some precision his epistemological state in trying to adjudicate between these positions. On these questions, Galen claims only to be able to offer 'a plausible conclusion' (*pithanon*), since he is aware that he does not have 'sure knowledge (*bebaian gnōsin*) of things of which I have no sure proof (*bebaian epideixin*)'.[244] The type of topics involved are those 'of which knowledge is not essential for the health of the body or the ethical virtues of the psyche but which, if they were known for certain, would be an additional adornment (or 'completion', *apoteloumena*)' to those more practical types of knowledge.[245] In adjudicating between these possible positions in ch. 15, Galen distinguishes between things that 'I know for certain', things that 'I do not claim to

[240] *QAM* IV.775, *SM* 2.38.9–18; also Hankinson 2006: 245–6. There is an obvious allusion to Plato's *Phaedo*, the classic text of Platonic dualism, which ends with Socrates expressing confidence in the immortality of the psyche shortly before he dies by hemlock poisoning (114d–118a).

[241] *QAM* IV.773, *SM* 2.36.15–16, also IV.776, *SM* 2.38.19–21. On the relatively unqualified statement of a physicalist view of the psyche in *QAM*, see also Donini 2008: 199–201.

[242] Chs. 7 and 14 are now available as part of the complete Greek text in Boudon-Millot and Pietrobelli 2005. Ch. 7 is a significant improvement on the Latin version previously available (in Nutton 1999) but ch. 14 is close to the Greek text in Nutton 1999.

[243] *Prop. Plac.*, IV.760–1, 14.2–3 Nutton, Boudon-Millot and Pietrobelli 2005: 187.24–188.6; on these positions and those among them which Galen is more inclined to accept, see Hankinson 2006: 248–9.

[244] *Prop. Plac.* IV.761, 14.4, p. 114.12–19 Nutton, trans. Nutton.

[245] *Prop. Plac.* IV.762, 14.5, p. 114.20–6 Nutton, trans. Nutton.

know for certain', and things that 'seem clear to me', as inferences made on the basis of things that Galen does claim to know.[246] Thus, he claims to 'know', presumably from his natural inquiries, that the basis of the make-up of our bodies is a mixture of the four elements (rather than being a result of the accumulation of atoms).[247] He does not claim to know whether the psyche 'governs animals by being mixed with the substances of the body, or whether the substance of the psyche has no existence per se [i.e. separate from the body]'.[248] However, 'it seems clear to me that even if the psyche (merely) takes up residence in bodies, it is subservient to their natures, which are, as I have said, derived from some mixture of the four elements... For the body has to be suitable for receiving the psyche and if it suffers some grave alteration in its mixture the psyche must depart from it immediately'.[249] The analogous section of ch. 7 states the same point even more forcefully.

> [I also think (*nomizō*) it is reasonable to suppose (*eulogon*)] that generation of the body comes from the relevant mixture of the four elements, and if the psyche is formed together with the body, its generation... derives from the very mixture of the four elements, and that the psyche has no other generation, and that there is not one kind of generation for the psyche and another for the perceptible body. The psyche surely does not have a substance (*ousia*) in itself... but it subsists (*huparchein*) as a certain form of the body.[250]

[246] *Prop. Plac.* IV.762–3, 15.1–2, p. 116.8, 23, 26–7 Nutton, trans. Nutton.

[247] *Prop. Plac.* IV.762, 15.1 Nutton; cf. the alternatives set out in p. 112.7–13 Nutton.

[248] *Prop. Plac.* IV.762–3, 15.2, p. 116.21–6 Nutton, trans Nutton, slightly modified. Cf. the fuller set of alternatives stated in IV.760–1, 14.2–3 Nutton, esp. 'others [think] that [the psyche] has no independent existence of its own, but that the individuality (*idiotēs*) of the body's substance is said to include the faculties of doing what it is born to do', p. 112.17–21.

[249] *Prop. Plac.* IV.763, 15.2–3, pp. 116.26–118.5, 10–14 Nutton, trans. Nutton, slightly modified. For the passages cited in text to nn. 244–9 above, see also Boudon-Millot and Pietrobelli 2005: 188.6–189.6.

[250] *Prop. Plac.*, ch. 7, Boudon-Millot and Pietrobelli 2005: 178, 29–35, my trans.; the gaps marked are those in the manuscript. The analogous part of the Latin version is this: 'and if the psyche arrives with the body, then it too is created with the four elements. But it is impossible that the psyche should come from one thing and the sensible body from another, because the essence of the psyche does not exist (independently) by itself but is found in conjunction with the appearance, I mean, the form, of the body' (7.2, p. 78.6–9 Nutton, trans. Nutton 1999, slightly modified).

Even so, Galen adds his customary qualification: 'I have shown what it is useful for a doctor to know, even though we are entirely ignorant of the substance of the psyche.'[251]

Can we sum up Galen's approach to this question? Clearly, he is drawn most strongly towards a physicalist account of the psyche, but seeks ways of formulating this account without surrendering his recognition that he does not engage in the kind of fully theorized philosophical analysis that would justify a firm conclusion. In *QAM*, he does this by offering a kind of interpretative reading of the implications of previous thinkers in the light of his own approach to natural inquiry, especially his analysis of living entities in terms of natural faculties and the four elements. In *Prop. Plac.*, the physicalist view is presented as a justified or necessary inference from Galen's account of natural entities (about which he does claim to have knowledge), though stopping short of a theoretical assertion about the nature of the psyche. Is this position tenable? Well, perhaps. But it is hard not to feel that Galen is trying to have it both ways, and to advance (indirectly or tentatively) a physicalist account of the psyche without having to mount a full-scale argument for this account. The stance he takes up, in which he contributes to debate on this subject (on the basis of his findings in natural inquiry) without engaging formally in this debate, is a delicate, and perhaps rather awkward, one. In effect, if not quite formally, Galen *is* engaging in this debate, if only by drawing out the inferences of his approach to natural inquiry. And, if he goes this far into the debate, one may well feel, why does he not go a bit further and adopt and argue for the view towards which he is inclined?

This is one of the points on which, I want to suggest, closer engagement with Stoic ideas might have helped Galen to make his position more clear-cut and cogent, and perhaps more consistent. The Stoic position is, in several ways, close to the one towards which he seems most inclined. Also some of the arguments offered by the Stoics for their position are more articulated versions of the kind of considerations that Galen offers for the view he favours. If Galen had

[251] *Prop. Plac.*, ch. 7, Boudon-Millot and Pietrobelli 2005: 179.2–3, my trans. See also Nutton 1999: 160, commenting on the analogous Latin section (7.2–3): 'This is Galen's strongest assertion of the corporeality of the soul', while he also notes Galen's reiterated agnosticism.

been prepared to go rather further than he does in advancing a formal position, the Stoics could, perhaps, have offered material useful for this purpose. As is clear from *QAM*, Galen, while approaching the question from a broadly Aristotelian standpoint, clearly favours a position that is more—or more explicitly—physicalist than that of Aristotle himself.[252] The Stoic position, as illustrated shortly, is an explicitly physicalist one. This, by itself, does not make it unusual in Hellenistic thought.[253] But, unlike Epicureanism, another physicalist theory in the Hellenistic period, Stoicism shares with Galen the features I have associated here with 'high naturalism'. These include (a version of) the features that Galen sees in *Nat. Fac.* as characteristic of the 'biological' conception of natural entities (by contrast with the atomic): the idea of matter as a fusion of the four elements underlying the idea that natural entities have inbuilt animation and constitute complexes of natural faculties.[254] The Stoic idea of psyche as 'natural breath' or 'connate *pneuma*' reflects this approach.[255] It has been suggested that Galen's reluctance to embrace physicalism more strongly than he does is motivated by the idea that this is associated with the kind of mechanistic-atomistic position he rejects in *Nat Fac.*[256] If this is so, the Stoic position on the psyche, which combines physicalism with Galen's 'biological' approach, should represent an attractive conceptual option for him.

There is a further, possibly yet more powerful, way in which Stoic thought might reinforce Galen's thinking about the psyche. A repeated strand in his thought is that it is difficult to make sense of psyche–body interaction, and of the impact of physical factors on the psyche, unless the psyche is itself physical. This underlies several points noted earlier, including the objection to Platonic psyche–body dualism noted earlier in *QAM* and the reservations about a non-physicalist conception of psyche in *Prop. Plac.*[257] The Stoics have a number of types of argument

[252] See text to nn. 232–3 above; Galen favours the more physicalist version adopted by Andronicus, and suggests that this is implied by Aristotle's own statements.

[253] On physicalism about psychology as the norm in Hellenistic thought, see Annas 1992: 2–7; on shared physicalist (and naturalist) assumptions held by several Hellenistic medical and philosophical theories and Galen, see von Staden 2000: 79–80.

[254] See Ch. 2 above, text to nn. 163–73.

[255] See LS 53 B, esp. (5–9) and G; also Annas 1992: 43–50.

[256] Hankinson 2006: 253–5.

[257] See text to nn. 239–40, 242–50 above.

for the physicalist view of the psyche;[258] and these include arguments about interaction that are quite close to those offered by Galen. One version of the 'sympathetic' argument, ascribed to Cleanthes, is this: 'no incorporeal interacts with a body, and no body with an incorporeal, but one body interacts with another body. Now the psyche interacts with the body when it is sick and being cut, and the body with the psyche; thus when the psyche feels shame and fear the body turns red and pale respectively. Therefore, the psyche is a body.'[259] A second type of argument ('contactual') attributed to Chrysippus, is similar in its point: 'death is the separation of psyche from body. Now nothing incorporeal is separated from a body. For an incorporeal does not even make contact with a body. But the psyche both makes contact with and is separated from the body. Therefore the psyche is a body.'[260] These arguments are close in type to the Galenic ones and also rely on principles that he too would accept. These are that nothing happens without a cause and that only bodies can act as causes.[261] Hence, for the Stoics, the interaction between psyche and body, which falls into the category of causal interaction, must constitute interaction between bodies.[262]

In Galen too, as Hankinson points out, similar considerations lead to the inference that the psyche is not immaterial: 'Such a consideration may in itself cast doubt on the [idea that] the essence of the psyche as a whole is non-bodily. If the psyche were not some quality, form, affection, or faculty of the body, how could it actually acquire a nature opposite to its own, just by association (*koinōnia*) with the body?'[263] Thus, both the position adopted by the Stoics, and the arguments they use to support it, are very close to those of Galen. In

[258] Long 1996: 235–6 identifies three main types of argument: (1) genetic (e.g. LS 53 C), (2) sympathetic, and (3) contractual; the last two turn on the question of interaction.

[259] Nemesius 78.7–79.2, LS 45 C (=*SVF* 1.518, in part), trans. LS, slightly modified. Cleanthes (331–232 BC) was the second head of the Stoic school (from 262 BC).

[260] Nemesius 81.6–19, LS 45 D (=*SVF* 2.790, in part), trans. LS, slightly modified.

[261] For the Stoic version of these ideas, see LS 55, esp. B (*SVF* 2.341). For Galen, see Hankinson 1991*a*: 203 (also 219 n. 60), referring to (e.g.) *PHP* V.389–90, 544, 567, *MM* X.36, 50.

[262] LS 45 A–C (also LS. vol. 1, p. 273); Annas 1992: 42.

[263] *QAM* IV.788, *SM* 2.20–5, trans. Singer 1997*a*: 160, slightly modified. The context is criticism of Platonic psyche–body dualism. See Hankinson 1991*a*: 203.

fact, the Stoic position and arguments are so close to his that it is in some ways surprising that Galen does not make use of them to support his case.[264] There is, of course, the difference that the Stoics engage, formally and explicitly, in philosophical debate about the nature or substance of the psyche, whereas Galen disclaims authority in this area. However, Galen does, even so, go some way in this direction; and the Stoics offer resources that he could have used to refine his stance or its grounds further—without claiming to be doing more than drawing out the inferences of his independent work in natural inquiry.[265]

This degree of congruence between the two theories raises the question—a recurrent one in this inquiry—why Galen does not go further than he does in engaging with Stoic thinking on this question. Apart from any broader conceptual differences that may bear on this question,[266] there seem to be some specific explanatory factors. One derives from a conclusion that Galen draws in *PHP* from an observation made in the course of his anatomical study of animal brains. After examining the effects of various types of partial damage to the brain, Galen infers that 'if the psyche is incorporeal, [the *pneuma* in the ventricles in the brain] is ... its primary dwelling-place, but if the psyche is a body, this very *pneuma is* the psyche.' He then continues:

But, when it occurs that, shortly after the ventricles have been closed up, the animal perceives and moves again, one can maintain that neither of these alternatives is true regarding the *pneuma*. It is thus better to suppose that the psyche dwells in the actual body of the brain, whatever it might turn out to be as regards its substance (*ousia*) ... and that its [the psyche's] primary instrument (*organon*) in regard to all the animal's sensation, and its voluntary movements as well, is this *pneuma*. For this reason when it is emptied out, and until it is collected again, the animal does not lose its life, but is rendered

264 Galen does, in fact, make some use of the Stoic view to support his case (see text to nn. 271–6 below); but this could have been taken much further.

265 The relative closeness of Galen's (tentative or implied) position to the Stoic one, by contrast with the Platonic or Aristotelian, might have made it easier for Galen to have adopted their approach without embarking on the kind of full-scale argument about the nature of the psyche that he, clearly, feels uneasy about mounting.

266 Such as the contrast between holistic ('structure') and part-based ('composition') conceptions of the part–whole relationship; see Ch. 1 above, text to nn. 40–51, and Ch. 4 below, text to nn. 42–55.

incapable of sensation and motion, whereas if it really were the substance of the psyche, the animal would die immediately it was emptied out.[267]

What, exactly, is Galen's line of reasoning? What Galen observes, presumably, is the escape of some kind of brain fluid from the ventricles, which he identifies with the *pneuma*. This is accompanied by a temporary loss of sensation and motion; but these functions return after the ventricles have been closed up again. The inference, then, is that the psyche is not identical with the *pneuma* (which has oozed out of the brain), but is somehow housed in the ventricles, enabling the psyche to reanimate when these are closed up again. Although this point is not explicit here, this implies that Galen rejects the Stoic view, that the psyche is actually identical with the *pneuma*, as distinct from being the first instrument (*organon*) of the psyche, a possibility Galen still leaves open. Galen may have elaborated these criticisms of the Stoic theory in the lost work (*On the Psyche*) that he refers to in *Prop. Plac.*, ch. 7, which is cited shortly after he notes the Stoic view that the psyche is *pneuma*.[268]

How cogent is Galen's reasoning here? There seem to be several gaps or oddities in his thinking. His conclusion depends on identifying the psyche, narrowly, with *that portion of brain fluid* that escaped during the period of observation. But, presumably, he supposes that the brain has the ability to generate more such fluid; otherwise, it is hard to explain why he continues to regard *pneuma* as the 'first instrument' of the psyche. In that case, what prevents us from concluding that the *pneuma* regenerated, like that lost, constitutes the psyche? Galen's response might be that this suggestion locates the animating power in the body of the brain (as the regenerating agent of *pneuma*), rather than in the brain fluid (identified with *pneuma*) itself; and that this animating power is what we are looking for when we try to define the psyche.[269]

[267] *PHP* V.606, 7.3.19–21, pp. 442.37–444.11 De Lacy, trans. Hankinson 2006: 235–6, slightly modified, cf. V.609, 7.3.30, p. 446.11–15. On this type of investigation, see Rocca 2003: 177–9.

[268] 'That he [Chrysippus], to my mind, entirely fails to express himself clearly on these subjects, I have shown in a book that I have written *On the Psyche*'; *Prop. Plac.*, ch. 7, p. 179, lines 26–8 (Boudon-Millot and Pietrobelli 2005), my trans. See also the preceding reference to the Stoic theory that the psyche is corporeal and identical with *pneuma* (ch. 7, p. 179, lines 18–19); also Boudon-Millot and Pietrobelli 2005: 200, n. 35.

[269] Presumably, this underlies his conclusion that 'the psyche resides in the actual body of the brain', and the (implied) demotion of *pneuma* to the status of 'first instrument', *PHP* V.606, 7.3.21, p. 444.5–7 De Lacy.

However, this still leaves open the possibility of a specification of psyche that gives a central role to *pneuma*, such as 'the brain's capacity to generate and regenerate *pneuma*'. No doubt, the implications of this observation might usefully be explored further. But what emerges, even from a brief discussion, is that Galen seems to be drawing very large conclusions from a limited set of observations and from rather incomplete arguments based on those observations. There is a striking contrast with the much more carefully formulated set of observations and arguments by which Galen sets about trying to invalidate the Stoic–Aristotelian belief that the heart serves as the organ that houses the ruling part of the psyche. Certainly, Galen does not define here alternative positions that can be tested by controlled and repeatable observations, the method which is used with such striking effect in the case of his research on the brain.[270] There is a further question about whether this set of observations has a bearing on *pneuma* as conceived by the Stoics (namely as fire or fire-and-air), which does not seem easy to identify with brain marrow.

Galen comments directly on the Stoic account of the psyche in the context of this question in a passage from *QAM* cited earlier. To what extent do his comments enable us to gauge his view of the Stoic theory and thus to explain why, in general, he does not go further than he does in engaging with their approach to this topic?

> [The Stoics] hold that the psyche, like nature [*phusis*] is a kind of breath (*pneuma*) but that of nature is more humid and colder, whereas that of psyche is drier and hotter. That is why this *pneuma* too is a kind of matter (*hulē*) appropriate to the psyche and the form (*eidos*) of the matter is such-and-such a mixture (*krasis*), consisting in a proportion of the airy and fiery substance (*ousia*)... It has, then, become clear to you now that in the view of the Stoics the substance of the psyche comes to be according to a particular mixture of air and fire. And Chrysippus has been made intelligent because of the well-tempered mixture of these two [elements], while the sons of Hippocrates... [have been made] swinish because of the boundless heat.[271]

As pointed out earlier, Galen's summary seems initially to give a reasonable account of the Stoic theory, while also introducing a

[270] See Ch. 2 above, text to nn. 101–10.

[271] *QAM* IV.783–4, *SM* 2.45.5–11, 21–4 (part of *SVF* 2.787), trans. Tieleman 2003*a*: 149–50, slightly modified; see also the translation of Singer 1997*a*: 157–8.

subtle but significant change of conceptual framework. The idea that modalities of 'tension' can be analysed in terms of 'mixture' (*krasis*) of elements answers to several key features of Stoic thinking, even if the Stoics themselves do not put the point in quite that way.[272] However, the presentation of this mixture as the 'form' (*eidos*) of the psyche and of *pneuma* as its 'matter' strikes a more jarring note. The form–matter distinction is an Aristotelian, rather than Stoic, one; and its Stoic analogue, between active and passive causes, functions rather differently in this case.[273] Air and fire (the components of *pneuma*) serve as the active cause and water and earth as the passive one (or 'matter').[274] To put it differently, *pneuma*, in its various modalities, informs and, in the case of animals, animates and activates the body (more precisely, the *rest of* the body).[275] Also, within a larger perspective, *pneuma* in a specific body is the localized instantiation of the cosmic active cause or god.[276] Hence, to characterize *pneuma* as 'matter', by contrast with mixture as 'form', is misleading. From the Stoic standpoint, *pneuma*, in its various modalities, including psyche, can be seen both as a formal principle, in so far as it is the active cause, and also as a material one, as a combination of fire and air. As elsewhere, Galen's characterization of Stoic thought recasts it in more Platonic or Aristotelian terms, and thus understates its radical holism, here the holistic combination in one entity, *pneuma*, of formal principle (essence or substance) and matter.[277]

Galen's view of the Stoic theory of psyche, as indicated here, may be linked with his conclusions about the idea of *pneuma* as psyche, and, more broadly, with his failure to draw out more fully the implications of Stoic ideas for his own thinking on this topic. Both in this passage in *QAM* and in the observation-based account in *PHP* 7, discussed earlier, Galen conceives *pneuma* in (purely) material terms, either as brain fluid or fire-and-air. In neither case does

[272] For relevant features of Stoic thought, see Ch. 2 above, text to nn. 202–3, 207–12.

[273] See LS 44, esp. B (D.L. 7.134 = *SVF* 2.300 and part of 2.299).

[274] See LS 47, esp. D, F, H–I.

[275] Cf. Long 1996: 235: 'Stoic animals . . . are compounds of . . . a flesh-and-blood body and a specific soul body'. See also LS 47 H, J, N, R; also LS vol. 1: 287–9.

[276] See LS 47 C (Cic. *N.D.* 2.23–5, 28–30), O (D.L. 7.138–9).

[277] See further Ch. 2 above, text to nn. 206–25, taken with refs in n. 266 above.

Galen envisage *pneuma* in Stoic mode, as a (unified or holistic) combination of a material entity and an active or substantial principle. Galen's recasting of Stoic ideas in Aristotelian form in the *QAM* may be significant for explaining why he does not see Stoicism as offering a distinctive conceptual alternative, which might be of special importance for the exploration or articulation of the kind of physicalist position to which he seems drawn. In *QAM*, the Stoic idea of psyche is cited simply as one of a number of theories supporting his core thesis about the psychological impact of the mixture of elements in the body.[278] In *Prop. Plac.*, the idea of psyche as *pneuma* is noted as one of a whole series of alternatives, but not given special emphasis as a preferred option.[279] But Galen seems not to register the point made here, that the Stoic conception of psyche should represent a specially important one for him. It is more physicalist than the Aristotelian one, while, unlike the Epicurean one, it shares Galen's 'biological' approach to natural entities. The fact that Galen, at least in part, translates the Stoic theory into more Aristotelian form, may be one of the factors that holds him back from engaging more fully with the Stoic theory than he does.

The second respect in which I think that Galen could have benefited by drawing more fully on Stoic thought is in the ethical conclusions that he draws from his main thesis in *QAM*, especially in the final chapter, 11 (IV.814–21). As has been pointed out, especially by Geoffrey Lloyd, Galen's thesis, 'that the faculties of the psyche follow [or 'depend on', *hepesthai*] the mixtures of the body', is ambiguous in its significance. It might be a very strong thesis (that the bodily state wholly determines psychological capacities) or a weak one (that the bodily state influences psychological capacities). The very wide range of material that Galen cites from earlier Greek medical and philosophical writing reinforces the ambiguity, since different texts support stronger or weaker versions of the thesis.[280]

[278] The *QAM* passage cited above (in IV.783–4) follows Galen's positive comments about Andronicus' version of Aristotle (IV.782–3), with no indication that it is seen as introducing a distinctive new idea. On the core thesis of *QAM*, see text to nn. 226–8 above.

[279] *Prop. Plac.* 7.4, p. 80.1 Nutton (*spiritus*), IV.761, 14.3, p. 112.16 Nutton; see also 7.5, p. 80.10–13 Nutton, referring to the passage on *pneuma* in *PHP* 7, discussed in text to nn. 266–70 above.

[280] Lloyd 1988: 33–9.

However, in ch. 11, it would appear that Galen sees his claim as a very strong one. He argues there that, even though our ethical character is determined—wholly, it seems—by our innate character and by other, physical influences, this does not invalidate ethical judgements of other people. We are all naturally inclined to respond positively to good and negatively to bad. So it is appropriate that we should find bad people repellent (and, if need be, punish or even kill them), regardless of whether their badness of character is due to innate character or their own choices.[281] In a related move, Galen argues against the Stoic view that all human beings are naturally capable of developing towards virtue and that their corruption is due to the influence of others or the lure of pleasure.[282] He argues that the Stoic view is inherently implausible and runs counter to the case that he has built up cumulatively in this essay, that psychological capacities depend on the mixtures of elements in the body, which are themselves a product of natural temperament combined with subsequent environmental and social influences.[283]

Galen's argument is mounted here with his customary vigour. As is sometimes noted, his conclusion seems to reflect the underlying aim of displaying the potential scope of medicine and natural inquiry (as distinct from ethical philosophy, as normally understood) on people's character and intellectual abilities.[284] However, the line of thought is problematic in a whole series of ways. There is ambiguity about whether inborn nature (combined with other external factors) is *wholly* determinant of ethical character or whether some scope is left for rational instruction and the agent's own choices.[285] There is also an apparent inconsistency between Galen's claim that *everyone*

[281] *QAM* IV.814–16, *SM* 2.73.3–74.21 (trans. Singer 1997*a*: 172–3).

[282] *QAM* IV.816–20, *SM* 2.74.21–78.7 (trans. Singer 1997*a*: 173–5).

[283] *QAM* IV.820–1, *SM* 2.78.7–79.6 (trans. Singer 1997*a*: 175–6).

[284] See esp. *QAM* IV. 767–8, *SM* 32.1–13, IV.807–8, *SM* 2.67.2–16. On Galen's project, see e.g. Lloyd 1988: 39–42; also Donini 2008: 199–202, Jouanna 2009.

[285] The former idea is stressed in *QAM* IV.814–15, *SM* 2.73.10–12. cf. IV.820–1, *SM* 2.78.8–12, 78.23–79.9. But *QAM* IV.815, *SM* 2.11–13 refers to a variety of factors (including teaching and choice, *prohairesis*), cf. IV.821, *SM* 2.78.21–3 (referring to education and opinions). Cf the ambiguity noted in the core thesis of the essay (text to n. 280 above). The deterministic element is stressed by Hankinson 1993: 215–20, whereas Lloyd 1988: 36–7 sees more scope for agency; Singer 1997*b*: 535–6 sees Galen's position as ambiguous.

loves the good and hates the bad and his assertion that some people, none the less, are irredeemably bad and need to be destroyed.[286] Galen's claims about the impact of inborn nature (and physical factors) on ethical character and about how we should respond to this fact are exceptional and non-standard, even in relation to the Platonic–Aristotelian framework of thinking the validity of which he assumes. A more typical view is that ethical character is the product of a combination of inborn nature, habituation, and the agent's rational choice (*phusis, ethos, logos*). It is also more typical to see scope for the improvement of rational understanding and ethical character even in adults, despite the recognition of the importance of nature and habituation.[287] This is, in fact, the assumption that Galen himself typically makes in his essays in practical ethics, including that on the passions of the psyche (*Aff. Dig.*).[288] It is also quite exceptional to suggest that moral judgements should not take any account of the degree of people's responsibility as agents for their character. Aristotle, in a well-known discussion (*EN* 3.5) offers a fine-grained analysis of this question.[289] Even the striking passage of Plato's *Timaeus* that seems to have greatly influenced Galen in this essay recognizes that, in so far as people's ethical character is shaped by their innate (body-based) nature, this should *exempt* them from the normal type of condemnation.[290] Plato also seeks to combine, in this

[286] *QAM* IV.815–16, *SM* 2.73.17–74.21. Contrast *SM* 2.73.17–19: it is natural (*huparchei*) for *all of us* (*pasin*) to love the good and hate the bad, with 2.73.13–21 (we rightly kill the irredeemably bad), also 2.73.10–12 (some are naturally good and some bad).

[287] See e.g. Plu. *Mor.* 2 A–B, 443 C–D, reflecting typical Platonic–Aristotelian ideas about development. See further Gill 2006: 231–2; also 412–21 on Plutarch's thinking about scope for change and correction in adult life.

[288] See 5.2 below.

[289] Aristotle's key point is that, even if we have an inborn tendency to develop in a certain way (and our character may have become irreversible) we are still 'co-responsible' (*sunaitioi*) as rational agents for the character we have developed. See esp. *EN* 1114^{a}3–21, ^{a}31–^{b}25.

[290] *Ti.* 86b–87b, which is striking both for presenting moral defects as a product of (primarily innate) body-based psychic illnesses and for arguing that those affected by these illnesses should not be blamed. Galen refers to this passage repeatedly in ch. 6 (IV.789–91) and also in ch. 10 (IV.812–13), immediately prior to ch. 11. On this passage, and ancient and modern readings of it, see Gill 2000, 2006: 200–3. As noted by Hankinson 1993: 219–20 n. 102, Galen is also strongly influenced by Pl. *Lg.* 731d, in his comments about punishment and irremediable character.

passage, the recognition of body-based influences on character with scope for education and rational agency in shaping our lives.[291] So, taken as a whole, Galen's argument is problematic both for its extreme stance (in relationship to the assumed intellectual framework) and for its potential inconsistency with his own project of improvement of character in his works of practical ethics.[292]

I suggested earlier that this is another topic on which Galen could have improved his argument by closer engagement with Stoic thought. This might seem to be an implausible suggestion since, here as often elsewhere, Galen frames his argument in the form of criticism of Stoic thought. Galen's critique of the Stoic theory of development (from a Platonic–Aristotelian standpoint) represents an exceptionally clear and explicit expression of the conflict between two competing conceptions of development in Hellenistic and Roman thought. I examine this conflict fully in Chapter 5, in connection with Galenic and Stoic ideas about practical ethics and the therapy of the emotions.[293] None the less, I think that there are aspects of Stoic thinking (of which Galen may have been aware) on which he could have drawn to render his own account more consistent and cogent. One of the assumptions that seems to underlie Galen's conclusions in *QAM* ch. 11 is that a physicalist approach necessarily means that psychological capacities and characteristics are seen as (wholly) determined from outside, by factors other than human agency. The dominant line of thought, especially towards the close of the essay is that innate temperament (mixture of elements) shapes both natural capacities and the way of life towards which people are drawn, which in turn accentuates our innate inclinations. The emphasis falls on differences of natural intelligence and emotional register (such as being sharp-tempered or cheerful).[294] But a similar line of thought supports his view that 'not all are born enemies of justice, not all its friends; each kind comes about through

[291] Pl. *Ti.* 86c–89c (also 90a–d); see further Gill 2000: 70–1, 2006: 200–1. Galen in fact cites this idea in *Ti.* 87b6–8 in IV.813, *SM* 2.71.22–72.2.

[292] Hankinson 1993: 212–20 argues strongly for the consistency of Galen's position. For a more critical reading, see Donini 2008: 200–2. See further on Galen's argument, taken in the larger context of his thinking about ethical development, Ch. 5 below, text to nn. 125–35.

[293] *QAM* IV.816–20; on these contrasting conceptions of development, see Gill 2006: 134–45.

[294] *QAM* IV.821, *SM* 2.78.23–79.24.

bodily mixture'.[295] The implication seems to be that a physicalist approach to psychological characteristics is also a determinist one, and that determinism negates ideas of personal agency and responsibility. However, as highlighted earlier, this is problematic in part because other features of Galen's argument presuppose scope for agency; and Galen himself elsewhere assumes that we can play a role as agents in shaping our own character as well as actions.[296]

It is on this point that reference to Stoic ideas might help Galen's argument. The Stoics, as Galen himself brings out, not only hold a physicalist approach to psychological characteristics, but also bring out how physical factors play a role in shaping and developing inborn ability or temperament.[297] The Stoics also maintain a determinist view of human character, at least in the sense that they see the development of good and bad character as an integral part of the seamless web of causation that determines all events. However, the Stoics also combine these ideas with the claim that all adult humans are, constitutively, rational agents, who are responsible for their actions and, in principle, for the shaping of their character. A key part of the theory that underlies this claim is the distinction between internal and external causal factors, more precisely between factors that do or do not reflect the nature of the person (or object) in question. A constitutive feature of adult human beings, for instance, is that they respond to events in a way that involves reason, in the form of rational impressions and assent to these. Hence, explanation of their actions and the development of their character needs to make reference to this feature (the 'internal' cause) as well as to the various influences ('external' causes) that have a bearing on their actions. This point is crucial for what is normally seen as their 'compatibilist' approach, combining determinism and responsibility. It also enables the Stoics to give weight to factors such as innate nature and environmental influence on character development, without denying

[295] *QAM* IV.814, *SM* 2.73.10–12, trans. Singer 1997*a*: 172; cf. the stress on innate qualities in children including generosity, meanness, compassion and meanness (IV.817, *SM* 2.75.12–15).

[296] See text to nn. 285–8 above.

[297] *QAM* IV.783–4, *SM* 2.45.9–46.1, cited in part in text to n. 271 above. For comparable ideas about the effect of the physical environment, see Cic. *De Fato* 8. See also Gill 2006: 178–9, and on the body-based strand in Stoic thinking about inborn and environmental factors, Tieleman 2003*a*: 146–66, 186–96.

scope for rational agency in this respect.[298] Since the Stoics are consistent physicalists in psychology, *all* such responses, including forming rational impressions and giving assent to these, are conceived as (physical) operations of psychic *pneuma*, managed by the (embodied) 'control-centre' (*hēgemonikon*).[299]

It is clear, perhaps, how the Stoics use these ideas as part of a conceptual framework that combines physicalist psychology with recognition of the causal role of rational agency; but what reason is there to think that Galen could have incorporated them in his approach? In fact, as pointed out earlier, Galen's thinking about causation seems to be strongly influenced by relevant features of Stoic theory. In particular, he gives a key role to the distinction between external (antecedent) causes and the disposition of the person responding to external factors, and sees events as explained by the *combination* of causes of this type. The application of this causal schema to the explanation of disease and likely cure is one of the key features by which Galen identifies his distinctive approach to medicine, in relation to other schools in his day.[300] Galen deploys this framework as part of a medical approach to (primarily) physical illness.[301] But there seems to be no reason in principle why Galen could not have applied this type of distinction in other contexts, including the discussion of *QAM* ch. 11, which explores the ethical implications of the thesis that psychological capacities and characteristics can be explained in physical, especially temperamental, terms. Galen too could have used the distinction between antecedent and dispositional causes to construct a physicalist account of character development that gave a role for rational agency and responsibility.

There is room for debate about exactly what form such an account would take for Galen. Clearly, any such account would have to be couched in the Platonic–Aristotelian terms that Galen presupposes, rather than the Stoic ones Galen rejects in *QAM* ch. 11. These terms include a part-based, rather than unitary, psychological model and

298 See LS 62, esp. C–D (Cic. *Fat.* 39–43 and Gellius 7.2.6–13); see further Bobzien 1998: ch. 6, esp. 290–301; also D. Frede 2003, and, in outline, Gill 2006: 183–4.

299 See further Long 1996: 233–4, 239–47, von Staden 2000: 100–3.

300 See Ch. 2 above, text to nn. 111–16.

301 On Galenic medicine and the psyche–body distinction, see 5.4 below.

analysis of development in terms of the interplay of (inborn) nature, habituation, and rationality.[302] However, a crucial point would be the use of the distinction between antecedent and dispositional (or external and internal) causes to analyse the formation of distinctively human (rational) psychological capacities and characteristics. This distinction could be applied at any given stage of a human life or to some, especially important, stages such as the start of adulthood, often seen in ancient thought as marking the emergence of rational agency.[303] Galen could use this distinction either to chart an ongoing interplay between external and internal factors in character development or to define a determinate stage at which a human being becomes a rational and responsible agent (with a stable disposition) and responds to external events on this basis.[304] As I have acknowledged, there is scope for argument about the form that such an account might take and also about how it might relate to other aspects of Galen's thinking in *QAM* and elsewhere. But my core point is that there is no fundamental conceptual reason why Galen could not have not combined (as the Stoics do) a physicalist approach to psychology and an analysis of character development in terms of the distinction between internal and external causes. This would have enabled Galen to maintain his main thesis in *QAM* about the (body-based) temperamental basis of psychological capacities and characteristics while still allowing scope for adult human beings to exercise rational agency and to have moral responsibility, including some kind of responsibility for their own character-development.

If we allow that Galen could have coherently adopted this Stoic distinction, along with their explicit psychological physicalism, how would this have improved his conclusions in *QAM* ch. 11? As stressed earlier, his analysis displays internal inconsistencies or at least tensions,

[302] On these as characteristic features of Platonic–Aristotelian (by contrast with Stoic, or Epicurean) accounts of character development, see Gill 2006: 134–6, (also on Plutarch) 231–2, 415–21.

[303] This is common ground to Platonic–Aristotelian and Stoic accounts, though differently conceived; see e.g. Pl. *R.* 402a, Arist. *EN* 3.5, and, on Stoic theory, Inwood 1985: 72–5, 79–80.

[304] Arist. *EN* 3.5 accentuates the idea that at a certain point in life one takes on responsibility, even if one loses the capacity for continuing modification; Stoicism stresses, rather, the idea of ongoing interaction between internal and external causes, see Bobzien 1998: 297, Gill 2006: 184, 377–9.

as well as being in conflict with most philosophical accounts of character development and ethical responsibility and, arguably, with Galen's own essays on character development.[305] More specifically, an account of the type just outlined would be more consistent, for instance, with those passages in *QAM* ch. 11 where Galen does give a role to rational instruction and choice (*prohairesis*) in character development.[306] More broadly, an analysis of this type might better meet the challenge he poses at the start of ch. 11, that of reconciling the stress in *QAM* as a whole on body-based temperamental factors with a credible account of ethical responsibility for actions and in some sense for character.[307] An analysis that incorporated *some* elements of Stoic theory—notably the distinction between internal and external causal factors—could be constructed within the Platonic–Aristotelian framework of thinking about character development Galen embraces in ch. 11. This move would have rendered unnecessary the awkward claim in Galen's present discussion of insisting that punishment (including capital punishment) should take no account of degrees of responsibility for one's actions or character.[308] A framework of this kind would also have been more consistent with Galen's project in the essays in practical ethics of appealing to the capacity of adult humans as rational agents to participate in the improvement of their own rational and emotional qualities.[309] Such an analysis might also be more consistent with Galen's body-based, teleological psychological framework, in which the rational part of the psyche, housed in the brain, is seen as having a directive role in human action. Indeed, an account of this type might also be more consistent with what seems to be Galen's underlying aim of promoting the role of the doctor in character development. The doctor will be better placed to influence the behaviour of his patients, as regards diet and regimen, for instance, if his analysis recognizes that they function in this regard as rational agents (that is as internal causes of a certain kind), able to vary their actions in response to rational considerations.[310]

[305] See text to nn. 287–8 above. [306] See text to nn. 285–6 above.

[307] *QAM* IV.814–15, SM 2.73.3–16.

[308] *QAM* IV.815–16, *SM* 2.73.16–74.21; on the contrast with the ideas found in Plato and Aristotle on this question, see text to nn. 289–91 above.

[309] See further 5.2 below, esp. text to nn. 28–56.

[310] On Galenic medical techniques, and on the extent to which this treats people as rational agents as well as bodies, see 5.4 below.

So one can argue that Galen has powerful reasons for adopting certain key features of Stoic thinking as a way of framing his conclusions in ch. 11 of *QAM*.

The suggestion that Galen could have improved his own argument by adopting relevant aspects of Stoic theory about ethical psychology in *QAM* ch. 11 is, clearly, more controversial than the previous suggestion that he could usefully have adopted Stoic physicalism as regards psychology. In *QAM* ch. 11, Galen argues explicitly against Stoic theory, though not the feature I have just highlighted, whereas his comments about the Stoic physicalist approach in *QAM* ch. 4 (IV.783–4) are positive ones. However, arguments can be mounted for both suggestions; and the second suggestion builds on the first. These suggestions complement the points made earlier about the potential relevance of Stoic thinking as regards Galen's psychological theory in *PHP* and *Foet. Form.* If these points are accepted, it is clear that, as regards Galen's thinking about psychology and the body, there could have been some substantial advantages in closer engagement with Stoic thinking—in spite of his intense criticism of some Stoic ideas in all three works. This raises in an acute form the question broached in ch. 1, why Galen did not in fact attempt to combine his ideas with Stoic ones. This is the first question addressed in the next chapter, before exploring a second strand in Galen's psychological thinking, in which the gulf between his ideas and those of Stoicism is yet greater.

4

Reason and Emotion: Parts and Wholes

4.1 THE GALEN–STOICISM RELATIONSHIP

This chapter has two interrelated themes. On the one hand, especially in this opening section, I return to the paradoxes highlighted in Chapter 1, which are reconsidered in the light of the intervening chapters. Why are Galen's most explicit and sustained responses to Stoicism so negative or critical, in spite of the fact that both theories express a naturalistic conception of psychology, by contrast, for instance, with Platonic psyche–body dualism, which was still a very live intellectual option in Galen's day.[1] In considering this question, I give close attention to another aspect of Galen's reactions to Stoicism, which forms the second main theme of the chapter, and is examined closely in sections 2–4. This is Galen's critique of Stoic thinking on psychological functions, especially emotion, in *PHP* 4–5. Why is this discussion so comprehensively negative, with virtually no indication of even potentially shared features?

The paradox underlined in Chapter 1 has been accentuated by the discussion of Chapters 2–3, which have brought out how much Galen already has in common with Stoicism, as well as pointing to areas of potential convergence. Earlier, I specified the kind of naturalism the two theories have in common (what I called 'high naturalism'), showing how this informs their respective thinking on psychology and on the development of the embryo.[2] An implication of the preceding chapters is that the combination of certain

[1] On this type of dualism, see Ch. 2, n. 41; Galen explicitly distances himself from this type of dualism in *QAM* (3.5 above, text to nn. 239–40).

[2] See 2.3 above, esp. text to nn. 212–25; also 3.4 above, esp. text to nn. 188–9.

aspects of both theories was intellectually possible, in terms of the thought-world of the period. In particular, the combination of an anatomical picture centred on the role of the brain and central nervous system and the Stoic psychological model, in which a unitary control-centre coordinates the work of a single communication system, would have constituted a more cogent and credible account than we find in either theory, or, arguably, in any other ancient theory of embodied psychology (3.2–3 above). Similarly, the combination of Galen's logico-empirical method, deployed effectively in connection with the location of the ruling part of the psyche, and Stoic theoretical rigour and coherence, applied to thinking through the implications of Galen's findings, could have constituted a uniquely powerful methodology.[3] For instance, Stoic thinking on psyche–body interaction and on the role of rational agents as causal agents could have been adopted by Galen in order to provide a more fully theorized and coherent version of the kind of physicalism that he is inclined towards (or that he could usefully adopt).[4] The suggestion that Galenic ideas could have been combined with those of another ancient theory is not merely fanciful. The project of *PHP*, or to a lesser extent *Nat. Fac.* or *UP*, is, explicitly, that of building on links between Galen's empirical findings or ideas and previous philosophical theories or approaches.[5] If Galen had chosen to make his masterwork on psychology *On the Doctrines of Hippocrates and Chrysippus*, this combination of ideas would have come about—and, as the preceding two chapters have indicated, this was by no means inconceivable. Also, as stressed earlier, examining this hypothetical, but unrealized, combination of ideas is not just an exercise in historical fantasy or wishful thinking. It serves to identify elements (in the two theories or in any one of them) which are conceptually consistent or inconsistent. It thus helps us to specify aspects of ancient theory about psychology that we, moderns, might wish to

[3] See 2.2 above, which also notes that Stoic ideas on logic and causation informed Galenic thinking and so helped him to formulate his method of natural inquiry (Ch. 2 above, text to nn. 117–24).

[4] See 3.5 above, esp. text to nn. 252–62, 294–304.

[5] On the project of *PHP*, see Ch. 3 above, text to nn. 13–25; on *UP* and *Nat. Fac.*, see Ch. 2 above, text to nn. 157–73.

adopt—or that are, in fact, already close to contemporary ideas or practices.[6]

In fact, of course, this combination of Galenic and Stoic thinking on psychology was not produced in antiquity. On the contrary, Chrysippus, in particular, in his works *On the Psyche* and *On Passions*, is a target for sustained criticism throughout *PHP* 2–5, a critique that also lies behind Galen's dissent from Stoic ideas in the much later work *Foet. Form.* What went wrong in this relationship? Why did Galen not see the scope for closer engagement of the kind that would have produced the powerful version of naturalistic psychology outlined here? Shortly, I review a number of possible explanations for this lack of closer engagement, with special reference to Galen's critique of Stoic psychology in *PHP* 4–5.[7] First, however, I look more closely at this critique. How does it fit into the larger objectives of *PHP* 1–6 and, more broadly, what light does it throw on the Galen–Stoicism relationship? In particular, how does this critique relate to the kinds of—at least partly—shared naturalism I have identified in the two theories?

If we look at the project of *PHP* 1–6, taken in the context of Galen's medical work in this period (which is especially focused on anatomy),[8] the psychological question to which Galen is best placed to contribute is that of the bodily location of the ruling part of the psyche. Why, then, do we have an extensive discussion of emotion in *PHP* 4–5, a topic for which Galen's medical work has not, it would seem, provided any independent basis in research or practice? In fact, Galen does mark the critique of *PHP* 4–5 as a digression, one extended to two books partly because of the decision to make fuller reference to Posidonius, a later Stoic thinker (*c.*135–*c.*50 BC) whom Galen presents as profoundly critical of Chrysippus.[9] However, as

[6] See text to nn. 19–23 below; also Ch. 6 below.

[7] See also the briefer comments on this subject in 3.1 above.

[8] The works completed in this period (Galen's first stay in Rome, 162–6), were in various ways centred on anatomy. They include *UP* 1 and works on the anatomy of veins and arteries and nerves (*Nerv. Diss.* and *Ven. Art. Diss.*), *On Bones for Beginners* (*Oss.*), as well as *PHP* 1–6; a first edition of *Anatomical Procedures* (*AA*) was written earlier (during 148–57). See the outline of Galen's works and dates in Singer 1997*a*: l–lii; also Ch. 2 above, text to nn. 11–18.

[9] See De Lacy 2005: 49, referring esp. to *PHP* V. 339, 3.7.17, p. 214.27–30 De Lacy; see also V.589, 7.1.8–9 De Lacy, V.652–3, 8.1.14 De Lacy.

Galen points out in this context, the two main topics of *PHP* 1–3, 6 and 4–5, respectively (that is, the location and the number of psychological parts or functions) are logically linked. There are also direct connections between Chrysippus' presentation, in *On the Psyche*, of reason and anger as functions of the unitary (heart-based) control-centre and his account, in *On Passions*, of passions or emotions (*pathē*) as (in adult humans) expressions of reason. Hence, it is natural for Galen to extend his critique of Stoic thinking on heart-centred psychophysiology to their theory of emotion.[10] There is a specific reason why Galen needs to address this aspect of their theory, as he himself indicates. The Stoics, like Galen and Plato in the *Timaeus*, see emotions such as anger as located in the area of the heart. Galen takes this fact as supporting his claim that there are three separate physical centres of psychological activity, whereas the Stoics see it as indicating the presence of psychological activity as such, including reason and emotion, in one central organ. So Galen needs to tackle their theory about the unified character of psychological functions, especially as set out in Chrysippus' *On Passions*.[11] In any case, as indicated earlier, Galen's intellectual programme in *PHP*, though one that evolved in the course of composition, was always conceived as an ambitious one, designed to include a range of ethical and psychological themes in its synthesis of medical and philosophical standpoints.[12] For instance, the theme of the virtues is sometimes presented as part of the intended subject matter, though it is not finally treated until *PHP* 7.[13] So Galen's large-scale assault in *PHP* 4–5 on the Stoic theory of emotions, which had

[10] In addition to the refs. in the preceding note, see *PHP* V.333–9, 3.6.1–7.19 De Lacy. On Galen's organization of the topic, taken in the light of ancient ways of subdividing the main topics of psychology (including location and number of parts), see Tieleman 2003*a*: 20–30. On Galen's (selective) reading of Stoic texts, including those by Chrysippus, see Tieleman 2003*a*: 51–8. On possible English translations of *pathos*, including 'emotion', 'passion', 'affection', see Tieleman 2003*a*: 15–16.

[11] *PHP* V.331–2, 3.5.42–7 De Lacy (also V.288, 3.5.1–2 De Lacy), continued in V.333–9, 3.6.1–7.19 De Lacy); also V.360, 4.1.1–4 De Lacy, V.428–9, 5.1.1–3 De Lacy. On Pl. *Ti.* 70a–b, and Galenic and (possibly) Stoic responses to this, see Gill 2006: 296–304.

[12] See Ch. 3 above, text to nn. 13–21.

[13] See *PHP* V.286, 3.1.6, p. 168.23–4 De Lacy, V.499, 5.7.73, p. 354.21–5 De Lacy, V.593–600, 7.1.23–2.17. See De Lacy 2005: 49 n. 1, Tieleman 2003*a*: 25–6.

already been criticized in rather similar terms by Plutarch,[14] is less surprising than it might seem initially.

What is the general form of Galen's treatment?[15] It is directed specifically at the main claims of Chrysippus' *On Passions*, although it does not follow what seems to have been the structure of that work.[16] Book 4 highlights the alleged inconsistencies and failings of Chrysippus' theory. The main thesis is that Chrysippus' highly unified and intellectualist psychology fails to explain the phenomena of emotions and psychic weakness that Chrysippus himself presents as being in some sense irrational. Galen maintains that Chrysippus cannot offer an effective explanation of these phenomena because he refuses to acknowledge the presence of non-rational functions in the psyche, unlike the later Stoic Posidonius (as Galen claims). Book 5 continues this theme, focusing on what Galen sees as problems in Chrysippus' use of the analogy between psychic and bodily health and beauty or proportion, a discussion examined later (4.4 below). Galen refers extensively to Posidonius' *On Passions*, arguing that the later Stoic's treatment of themes such as childhood development and the cause of passion constituted a radical critique of Chrysippus' theory. Book 5 closes with Galen's endorsement of Plato's argument for separate and independent psychic parts in *Republic* Book 4, which precedes Galen's more detailed account of the linkage between Platonic and 'Hippocratic' psychophysiology in *PHP* 6.[17]

Galen's discussions in these two books, and the evidence they provide for Chrysippus' treatise on the passions and that of Posidonius, have been examined in depth by Tieleman (2003*a*). I have also considered this material in some detail, especially with a view to bringing out the combination of psychological and psychophysical holism and Socratic-style radical ethical claims expressed in the Stoic theory.[18] My focus here is on locating *PHP* 4–5 within the larger

[14] In *On Ethical Virtue* (*Mor.* 440 D–452 D); see Gill 2006: 219–29.

[15] The following paragraph is similar in content to Gill 2006: 245–6.

[16] For an outline analysis of *PHP* 4–5, see Tieleman 2003*a*: 30–3; and for the probable structure of Chrysippus' treatise, see Tieleman 2003*a*: 325–6, Gourinat 2005.

[17] See *PHP* V.479–501, 5.7.1–18 De Lacy, referring to Pl. *R.* 435–41.

[18] Gill 2006: ch. 3, esp. 238–90; I draw on parts of this analysis in 4.2 below. See also Gill 1998 and 2005.

exploration of Galen's relationship to Stoicism. For instance, how, if at all, does the critique bear on the question of their shared naturalism of approach and the paradox that this naturalism is not developed by Galen into the basis for intellectual synthesis, of the kind attempted with other thinkers notably Plato and Hippocrates? On the face of it, *PHP* 4–5 is a self-contained treatment of psychological functions, especially reason and emotion, with little explicit linkage with the questions about psychophysiology and the philosophy of nature that I have discussed so far. It is also a uniformly negative or critical treatment of—at least—Chrysippus' theory, with none of the indications of actual or potential convergence that I have underlined in other contexts. Indeed, this consistently negative response on Galen's part forms the basis for the first conclusion I want to draw for my larger inquiry. It seems likely that Galen's sustained negative response to their theory of emotion, taken with his serious disagreement over the location of the ruling part of the psyche, constituted one of the decisive factors that ensured that in other contexts Galen never engaged with Stoicism subsequently in great depth, despite their potential points of contact. Indeed, as Tieleman has suggested, after his intensive study at this time of (at least parts of) Chrysippus' *On the Psyche* and *On Passions*, along with Posidonius' *On Passions*, Galen may never have conducted detailed examination of Stoic treatises again.[19]

But why, exactly, is Galen so negative about the Stoic theory of emotions? And does his response have nothing to do with the question of 'naturalism' in psychology, as so far considered here? There is, of course, a specific linkage between the theme of *PHP* 4–5 and Galen's psychophysiology in *PHP* 1–3, 6, highlighted earlier;[20] and this linkage has further implications for the question of Galen's stance in *PHP* 4–5 which are considered shortly.[21] But in a broader sense, Galen's fundamental objection to the Stoic (or as he presents it, Chrysippus') theory of emotions is that it is *unnatural*. More

[19] Tieleman 2003*a*: 149 n. 44, 2009: 297. On the texts Galen cites, which include Chrysippus' *On the Psyche* 2 (but not 1), Chrysippus' *On Passions* 1, 2, 4 (but not 3), Posidonius' *On Passions* (but not Zeno's), see Tieleman 2003*a*: 51–8, 85–8. On Galen's earlier study of Stoic logic during his education at Pergamon, see Tieleman 2009: 284–6.

[20] See text to n. 11 above.

[21] See text to nn. 55–6 below.

precisely, he regards the idea that emotions, in adult humans are (crucially at least) beliefs, rather than non-rational functions, as essentially misguided, perverse, and in conflict with any psychologically credible account of human nature. This reaction underlies his attempt to drive a wedge between Chrysippus' theory and that of Zeno and, still more, Posidonius. Chrysippus' account, as Galen claims, placed a special, even exclusive, emphasis on the idea that emotions are beliefs, ignoring the non-rational dimension recognized even by other Stoic thinkers. This assumption about the unnatural character of the Chrysippean theory underlies the whole critique of *PHP* 4–5. There is no theorized statement about what should count as a 'natural' account of psychology; but Galen's assumptions are indicated in his presentation, here and throughout *PHP* 1–6, of Plato's tripartite psyche as a clear expression of a more inherently credible account of human psychology.

Galen's view that the Stoic theory offers an implausible account of human nature is far from exceptional in ancient or modern thought. But it is, none the less, highly problematic for several reasons. One is that, as Tieleman has brought out very clearly, Galen gives what is, arguably at least, a seriously distorted picture of the relationship between the accounts of emotions offered by the various Stoic theorists. Also, Galen's account of Chrysippus' theory—which is, essentially, I think, *the* Stoic theory, shared with other Stoic thinkers—is profoundly misleading, and can be corrected, in part, by drawing on the full quotations that Galen himself provides. Viewed more sympathetically, we can see the Stoic theory not only as much more plausible than Galen suggests but also as 'natural', in several senses. It reflects, for instance, key features of the naturalism we have already considered, including their physicalism about psychology and their causal theory, on which Galen himself draws in forming his methodology of natural inquiry. Their psychology also expresses what I described as the 'high naturalism' shared with Galen, according to which humans and other animals are seen as structured complexes of natural faculties, which constitute an integral part of the physical universe, conceived from a teleological standpoint. These points apply to their thinking about animal (including human) motivation and development, which underlies their account of emotion. By contrast, Platonic psychology, which Galen takes as his paradigm, expresses in certain respects an idealist or transcendental outlook, especially as regards the role of reason or mind, a dimension which is quite remote from Galen's more naturalistic approach and which he largely ignores.[22] However, the Stoic theory of emotion, alongside these kinds of naturalism, also expresses a radical holism and revisionism (in relation to previous theories of emotion), and these features give the theory a provocative, and sometimes paradoxical, character. There are close and important links between their ethical ideals and the psychology of emotion (and their theory of human development) that reflect in various ways the radical holism of Stoic theory.[23] It is, I suspect, these features of the theory against which Galen, like some other ancient or modern thinkers, principally reacts. But his criticism is directed explicitly at more basic or fundamental aspects of the theory, its coherence and credibility (that is, in effect, its unnatural view of human psychology), rather than these more advanced or complex features.

There is a further aspect of the naturalism of the Stoic theory to which Galen could have responded positively if he had recognized its relevance for his own thinking. Earlier, I suggested that Galen's anatomically based picture of the workings of the brain and nervous system would have fitted better with the Stoic idea of a unified control-centre than with Galen's idea, adopted from Plato, of a three-centre psychophysiological model.[24] If Galen had adopted a view of that kind, he might also have taken a much more positive attitude towards the Stoic idea that emotions as well as reasoning are based in a single organ, which would have been, for Galen, the brain. As Tieleman points out, Galen himself notes some phenomena that might have led him to that view. For instance, he cites cases where sacrificial cows were still able to run away in a panic-stricken way, while their hearts were beating on the altar. Galen takes this example as showing that the functions of respiration and motion are controlled by the brain and nerves; but it could also be seen as implying that feelings, such as the cow's panic, are based in the brain.[25]

[22] See e.g. Pl. *R.* 611d–612a, *Phd.* 78d–84b; see further Gill 2006: 5–6, Gerson 2002. The contrast between this side of Platonic thought and Galen's approach becomes evident in *QAM*; see Ch. 3 above, text to nn. 239–41.

[23] See text to nn. 100–33 below.

[24] See Ch. 3 above, text to nn. 91–115.

[25] *PHP* V.238–9, 2.4.45–9 De Lacy. Tieleman 2002: 264–5, 269–70, which also refers to *PHP* V.234–5, 2.4.33 De Lacy, where certain affections (or emotions, *pathē*) are linked

As Tieleman also notes, the idea that feelings as well as reasoning were functions of the brain had appeared earlier in Greek thought, notably in Hippocrates' *On the Sacred Disease* (chs. 14, 17) and in Galen's predecessors in medical research on the brain, Herophilus and Erasistratus.[26] So it would have been conceptually possible, in the context of ancient thought, for Galen to have adopted something more like the Stoic idea that both emotions and reasoning are based in a single centre. It does not follow, of course, that Galen would also have adopted this view in the highly unified form it takes in Stoicism, in which emotions are understood as directly informed by reason, an idea similar to modern 'cognitive' theories of emotion. Modern theorists of emotion, while assuming that emotions are based in the brain, do not necessarily also adopt a Stoic-style cognitive theory of emotion.[27] But a more constructive and less polemical response to the Stoic theory might have led Galen to question, at least, his three-centre psychophysiological model, and to think more positively about the idea of locating emotions in a unitary control-centre.

The last point, in particular, gives force to the question why Galen adopts a Platonic view on psychology in *PHP* and assumes that the Platonic view gives a more plausible account of human nature than the Stoic one. Galen is sometimes supposed to have had at least a broad philosophical affiliation to Plato; and it is certainly true, as noted earlier, that he gives a special status to Plato among philosophers, just as he gives a unique authority to Hippocrates among doctors. But this point needs to be taken together with Galen's consistent intellectual independence; although he forms alliances with various earlier thinkers in different contexts, the underlying medical–philosophical programme is very much Galen's own.[28] Although Galen adopts some views on psychology that seem to be

with 'forced' inhalation that is presented as dependent on the nerves, and thus the brain.

[26] See further Solmsen 1961: 155, also 196–7 (on Herophilus and Erasistratus), and von Staden 1989: 249. Mansfeld 1991: 125 suggests that the presence of this idea in the Hippocratic work may explain why Galen claims it is not an authentic work.

[27] The two issues are distinct, though they can be linked e.g. by theories about the workings of different parts of the brain and nervous system. See 6.2 below.

[28] On this point, see Ch. 2 above, text to nn. 30–47.

common in first- and second-century Platonism,[29] he is not a typical Middle Platonist in the issues he addresses or the positions he adopts, as Riccardo Chiaradonna (2009) has recently shown. As we have already seen, Galen is capable of embracing Stoic ideas where they match his agenda and also of dissociating himself from sides of Plato's thought that he finds uncongenial.[30] So the question remains an urgent one: what makes Platonic psychology so compelling to him, rather than Stoic ideas—in spite of the problems this raises for the coherence of this overall theory in *PHP* 1–6 (underlined in 3.2–3 above)?

If we focus on *PHP* 1–6 as a whole, especially the debate about the ruling part of the psyche in Books 1–3, 6, the answer is relatively clear. What Galen surely values above all is the support Plato gives in the *Timaeus* to the idea that the ruling (for Plato, the rational) part of the psyche is located in the head rather than the heart. In assessing the importance of this point for Galen, we need to recognize the general tendency in post-Hellenistic philosophy (that is, the period from the first century BC to the second century AD) to seek support for one's own position by reference to the authority of earlier, sometimes much earlier, thinkers. Also, although there was no real consensus on this question in previous philosophy, several highly influential theories, including the Aristotelian, Stoic, and Epicurean, continued to favour the heart as the seat of the control-centre. A robust restatement of the case for a heart-centred psychological picture was made shortly after Galen's time by the important Aristotelian thinker, Alexander of Aphrodisias.[31] Galen's brain-centred view was, as he makes plain, based on independent anatomical work, developing the observation-based findings of Herophilus and Erasistratus. Galen appeals to the outcome of empirically based natural inquiry, which in modern thought (in the form of scientific method) is seen as having a unique kind of authority. But this kind of appeal was much more innovative and debatable in the second century AD, even though Galen's formulation and presentation of his

[29] See text to n. 33 below.

[30] Both moves are made in *QAM*, for instance: see 3.5 above.

[31] Alex. Aphr. *De An.* pp. 94.7–100.17 Bruns, e.g. 94.17–20, cf. Arist. *GA* 2.4, 740[a]18–23. See further Tieleman 1996: xxvi and 73–6.

logico-empirical method was an important move in that direction. The support of a famous and influential early philosopher was just as important for giving credibility to one's claims, especially when, as in this case, most of the main philosophical schools supported a competing view. This factor, above all, must explain Galen's enthusiastic adoption of Plato's tripartite psychology, especially as presented as *Timaeus* 69–72, and the attempt to merge this with the ideas of 'Hippocrates', which are in substance, Galen's own ideas about anatomy and physiology.

On the face of it, all Galen really needed from Plato was support in locating the directing part of the psyche in the head; but in practice, he takes over much more of Plato's psychology, from the *Republic* as well as the *Timaeus.* As emphasized in 3.2–3 above, this merger led to some serious incongruities in Galen's theory, especially the tension between his brain-centred anatomical account and the Platonic idea of three separate physical centres of psychological agency. A further awkwardness, underlying *PHP* 1–3, is that Galen's brain-based 'ruling part' (*hēgemonikon*) is, as in most earlier medical thought, the centre of sensation and action, whereas Plato's head is the location of the 'rational part' (*logistikon*), whose functions only partly overlap with Galen's 'ruling part'.[32] None the less, having adopted the Platonic tripartite account in *PHP* 1–3 (and 6), Galen continues to use this account as a reference point in *PHP* 4–5, in his critique of the Stoic psychology of emotion. Although Galen sees this debate as being, in one sense, a digression, he also sees it as a logical continuation of the argument against the heart-centred picture in *PHP* 1–3, and, so to speak, another battle that Galen had to win to shore up his brain-centred account. This is, probably, the main factor underlying Galen's uniformly negative and polemical response to the Stoic theory of emotions and psychological functions more generally in

[32] Galen shares the assumption, standard by his time, that the ruling part of the psyche (or *hēgemonikon*) is the seat of perception and volition (see Tieleman 2002: 260–2, referring to *PHP* V.220, 2.3.4–7 De Lacy, V.649–50, 8.1.2–4 De Lacy), whereas for Plato it is the locus of reasoning and knowledge (*R.* 436a, 441e, *Ti.* 71a1–3); common to both Plato and Galen is the idea that this part is the seat of agency and direction. This may reflect what Steel 2001 presents as a fundamental difference between Plato's essentially moral aim in his account of the human body in *Ti.* 69–72 and Galen's focus on empirically based natural inquiry.

PHP 4–5. His assumption seems to be that, if the Stoic unified psychological account was not removed from serious consideration, it could be used by one of Galen's opponents on some future occasion as an independent argument for the (unified) heart-based psychophysiology attacked with such vigour in *PHP* 1–3.

However, despite these links between the two debates, there are also some independent factors that may have intensified Galen's uniformly negative response to this aspect of Stoic psychology. By contrast with the debate on the location of the ruling part of the psyche, where Galen was relatively isolated, as regards philosophical allies, he might feel more strongly supported on the question of the psychology of emotion. Plutarch, in an essay that Galen presumably knew, had already mounted a vigorous attack on the Stoic theory. Plutarch uses as a counterweight against the Stoic unified psychology a part-based (bipartite or tripartite) psychology based on a combination of Platonic and Aristotelian strands in ethical psychology, a combination sometimes found elsewhere in post-Hellenistic Middle Platonic thought.[33] Galen, in *PHP* 4–5 adopts the same approach, thus supporting his view by an appeal to something resembling a philosophical consensus, in a way he cannot do in the case of the location of the ruling part of the psyche in *PHP* 1–3. Galen's attempt to drive a wedge between Chrysippus' position and that ascribed to the earlier Stoics Zeno and Cleanthes, as well as the later Stoic Posidonius, who is presented as re-adopting the Platonic view, represents an extension of this move. Also, as Tieleman suggests, the probable use by Galen, as by other post-Hellenistic thinkers, of doxographical (handbook) summaries of earlier positions in psychology accentuated this standpoint. Although such handbooks were, in principle, neutral and simply set out the main theses, in practice, Platonic and Aristotelian views tended to dominate the range of options. The Stoic position, with its radical unification of psychological functions in a single control-centre,

[33] On relevant features of Plutarch's *On Ethical Virtue* (*Mor.* 440 D–452 D), see Gill 2006: 219–38. Although there are no explicit references in Galen to this work, as far as I am aware, the general approach is so similar that it is reasonable to suppose Galen had read it. Galen alludes to Plutarch's ethical writings in *Indol.* (written later than *PHP* 4–5); see Boudon-Millot 2007*b*: 76, and Nutton 2009: 32 (on Galen's reading in general see Nutton 2009).

set against this philosophical background, seemed relatively exceptional and therefore an easier target for criticism.[34]

A further probable factor, though one whose effect is more difficult to assess precisely, is that on this topic, by contrast with the debate about psychological location in *PHP* 1–3 and 6, Galen does not actually have any independent contribution to make, based on his medical practice and natural inquiry. In effect, Galen is simply playing off one (already formulated) set of ideas against another. Galen's main contribution, as he might see it, is his introduction of greater logical rigour to the inquiry, a respect in which he sees himself as building on the path-breaking arguments of Plato for psychic parts in book 4 of the *Republic.*[35] Hence, Galen's criticism of Stoic psychology in *PHP* 4–5 is, typically, couched as logical analysis, designed to uncover inconsistencies and defective forms of classification in Chrysippus' account of emotion. This is a method that accentuates further the negative character of Galen's response to the Stoic theory, as brought out later. By contrast with *PHP* 2–3, we do not have the positive element of Galen's anatomically based account of psychophysiology—an account which could have been effectively combined with the Stoic psychology that Galen criticizes there, as argued earlier (3.2–3 above).

However, in fact, Galen's critique is not a merely logical one; for his arguments to work, he presupposes a certain kind of psychological framework. Galen's arguments assume the validity of a part-based, rather than unified, psychological model. More precisely, they assume that psychic parts constitute independent, and potentially conflicting, sources of motivation, an idea which Galen adopts from Plato's arguments in *Republic* book 4 in particular. On the Stoic side, by contrast, we have a strongly unified or holistic account, in several respects. The theory of emotions and emotional dispositions is couched, in part, in psychophysical terms that reflect the prevalent Stoic holism about psyche–body relations. A further, very marked, feature is the psychological holism, according to which, in adult humans, all psychological processes, including emotions, are seen

[34] See Tieleman 2003*a*: 34–9, 61–88; 2003*b*.

[35] On the relatively derivative character of Galen's thinking on ethical psychology, see also 5.2 below.

as reflecting the rationality that is a constitutive part of being a developed human being. A less obvious, but also important, dimension of Stoic thought about emotions is the linkage with their thinking about ethical development and related ideas about the character of the good (fully developed) person and the defective (incompletely developed) one. This reflects the standard Stoic view that only the wise person, the ideal outcome of ethical development, has a fully stable and coherent character and that all non-wise people are more or less incoherent in character. This aspect of their thinking, despite initial appearances, is consistent with their psychological and psychophysical holism. It also reflects holism of a different kind: holism about knowledge and the interconnections between branches of knowledge. The most prominent version of this type of holism is their conviction that, ideally or ultimately, the three main branches of knowledge (logic, ethics, and physics) constitute a unified whole, an idea I have elsewhere termed 'rich naturalism'.[36] But their belief in the unified character of knowledge is evident also in their thinking about emotion. Their ideas about ethics, for instance about the wise person as a norm, and about the psychology of action and character are thoroughly interconnected in a way that reflects their larger holistic approach to knowledge. It is the latter type of holism, together with the other types (holism about psychological and psychophysical unity) that does much to make Stoic thinking about emotion revisionist, when viewed in relation to previous theories, and also paradoxical, when viewed in relation to conventional thought on this topic.[37]

The distinction just drawn between the psychological frameworks assumed by Galen and Stoicism can usefully be characterized in terms of the contrast drawn in Chapter 1 between two different patterns of thinking, those of 'composition' and 'structure'. I restate the main features of the contrast here. Broadly stated, in the first pattern ('composition'), the focus is on the parts and in the other ('structure') it is on the whole. More precisely, the contrast is between seeing the whole as identical with, and defined by, the combination of its parts and seeing the whole as the primary locus of identity, to which the parts are subordinate. In the first pattern ('composition'),

[36] See Gill 2006: 145–66, 199–200.

[37] See text to nn. 100–33, 257–68 below.

the parts are identifiable independently of the whole, and in the second ('structure'), the parts are identifiable only in the context of the whole. In the first pattern, we can say that the whole *has* structure (understood as the combination of its parts), in the other, the whole *is* structure (which gives the parts their identity). In using this contrast I am redeploying ideas used by Verity Harte's study to analyse Plato's conception of the part–whole relationship.[38] Here too, especially in connection with one passage in *PHP* 5, I use the distinction to define competing Galenic and Stoic accounts of the part–whole relationship.[39] But I think the contrast can also serve as an effective way of defining the conceptual differences between their ways of thinking about emotions in *PHP* 4–5.

In introducing this contrast into the interpretation of the Galen–Stoicism debate on emotions, I am not suggesting that Galen or the Stoics necessarily formulated their positions in quite those terms. The 'structure–composition' contrast is designed as an interpretative or conceptual device to enable us (modern thinkers) to analyse more effectively the relationship between these two ancient patterns of thinking about emotion. However, I do think that the contrast serves to identify salient features that Galen and the Stoics would have recognized in their respective approaches. For instance, on Galen's side, the contrast underlines the crucial importance of his view that psychic parts constitute separate and potentially competing sources of motivation. Psychic harmony is therefore a matter of imposing order on elements that have their own independent character; the parts are prior to the whole in this sense. On the Stoic side, the contrast helps to underline the importance of their view that emotions are seen as an integral part of a unified process of motivation and that the occurrence of emotions reflects the overall (whole) character state of the person experiencing the emotion. The seemingly paradoxical Stoic ideas that emotions are beliefs and are informed by rationality and that emotions express an unstable or 'sick' character are aspects of this view. In other words, for Stoicism, although emotions form what are in one sense 'parts' of the overall psychological state of a person, it is the overall state (the whole) that

[38] See Ch. 1 above, text to n. 40; the summary given there is based on Harte 2002: 158–67, 267–81. [39] See 4.4 below, text to nn. 257–68.

is conceived as the prior entity and the emotion as a subordinate or derivative aspect of this whole.

If I am right to suggest that the contrast between 'composition' and 'structure' approaches can serve to define salient features of the Galenic and Stoic ways of thinking about emotions, the question arises of how these patterns emerged. In a previous study of ethical psychology in Hellenistic and Roman thought, I suggested that the contrast between holistic and part-based psychological theories was useful for differentiating the approaches between Stoic (and Epicurean) theory, on the one hand, and (at least some) Middle Platonic theory on the other. The Middle Platonic pattern reflected certain prevalent patterns in Plato and Aristotle, although different strands in both Platonic and Aristotelian thought offered ideas that seem to have shaped both the competing later ancient approaches (that is, the holistic and part-based ones).[40] I also suggested that the contrast between unified or holistic and part-based psychological theories became articulated in a more explicit and self-conscious way as an issue of intellectual controversy in the course of the Hellenistic and post-Hellenistic periods. Hence by the first and second centuries AD, we find in Plutarch's essay *On Ethical Virtue* and Books 4–5 of Galen's *PHP* full-scale debates on this topic, of a kind that are not found in earlier thought.[41] The contrast drawn here between 'structure' and 'composition' approaches is a more theoretically formulated version of the contrast that is central to my earlier study, between holistic and part-based conceptions of psychology. In terms of the history of ideas, my suggestion is that Galen's sustained critique of the Stoic theory of emotion, together with the contrast between approaches embodied in that critique, reflects a progressively emerging conceptual dichotomy, with Plutarch as a key predecessor and, presumably, influence.

However, this analysis raises a further important question: how far does this contrast in conceptual approaches reflect the predominant patterns to be found in the Stoic and Galenic theories, particularly as so far discussed in this book? Should we say that, in general, Stoic thought reflects a holistic ('structure') approach

[40] See Gill 2006: ch. 1, esp. pp. 3–29; also Ch. 1 above, text to nn. 37–9.

[41] See Gill 2006: 207–19.

and Galenic thought a part-based ('composition') one; or is the contrast in thinking confined to this one area, that of the psychology of emotions? As far as Stoicism goes, as suggested in Chapter 1, their approach can reasonably be analysed as the systematic expression of a 'structure' or holistic approach. In a number of aspects of their theory, they take the whole as the primary element and conceive parts in relation to the whole. This holds good, for instance, for their thinking about the status and nature of the psyche both as a fundamentally embodied entity (a psychophysical whole) and as a coherent nexus of (embodied) functions, which, in adult humans, are informed by reason.[42] Other aspects of their theory that can usefully be interpreted in these terms include their thinking about the *scala naturae* (the spectrum of natural kinds), in which all entities in the universe, and not simply living creatures, are conceived in terms of the operation of *pneuma* or active and passive causes or as modalities of 'tension'.[43] A further relevant dimension, already noted, is their view that knowledge as a whole, characterized as a combination of logic, ethics, and physics, ideally constitutes a unified or structured synthesis and whole.[44] The revisionism, which I have noted as a characteristic feature of their thought, is partly bound up with their thinking about the integrated nature of knowledge. What underlies—and to some extent justifies—their innovative theses in any one area, or on topics that span different areas—is the claim that the thesis is, or could be, supported by the integration of knowledge of different kinds.[45] Thus, in a series of ways, their thinking in general can be seen as consistently expressing a 'structure', by contrast with 'composition', approach, and their views on the psychology of emotions constitute just one expression of this tendency.

[42] See Ch. 2 above, text to nn. 71–6, Ch. 3 above, text to nn. 38–44; also 4.2 below.

[43] See Ch. 2 above, text to nn. 206–12.

[44] See LS 26, esp. B (=D.L. 7.39–41). The complete understanding of this whole body of knowledge is only achieved by the ideal wise person (LS 26 F (=Sen. *Ep.* 88.25–8), cf. LS 41), but it remains a valid target for human aspiration.

[45] Stoic revisionism is compatible with the belief that all human beings are constitutively capable of forming valid or true 'preconceptions' (*prolēpseis*); see LS 40, esp. N, R–T, also, on related ideas implied in the Stoic methodology of inquiry, Ch. 2, above, text to nn. 141–8.

Where does Galen stand in this respect? As indicated earlier, the position is more mixed or ambiguous in his case;[46] and the discussion of Chapters 2–3, as well as the subsequent treatment in this chapter, illustrates this point. In *PHP* 1–6, especially 2–5, his disagreement with the Stoics can be seen as centring on the question whether the psyche is conceived, primarily, as a whole to which the parts are essentially subordinate or as a collection of separate and independent parts whose interrelations determine the character of the whole. This point applies to Galen's thesis in *PHP* 1–3 that the three main psychological functions are housed in spatially separate locations, which serve as the locus of distinct and independent psychophysiological systems, those of nerves, arteries, and veins. It also applies to his assumption in *PHP* 4–5 that reason, anger, and appetite constitute independent and potentially conflicting sources of motivation, by contrast with the Stoic thesis that they function in a fundamentally integrated or unified way. A particularly illuminating section of *PHP* 5, examined in 4.4 below, centres on the question whether the Stoics (especially Chrysippus) are entitled to use the notion of psychic *parts* at all, given their unified account of the psyche. So in *PHP* 2–5, especially 4–5, as suggested earlier, it seems plausible to see Galen's dispute with the Stoics as expressing the clash between two profoundly different conceptual frameworks, with divergent conceptions of the part–whole relationship.

On the other hand, other aspects of Galenic thinking seem to express a more holistic approach that is much more akin to that of Stoicism. Galen's anatomical theory, centred on the brain and nervous system, if stripped of the linkage with the Platonic tripartite model, presents animal psychophysiology as constituting a unified structure, in which the parts make sense in terms of the whole unit (3.3 above). His view of the natural world, as uniformly shaped by design—an idea he actually pushes further than any previous thinker—seems to reflect a similarly holistic outlook.[47] Similarly, his account of natural entities as consisting, ultimately, of compounds or mixtures of the four elemental qualities implies a similar

[46] See Ch. 1 above, text to nn. 48–50.
[47] See Ch. 2 above, text to nn. 157–62.

approach.[48] Galen deploys a single *scala naturae* running from basic to advanced forms of natural and psychological function.[49] He also aims at offering an account of knowledge that is both extraordinarily comprehensive in certain ways and is also closely integrated, with a single overall objective, that of providing the most effective form of medical practice.[50] All these features of his thought and work seem to express an outlook that is fundamentally unified and holistic.

Does Galen go as far as the Stoics in achieving, or aiming at, a unified or holistic outlook, in these areas at least? In some cases, this does seem to be so, if we set aside other variations in the way the two theories approach similar topics. For instance, as just noted, Galen's teleological approach is applied in an exceptionally uniform and systematic way to natural entities, especially the animal body.[51] Similarly, his analysis of the material basis of matter in terms of mixtures of the four elements is applied in a way that is—virtually at least—as complete and systematic as we find in Stoicism.[52] Admittedly, in considering earlier their respective accounts of the philosophy of nature, I noted some respects in which the Stoic version is yet more unified, and, similarly, more revisionist of previous or accepted ideas. For instance, the Stoic version of the *scala naturae*, centred on the operation of *pneuma* and modalities of 'tension', embraces *all* entities, not simply natural ones, as well as extending to forms of rationality.[53] The Stoic conception of the unity of knowledge is both more systematic, both as regards the broad mapping of the spheres of philosophy (in terms of logic, ethics, and physics) and as regards the—at least ideal—outcome of their integration.[54] Also, the achievement of a systematic framework of

[48] See Ch. 2 above, text to nn. 163–9.

[49] See Kovačić 2001: 195–209.

[50] His treatises (extant and lost) embraced virtually all aspects of ancient medicine (including much natural inquiry), e.g. anatomy, physiology, pharmacology, dietetics, therapeutics, as well as logic and (practical) ethics; see Galen's own résumé in *Libr. Prop.*, trans. Singer 1997*a*: 3–22. On the overall practical objective, see M. Frede 2003: 77–9.

[51] See Ch. 2 above, text to nn. 157–62.

[52] On one reservation, whether there is a total mixture of the elements (as the Stoics maintained) or only mixture in the qualities (as Aristotle thought), see Ch. 2 above, text to nn. 202–5. This might be thought to express a marginally less unified or holistic conception of the material world than that supposed by the Stoics.

[53] See Ch. 2 above, text to nn. 197–205.

[54] See nn. 44–5 above.

theoretical understanding, without gaps or reservations, is a central objective for the Stoics, whereas Galen, as noted earlier, refrains from tackling some fundamental theoretical questions.[55] Even so, if we leave aside questions of psychology, especially as formulated in *PHP*, there are grounds for attributing to Galen, as well as the Stoics, a broadly holistic or unifying approach in a number of analogous areas, even if Galen does not push this approach as far as the Stoics do.[56]

This raises in another way the question why Galen's standpoint in psychology seems to have a different character in *PHP* 1–6 and especially in *PHP* 4–5. In 1–6 taken as a whole, as already emphasized (3.3 above), we can at least see a tension between a unified anatomical picture, centred on the brain and nervous system, and the Platonic-style part-based psychological model. But in *PHP* 4–5, the debate focuses exclusively on the contrast between the unified Stoic (especially Chrysippean) psychological model and the part-based one. If Galen does not, typically or systematically, apply a 'composition' approach, why is this approach so prominent in *PHP* 4–5? Should we suppose that there is some feature of this topic, or of the way Galen interprets it, that makes this standpoint seem more appropriate in this case than others? As suggested earlier, one factor may be the influence of Middle Platonist patterns of thought, as exemplified most clearly by Plutarch, and of the conceptual contrast embodied in the ongoing controversy between Platonic–Aristotelian (part-based) and Stoic (holistic) conceptions of emotion and psychological functions generally. However, the question still remains: why does Galen's approach reflect this influence so strongly here, in a way that produces a more pronounced pattern of part-based ('composition') thinking than is evident elsewhere in his writings?

Although Galen's motives, in the absence of an explicit statement on his part, must remain to some extent conjectural, I think we can construct a plausible line of explanation, based largely on points

[55] See also Ch. 2 above, text to n. 4, Ch. 3 above, text to nn. 208–14.

[56] M. Frede 2003: 77–81, argues that physics, understood as a theoretical analysis of the principles of nature, is absent from Galen's programme of inquiry, reflecting his fundamentally practical objectives. If so, this marks a rather important gap in the kind of unified knowledge he aspires towards.

made already. As suggested earlier, Galen's uniformly negative view of the Stoic theory of emotion seems to reflect the linkage that he sees between this question and that of the location of the ruling part of the psyche. He believes that the Stoic theory needs to be removed from serious consideration to prevent its being used in support of the heart-centred theory that he has worked so hard to undermine in *PHP* 1–3. By contrast with *PHP* 1–3, where he is able to offer arguments based on his independent anatomical work and the methodology he has evolved for this purpose, Galen has to rely on the ideas of others, in particular, Plato's tripartite account and, more broadly, Platonic–Aristotelian psychological theory. He also needs to interpret his competing part-based model in a way that differentiates it sharply from the Stoic unified account. Hence, he adopts and accentuates the conceptual contrast already embodied in the post-Hellenistic debate about emotions, as illustrated by Plutarch, for instance, in order to sharpen his opposition to the Stoic theory. The resulting debate, in *PHP* 4–5 thus represents a starker version of the contrast between 'structure' and 'composition' approaches than we find elsewhere in Galen's works, even in *PHP* 2–3, where there are competing dimensions in Galen's psychophysiology. This stark conceptual conflict is the product of Galen's need—as he sees it—to find a counterweight to the Chrysippean holistic psychological account. The starkness of the contrast in this context does not reflect Galen's thinking elsewhere, which is, typically at least, more holistic. Rather, it reflects Galen's chosen strategy, in this context, of bringing out the inadequacy of the Stoic psychological theory. In other words, the sharpness of the conceptual contrast expresses the needs of Galen's dialectical debate with Stoicism, at this stage of the argument of *PHP*, rather than a more prevalent conceptual divide between Galenic and Stoic thought.

In the rest of this chapter, I examine Galen's critique of Stoic thinking in *PHP* 4–5 in the light of this hypothesis. I begin by examining the kinds of criticism he makes of the Stoic theory of emotions (4.2). His criticisms, mainly directed at the methodology of the Stoic approach are consistently negative and polemical in tone. Their effectiveness as criticism depends on accepting Galen's (part-based or 'composition') psychological assumptions. I offer a more sympathetic account of the features of Stoic theory that Galen criticizes. Although there are substantive differences of approach from Galen's assumed framework (the Stoic framework is consistently holistic or 'structure'-based), the Stoic theory emerges as a powerful alternative account of emotion and not the botched or implausible theory that Galen presents. Subsequently (4.3), I examine more closely the psychological assumptions that inform Galen's critique. These emerge indirectly, from Galen's reading of Plato's argument for separate parts of the psyche in book 4 of the *Republic*, and from his comments on Posidonius' ideas about ethical development, which he presents (I think, misleadingly) as constituting a rejection of Chrysippean theory by the later Stoic thinker. These discussions enable us to form a view of Galen's psychological framework, which represents a version of the Platonic–Aristotelian part-based one, with clear points of contrast from the Stoic holistic account. Finally (4.4), I examine Galen's discussion in *PHP* of the sense in which Chrysippus is entitled, given his unified psychological theory, to use the notion of psychic parts at all. This discussion enables us to pinpoint the key differences between the Galenic and Stoic psychological approaches and also to show how this embodies a contrast between two ways of understanding the part–whole relationship, those associated here with the contrast between 'composition' and 'structure' approaches.

4.2 GALEN'S CRITIQUE OF STOIC EMOTIONS

In this section, I consider salient features of Galen's critique of the Stoic theory of emotions in *PHP* 4–5. I also offer what seems to me a more credible account of the aspects of Stoic thinking criticized by Galen. My concern, in this context, is not just with trying to recover from Galen's evidence a more plausible picture of Stoic theory than Galen himself offers[57]—though this is part of what I want to do. I want to bring out the differences between Galen's psychological assumptions and those of Stoicism and to gauge how deep these

[57] This is my main aim in Gill 2006: 244–90; see also Tieleman 2003*a*.

differences go. Also, I consider whether, along with the obvious differences, there are common features that could have been developed, along with other, actual or potential, shared features, to construct a shared naturalistic conception of psychology.[58] Thus, I want to get behind Galen's explicit critique—which is intense, sustained, and consistently negative—to a more illuminating and considered view of the relationship between the two theories in this area. In fact, the scope for common ground between the two theories on this topic is markedly less than on other aspects of their thinking. I have already suggested why this is the case (by reference to Galen's dialectical objectives in *PHP* as a whole),[59] and I return to this question in the final section.[60] In this way, I continue my exploration of the paradox highlighted in Chapter 1 above, that Galen is so consistently negative, especially in *PHP* 4–5, about the psychological ideas of a theory with whose naturalistic approach he has much in common.

For anyone trying to form a fair-minded and reflective view of the relationship between Galenic and Stoic thinking on psychology, Galen's critique offers rather frustrating material. Much of his response, especially in Book 4, consists of a highly polemical attack on Chrysippus' theory of emotion. This often takes the form of maintaining that Chrysippus' theory is inconsistent on important points either with itself or with other Stoic theories, notably that of Zeno or Posidonius. As brought out shortly, this critique is, in my view, very misleading both in its claims about Chrysippus' self-contradictions and about the alleged inconsistencies with other Stoics. However, what underlies these charges is, I think, a specific line of criticism on Galen's part. The underlying objection, as suggested earlier, is that Chrysippus' theory offers a very *unnatural* and implausible account of human psychology, and that the unnatural character of the theory leads him into insoluble problems and contradictions. Although this type of critique of Stoic theory is not without parallels in both ancient and modern thought,[61] it is, I think, unjustified. The Stoic theory is no more unnatural in its

[58] See text to nn. 110–15, 155–7 below.

[59] See 4.1 above, esp. p. 188.

[60] See esp. text to nn. 268–9 below.

[61] For some partly parallel criticisms by Antiochus and Plutarch, see Gill 2006: 168–9, 225–7; also, among recent treatments, see Sorabji 2000: chs. 1–2.

picture of human psychology than Galen's preferred approach. Though different in crucial respects from Galen's picture, it offers an account we can appropriately describe as 'naturalistic'. Indeed, as suggested later, we can see indications in the theory of some of the types of naturalism that are at least partly shared with Galen, namely certain aspects of what I am calling 'high naturalism', also a physicalist approach to psychology, and a causal analysis similar to that incorporated by Galen into his medical methodology.[62]

What is Galen's competing psychological framework, and how far does this explain his negative response? And what are the really important differences between the two approaches, if we dig beneath the surface of Galen's polemics? Galen's mode of presentation does not make it altogether easy to answer these questions, because he focuses on the alleged defects of Chrysippus' account, especially in *PHP* 4, and he does not offer an analytic account of his own assumptions. But salient differences emerge in *PHP* 5, in Galen's discussion of Plato's arguments for separate psychic parts, as well as his treatment of ethical development, and, in particular, psychic parts and wholes.[63] In many respects, the difference can be characterized as that between a theory that focuses on the role of distinct psychic parts, especially on the difference between rational and non-rational parts, and one that focuses on psychic wholes. The difference can be more precisely defined, as indicated earlier, by using the distinction between 'composition' and 'structure' conceptions of the part–whole relationship.[64] Indeed, the contrast between the Galenic and Stoic standpoints is a striking example of a type of contrast (between part-based and holistic psychological theories) that is recurrent, in different forms, in ancient thought, and that has some important analogues in modern thought.[65] But also, as brought out later, the Stoic theory combines radical holism, of various kinds, with certain strongly revisionist features. These features derive especially from their theory about the final stages of ethical development and from related ideas about the contrast between the psychological coherence of the wise person and the incoherence and instability of non-wise

[62] See text to nn. 90–3, 97–100 below. [63] See 4.3–4 below.

[64] See Ch. 1 above, text to n. 40, and nn. 257–68 below.

[65] On some parallels with modern thought, see Ch. 6 below. See also (on ancient part-based and holistic psychological theories), Gill 2006: ch. 4.

people.[66] These features are, certainly, controversial, and are in some ways more obvious targets for criticisms than the grounds on which Galen does actually attack the theory. Perhaps a reaction against these strongly revisionist features *does* underlie Galen's criticism, though, if so, he fails to discuss them in analytic form or to mount an effective challenge to them. But these revisionist features are important both in their own right and because they underlie Stoic thinking on emotions and on the relationship between psychological and physical sickness.[67]

A typical move made by Galen in his critique of the Stoic theory, especially in *PHP* 4, is to maintain that Chrysippus' presentation is undermined by the failure to observe some elementary logical or categorical distinctions. Galen's claims often seem rather inadequately argued or even arbitrary; and, indeed, I think, they are not convincing unless we combine them with certain assumptions about what constitutes a valid psychological framework—that is, one that involves both rational and non-rational parts. For instance, early in Book 4, Galen argues that Chrysippus' analysis of emotion fails to observe an important basic 'division' (*diairesis*) or distinction: 'An emotion such as love is either a judgement or supervenes on judgements or is a runaway movement of the appetitive faculty. Similarly, bitter anger is also either a judgement or some irrational emotion following on this judgement or a violent movement of the spirited faculty.'[68] Galen seems to imply that there is some formal or classificatory principle requiring that an emotion should be defined as (only) one of these notions.[69] However, his objection is really to the idea of combining (1) judgement with either (2) supervening reaction or (3) violent or runaway movement. Hence, he presents Chrysippus as contradicting himself because he defines emotion at one point as a belief (that something bad is present or expected) and at another point as a reaction that supervenes on judgement (for instance, 'a shrinking at what is thought to be a thing to avoid').

[66] See text to nn. 115–33 below.

[67] See text to nn. 146–54 below, and Ch. 5 below, text to nn. 267–81.

[68] *PHP* V.365, 4.1.16, p. 238.15–19 De Lacy, trans. De Lacy, modified.

[69] *PHP* V.366, 4.1.17, p. 238.19–20 De Lacy, trans. De Lacy: 'But although the question admits of being divided three ways, he [Chrysippus] does not handle the argument thus.'

He also sees a contradiction between defining emotion as a belief and as a runaway or violent movement, which he presents as being that of an irrational faculty.[70] The implication is that there is some logical or categorical contradiction involved; but the contradiction depends on a Galenic assumption, which is clearly implied in the context. The assumption is that psychological states must be either (1) functions of a rational faculty, such as beliefs or (2) functions of an irrational faculty, such as affective reactions. A correlated assumption is that the psyche consists of parts, either two or three, that have only one type of function, rational or irrational. In fact, as Galen must have known, Chrysippus and other Stoics offer definitions of emotion that combine all three kinds of psychological phenomenon. They do this, on the premise that the psyche functions as a whole, and that all the psychological states of adult humans are informed by rationality.[71] Galen wants to reject this picture; but he does so, not by analytic argument about the merits and disadvantages of his theory and the Stoic one, but by maintaining that the Stoic version is inconsistent—meaning, actually, inconsistent with his preferred picture.

Galen responds in a similar way to Chrysippus' attempt to specify the kind of irrationality involved in an emotion.[72] His criticism is directed at passages such as the following, which Galen cites from Chrysippus:

> Therefore some people say not inappropriately that an emotion of the psyche is a movement contrary to nature, as in fear and desire and the like. All such movements and states are disobedient to reason and reject it: accordingly we say that such persons are moved irrationally (*alogōs*), not in the sense of reasoning poorly, as one might speak of someone who reasons the opposite of well, but in the sense of the rejection of reason (*tou logou apostrophē*).[73]

[70] *PHP* V.366–7, 4.2.1–7, De Lacy, esp. p. 240.4, cited, trans. De Lacy. See also V.361–5, 4.1.5–14 De Lacy: Chrysippus' citation of Homeric lines describing emotions (and placing emotions in the breast) in *On the Psyche* is presented as implying that Chrysippus adopts the Platonic tripartite psyche, whereas in *On Passions* (Galen alleges) Chrysippus rejects the Platonic theory while still sometimes saying things that imply it.

[71] See further text to nn. 100–6 below.

[72] The following paragraph is a modified version of Gill 2006: 250.

[73] *PHP* V.385, 4.4.16–17, p. 254.13–19 De Lacy, trans. De Lacy, slightly modified.

Galen suggests that Chrysippus, here and elsewhere, is drawing a distinction between the kind of irrationality involved in emotion and that involved in other kinds of error in reasoning or ethical mistake (*hamartēma*).[74] But Galen claims that Chrysippus is unable to define this category effectively, because of his failure to recognize the existence of functions of a non-rational part of the psyche. Galen argues that there are two—and not more than two—possible senses of 'irrational' (*alogon*) in Greek. These are (1): the defective use (*kakōsis*) of rationality and (2) the complete absence (*sterēsis*) of rationality. He then argues that if a mistake constitutes the defective use of rationality, the only sense left for emotion is that of the complete absence of rationality. But, he points out, this sense is ruled out by Chrysippus' key claim that emotions, which occur only in adult humans, are judgements (*kriseis*) and do not arise in a non-rational part of the psyche, because there is no such part. He concludes that Chrysippus' attempt to define the kind of irrationality involved in emotion, by contrast with other kinds of mistake, is a failure. But this conclusion only holds good if you assume the falsity of Chrysippus' assumption that emotions involve rationality of some sort. If you allow this assumption, emotions can be seen as the defective use (*kakōsis*) of rationality, but different in kind from other types of error or mistake. In other words, Galen's argument only works if you assume the validity of a specific type of psychological framework, namely one containing a non-rational part. One may also wonder what the basis is for Galen's claim about the possible senses of 'irrational'; why are these two senses the only possible ones? One may also question whether this twofold distinction leaves room for the kinds of irrationality found in a part-based psychological framework, of the type Galen favours. For instance, should we describe the struggle of appetite against reason in Plato's arguments in *Republic* 435–41 as either the defective use of rationality or its complete absence? Neither description seems really

[74] This formulation for the distinction seems to be Galen's own (cf. Hankinson 1993: 189–90, 192–7), but used to analyse Chrysippus' attempt to define the specific kind of irrationality involved in emotion. See e.g. V.369, 4.2.12, p. 240.26–7 De Lacy (discussed by Galen in V.371–2, 4.2.24–7 De Lacy), V.385, 4.4.17, p. 254.17–19 (discussed by Galen in V.386–7, 4.4.23 De Lacy).

adequate.[75] Again, Galen is attacking the Stoic theory in terms of logical or classificatory principles, and ones of doubtful validity, instead of arguing in general terms about the merits of different kinds of psychological theory.

A related move made by Galen is to maintain that Chrysippus' theory is inconsistent with that of other Stoic theorists, namely Zeno and—especially—the later Stoic Posidonius.[76] The inconsistency arises, Galen maintains, because these other Stoics, unlike Chrysippus, acknowledge the fact that emotions are non-rational and are functions of a non-rational part of the psyche. As far as Zeno is concerned, the alleged difference is that 'Chrysippus thought that the emotions *actually were* the judgements . . . whereas Zeno and many other Stoics thought the emotions occurred on the occasion of (*epi*) judgements, but (in the case of distress and pleasure at least) *actually were* the contractions and expansions', that is the 'impulses' that follow from the judgements.[77] As regards Posidonius, Galen's claims are much more extensive, detailed, and emphatic. He maintains that the later Stoic explicitly rejected the unitary psychological model altogether and adopted Plato's tripartite picture, except that he saw the psychic parts as functions of a single control-centre.[78] Galen's intention is to suggest that the Chrysippean belief-based account of emotions is isolated even within the Stoic school, thereby underlining its (allegedly) implausible and unnatural account of human psychology.

This move, like the complaints about Chrysippus' failure in classification, is highly questionable. As regards the relationship with Zeno's theory, recent scholarship tends to view Galen's claims with scepticism. After a thorough review of the available evidence, Anthony Price concludes that there was, at most, only 'a fine point of

[75] If appetite is defined as non-rational (different from reason), its struggle cannot be the defective use of reason; but the ability of appetite to compete with reason seems to imply some degree of rationality. On Plato's argument and its implications, see Gill 2006: 310–13, also text to nn. 161–84 below.

[76] Posidonius (*c.*135–*c.*50 BC), was a pupil of the last head of the Stoic school, Panaetius, and a leading Stoic thinker and writer.

[77] The formulation of Galen's views is taken from Sorabji 2000: 34–5, referring to *PHP* V.367, 377, 429. 4.2.5–6, 4.3.1–2, 5.1.4 De Lacy.

[78] See e.g. *PHP* V.429–30, 5.1.4–7 De Lacy, V.454–5, 5.4.2–3 De Lacy, cited in Ch. 3 above, text to n. 67.

divergence between the two thinkers: Zeno might have identified opinions with causal complexes wherein contractions and the like follow upon opinions, whereas Chrysippus might have thought that opinion of a kind constitutes emotion even before it causes (even if it always *does* cause) contraction or the like'.[79] In standard Stoic definitions of emotion, we find a combination of (and a close causal link between) belief and motivational response (*hormē*) with no indication that this represented an area of controversy or divergence within the school.[80] As Tieleman points out, at the end of his account of Stoic thinking on emotion, Galen presents it as an open question exactly what view Zeno held about this question—despite his confident assertions earlier. It seems, to judge from Galen's normal reading practice, as far as we can establish this, that he has probably not consulted Zeno's treatise *On Passions* at all, and is relying on inferences that he draws from what is said by Chrysippus and Posidonius about his views.[81] Given these points, it seems that Galen's attempt to drive a wedge between Zeno and Chrysippus on this point is just a debating tactic, designed to reinforce the supposed implausibility of Chrysippus' theory.

The case of Posidonius is more complex. Galen's argument on this topic is more specific, reiterated, and is supported by extensive quotations and summary of his treatise. Indeed, it has been normal until recently to accept Galen as an accurate reporter of Posidonius' theory of emotions.[82] However, here too there are grounds for strong scepticism about the reliability of Galen's account. The issues are quite complex, and have been fully examined in some recent treatments;[83] I outline here some salient points. Galen is, in fact, the only ancient source that maintains that Posidonius rejected the standard

[79] Price 2005: 473–4; for similar views, see Inwood 1985: 130–1, Inwood and Donini 1999: 699, Graver 2007: 28–34. However, Sorabji 2000: 34–6 accepts that Galen's report is broadly accurate. [80] See text to nn. 100–4 below.

[81] *PHP* V. 477–8, 5.6.40–2 De Lacy. See Tieleman 2003*a*: 85–6, also 48–9 on Galen's apparent reading practice as regards Stoic treatises. Chrysippus and Posidonius seem to have followed the usual practice in Stoic treatises in starting from discussions of Zeno's definitions on the relevant subject.

[82] See e.g. Kidd 1971, 1988, 553–625, and LS, vol. 1: 421–3; also Sorabji 2000: 93–108.

[83] See Fillion-Lahille 1984, part 3, chs. 1–3, Cooper 1998, Tieleman 2003*a*: ch. 5; also Gill 1998: 124–30, 2006: 266–90.

Stoic (that is, Chrysippean) view and adopted a Platonic tripartite account of psychology. Galen himself records some evidence showing that Posidonius also thought that emotions in adult humans were based on beliefs.[84] The one securely attested innovation in Posidonius' theory is the idea of 'emotional (or affective) movements' (*pathētikai kinēseis*). This idea seems to be designed to identify and explain the motive force of non-rational affective impulses in non-human animals and human children and belief-based emotions in adult humans.[85] Though this idea is a new feature, at least in terminology, it may represent little more than an extension of Chrysippus' idea that emotions constitute a type of 'runaway' movement of the psyche and are like 'running legs'. That is, it may be another way of expressing the idea of psychological or psychophysical inertia, which is strongly marked in Chrysippus' thought.[86]

However, if (at least) some modern scholars see so little innovation in Posidonius' thought, what is the basis for Galen's assertions that Posidonius criticized Chrysippus heavily and that he adopted Plato's ideas about psychology? Tieleman addresses these questions with a thorough examination of Galen's presentation of Posidonius' comments and views, in the light of Galen's practice elsewhere in *PHP* 2–5. What he suggests is that Galen ignores or misrepresents the fact that Book 2 of Chrysippus' *On Passions* consisted of 'problems' (*aporiai*) about the detailed implications of the Stoic theory, dealing especially with cases where beliefs, or different types of belief, and impulses appear to come apart and offering solutions to these cases. Posidonius developed this theme, suggesting in some cases variations on these

[84] *PHP* V. 463, 5.5.21, p. 320.23–8 De Lacy; also [Plu.] *Whether Appetite and Desire Belong to the Soul or the Body*, ch. 6, Posid. fr. 154 in Edelstein and Kidd 1972/1989. See further Cooper 1998: 87–8, Tieleman 2003*a*: 231–42, 278–9, Gill 1998: 126–7, 2006: 269–73.

[85] See e.g. *PHP* V. 422, 425, 4.7.28, 37 De Lacy, V.429–30, 5.1.5, p. 293.23–5 De Lacy. In *PHP* V.463, 5.5.21, p. 320.25, 29 De Lacy, 'emotional movements' are combined with beliefs in causing emotions, thus counteracting Galen's claim that Posidonius' new idea replaced the belief-based analysis.

[86] See further Cooper 1998: 84–90 (also 94–9), who sees some modification of Chrysippus' theory, though Posidonius retains the core Stoic idea that emotions depend on beliefs; and Tieleman 2003*a*: 202–6, 231–42, 284–7, who sees at most terminological innovation in the idea of 'emotional movements'. See also Gill 1998: 124–8, 2006: 268–75. On 'runaway motion' in Chrysippus, see text to nn. 127–37 below.

explanations, which Galen presents as constituting a root-and-branch critique of Chrysippus' theory. However, the quotations that Galen actually provides do not bear out this picture of Posidonius' aims. A more plausible reading of these passages is that Posidonius is offering alternative ways of explaining these puzzles within the same belief-based theory of emotion.[87] What about Galen's claim that Posidonius adopted Platonic theories on psychology and development? On this point, Galen ignores a marked difference between the apparent practice among early Stoics, including Zeno and Chrysippus, and later (post-Hellenistic) Stoics, especially Panaetius and Posidonius. The early Stoics, though almost certainly influenced by earlier philosophers, including Plato, focused on setting out their own theories, for the most part without referring to those earlier thinkers. In the later Hellenistic period, along with the growth of a commentary tradition, Stoic thinkers, like those in other schools, such as Antiochus, discuss explicitly the relationship between their ideas and those of earlier thinkers, both in agreement and disagreement.[88] If we look at the comments on Plato reported by Galen, bearing this tendency in mind, it seems most likely that Posidonius is simply commenting explicitly on the relationship between Platonic and Stoic ideas, and may well be recruiting Platonic ideas in support of Stoic theory or translating them into Stoic form.[89] This would help to explain why Galen is alone in claiming that Posidonius made a radical break with earlier Stoic theory on emotion and adopted the Platonic approach instead. On this view, then, which I accept, Galen, whether misunderstanding or deliberately misrepresenting Posidonius' practice, offers a highly misleading picture of the relationship between Chrysippus' thinking and that of Posidonius,

[87] Tieleman 2003*a*: 250–64 (also 122–32), Gill 2006: 276–8; see e.g. *PHP* V.396–403, 4.5.19–46 De Lacy, V.416–26, 7.1–44 De Lacy. For a different reading of this evidence, following Galen in seeing a more serious critique of Chrysippus by Posidonius, Sorabji 2000: chs. 7–8.

[88] On this contrast, see M. Frede 1999*a*: 774–8, 783–4, Sedley 2003: 20–4, Gill 2006: 213–14, 281–2.

[89] See Tieleman 2003*a*: 206–30, also Gill 2006: 282–90; see e.g. *PHP* V.465–7, 5.5.30–5 De Lacy, V.469–70 5.6.4–8 De Lacy. A similar approach to Plato's theory is ascribed to Antipater, head of the Stoic school *c.*159–*c.*129 BC (Clement, *Stromateis* 5.97.6 =*SVF* 3.56); see Tieleman 2003*a*: 225.

with a view to undermining Chrysippus' belief-based analysis of emotion.

I now offer an alternative account of the features of Stoic thinking about emotions that Galen criticizes. I aim especially to explain the combination in their analysis of emotion of (1) belief, (2) impulse, and (3) 'irrational' response such as the 'rejection of reason'. I also seek to explain the sense in which an emotion can be seen as the 'defective use' (*kakōsis*) of rationality. My focus is on Chrysippus' theory, although I think that this is substantially shared with other Stoic thinkers. To make sense of these features of Stoic thought about emotion, we need to place them in a broader context, referring especially to their theory of ethical development. Closer examination of the Stoic theory brings out both (actual or potential) common features with Galenic thought and important differences of approach. The main common features are these. (1) The Stoic theory of development reflects key features of the 'high naturalism' shared by Galen and Stoicism. In particular, it reflects a strongly teleological picture of animal (including human) development. It also expresses a view of humans and other animals as unified or structured complexes of natural faculties.[90] (2) A second shared feature is the physicalist approach to psychology that is shared by Stoicism and Galen—up to a point at least—and which separates both theories from the psyche–body dualism in Plato and much later Platonism. This feature comes out in the strongly physical account of emotions, as temporary or occurrent states, and of longer term emotional states (or psychic illness).[91] (3) The Stoic theory also reflects the same type of causal analysis that we find in their theory of determinism, namely that based on the combination of an antecedent (external) cause and a 'sustaining' cause, which is 'internal' and which reflects the character of the agent. The judgement—more precisely, the two kinds of judgement—involved in an emotion constitute a response based on how something 'appears' at the relevant time (antecedent cause) and on the underlying character of the agent.[92] Galen adopts

[90] For these common features, see 2.3 above, and text to nn. 97–100 below.

[91] See 3.5 above; also text to nn. 111–15, 147–54 below.

[92] On this feature of the Stoic theory of emotion, see Tieleman 2003*a*: 108–13 (also 124–5 on the two kinds of judgement). On the Stoic theory of determinism, see Bobzien 1998, esp. ch. 6, and D. Frede 2003. See further text to nn. 101–4, 134–6, 155–7 below.

this general causal analysis, which forms a key part of his conception of sound medical practice.[93] Thus, despite Galen's overwhelmingly negative picture of the Stoic theory, there are some actual or potential shared elements in Galenic and Stoic thought on this topic. However, as suggested earlier, there are also substantial conceptual differences, deriving from the combination in Stoic theory of radical holism and revisionism. Their holism (or 'structure') approach is strongly at odds with Galen's part-based ('composition') approach to psychology, while their revisionism involves a rejection of ideas that are firmly embedded in the Platonic–Aristotelian framework that Galen assumes. I underline these features of the Stoic theory, which form an important part of the explanation for Galen's uniformly negative and unsympathetic response.

Before turning to the content of the Stoic theory, I summarize the treatise that Galen took as his main target in *PHP* 4–5, namely Chrysippus' *On Passions*, as reconstructed by Tieleman, in large measure from Galen's own evidence.[94] The treatise consisted of four books, of which the first three seem to have been theoretical in character, while the fourth ('therapeutic') book was more practical in its objectives, though still based firmly on Stoic theory.[95] The first book seems to have centred on Chrysippus' elaboration of Zeno's account of emotion or passion (*pathos*), especially the definition of the four basic emotions (pleasure, appetite or desire, distress or grief, and fear) and subdivisions of these. Although it seems clear that the idea that emotions involve judgements was fundamental for both Zeno and Chrysippus,[96] both thinkers also stressed that emotions constituted psychophysical reactions, such as contractions or expansions of *pneuma* in the control-centre, which were correlated with judgements. Book 2 seems to have consisted of discussion of 'problems' (*aporiai*), including the question how to explain cases when the two types of judgement associated with emotion apparently come apart from each other or from the usual psychophysical reactions. Another topic that seems to have been treated here is the source of

[93] See Ch. 2 above, text to nn. 111–16, 122–4.

[94] This paragraph is based on Gill 2006: 245. For an outline of topics in Chrysippus' treatise and the sources on which these are based, see Tieleman 2003*a*: 325–6.

[95] On book 4, see Tieleman 2003*a*: ch. 4 and 5.3 below.

[96] See text to nn. 79–81 above.

the corruption of human judgements that leads to the occurrence of emotions. There is no evidence indicating the contents of book 3. The fourth ('therapeutic') book seems to have discussed several topics, including the analogy between psychic and bodily health or sickness, weakness of character and the rejection of reason, emotion as madness, and practical techniques of therapy of the emotions.

Galen criticizes especially two aspects of the theory, the linkage between belief, impulse, and ideas such as 'rejection' of reason, and the idea that emotion is a 'defective use' of rationality. In seeking to provide an explanatory framework for these ideas, I focus first on the (relatively straightforward) linkage between belief and impulse and then on the rather more complex and revisionist idea that emotion constitutes a rejection of reason and a defective use of this. Fundamental to the Stoic analysis of emotion, as to much else in Stoic psychology and ethics, is their theory of development as 'appropriation' or 'familiarization' (*oikeiōsis*).[97] This theory strongly reflects the 'high naturalism' common in different ways to both Stoics and Galen. Human beings and other animals, conceived as coherent psychophysical entities and complexes of natural faculties, are also seen as naturally motivated to seek what promotes their own welfare (what is 'appropriate' for them, *kathēkon*) as well as the welfare of others of their kind. This is a key feature of the Stoic teleological picture of human beings, viewed as an integral part of the natural world.[98] Their theory of animal (including human) motivation can be linked with this view of development. Animals are seen as instinctively motivated to seek what is appropriate for their welfare, and to do so in a highly unified way, both psychologically and psychophysically. This seems to underlie the distinctive Stoic analysis of motivation as a reaction ('impulse', *hormē*) that responds directly to an 'impression' (*phantasia*) that it is 'appropriate' to want or not to want *x* or *y*, or that *x* or *y* is good or bad and worth wanting or not worth wanting. As it is put in one source,

[97] On the theory of 'appropriation', See further LS 57 and 59 D, Pembroke 1971, Inwood 1985: ch. 6, Engberg-Pedersen 1990, Striker 1996: ch. 13, Inwood and Donini 1999: 677–82, 727–31.

[98] See e.g. D.L. 7.85 (LS 57A(2)), Cic. *Fin.* 3.16, Hierocles, *Elements of Ethics* 1.37–8, 51, 54, 2.1–9 (LS 57 C); also Gill 2006: 37–9. On 'high naturalism' in Galen and Stoicism, see 2.3 above.

'What activates impulse ... is precisely an impression capable of directly impelling an appropriate action'.[99] This pattern of motivation is common to all animals, including human beings. However, as human beings pass from childhood to adulthood, they function in more structured and complex ways, which include mastering language as a system; and a corollary of this development is an important shift in motivation. There are two main changes: impressions become 'rational' in the sense that they express these more complex and organized ways of thinking (above all, the use of language), and they require 'assent' (*sunkatathesis*) before they stimulate an 'impulse' to act or react in a given way. A related change is that adult humans do not merely pursue instinctively or automatically things that are appropriate (*kathēkonta*); they 'select' them and 'reject' their opposites in an increasingly coherent and structured way.[100]

The Stoic theory of emotion forms a subdivision of their theory of motivation generally. As just stated, motivational responses in animals are seen as reactions to what is beneficial or harmful in a given situation. But the responses of adult humans, as rational animals, have certain distinctive features. A motivational response (*hormē*) requires 'assent' to a 'rational impression'; in more conventional terms, it involves belief or judgement. The relevant kinds of judgement (or 'rational impression') are (1) that something is good or bad and (2) that it is therefore appropriate (*kathēkon*) to act or react in a certain way.[101] This analysis applies to all motivational responses; emotions or passions constitute a specific type of motive, marked by a certain type of belief and by certain additional features, which indicate the defective character of emotional states. Stoic definitions of emotion, of the kind offered by Stoic theorists from Zeno onwards, refer to all three aspects. These three aspects are (1) the judgement that *x* is good or bad and that it is appropriate to react in a certain way accordingly, and (2) the motivational response

[99] Stobaeus 2.86.17–18 (LS 53 Q(1)), LS trans., slightly modified; see further Inwood 1985: 224, Brennan 2003: 268–9, Gill 2006: 138–9, Graver 2007: 24–8.

[100] See LS 33 C (*SVF* 2.187), I (*SVF* 3.171), Cic. *Fin.* 3.20 (LS 59 D(3)); also Inwood 1985: 72–91, Gill 2006: 140–1.

[101] See further Brennan 2003: 260–9, referring e.g. to Epict. *Diss.* 1.18.1; also Inwood: 1985: ch. 3, Sorabji 2000: 29–24. Gill 2006: 138–9.

(*hormē*) which is triggered by the judgement. (3) The—defective and problematic—character of the emotional response is characterized in several ways, including that of 'runaway motion', 'excessive impulse', or 'rejection of reason'. The first two aspects are brought out in standard Stoic definitions of emotion, for instance, those of the four main emotions (fear, pain, appetite, and pleasure). Thus, for example: 'Pain (or distress, *lupē*) is an irrational contraction, or a fresh opinion that something bad is present, at which people think it appropriate to be contracted [i.e. depressed]'.[102] Another version of this definition spells out even more clearly the causal link between the belief and the motivational response (*hormē*), in this case, being contracted. 'Pain is a contraction of the psyche disobedient to reason, and its cause is believing that a "fresh" bad thing is present, for which it is appropriate to suffer contraction in the psyche.'[103] The second definition underlines the integral connection between the three features noted earlier, namely belief or judgement, the resulting impulse (such as 'contraction' of the psyche), and the evaluative description of the state of mind involved, here as being 'disobedient to reason'.[104]

Although the third aspect of these definitions needs to be explored further, this outline of Stoic thinking on emotion is sufficient, I think, to bring out the coherence and credibility of the linkage involved between beliefs and impulses. The underlying Stoic claim is that adult humans, though not animals or human children, are constitutively adapted to act and feel on the basis of beliefs.[105] Although, of course, one can argue against this claim, and against the associated distinction between the motivational process of adult humans and other kinds of animal, this claim does not involve the kind of elementary logical or classificatory error that Galen asserts.[106] What it does involve are certain 'holistic' assumptions about psychological processes, which are outlined shortly. These holistic assumptions run counter to the part-based (or 'composition') framework that Galen applies to psychology in *PHP* 4–5. But the fact that the

[102] Andronicus *On Passions* 1 (*SVF* 3.391), LS 65 B(1), trans. LS, slightly modified.

[103] Stobaeus 2.90.14–16 (*SVF* 3.394), trans. Inwood and Gerson 1997: 218, slightly modified. On the significance of 'fresh', see n. 132 below.

[104] See further Brennan 1998: 22–39, 2003: 269–74.

[105] On analogous modern ('cognitivist') theories of emotion, see Ch. 6 below, text to nn. 31–5.

[106] See text to nn. 68–75 above.

two theories apply different frameworks does not make either of them therefore incoherent, defective, or implausible in their account of human psychology, despite Galen's strongly negative presentation of the Stoic theory.

There are two main types of holism implied in the Stoic theory, as so far outlined. The most obviously relevant type is psychological holism. Aspects that in a different framework—notably that presupposed by Galen—would be regarded as substantially different in kind are seen here as integrally linked.[107] Thus, the 'rational' aspect (belief or judgement) and the 'emotional' aspect (the motivational response) are seen as causally interlinked. As expressed in one source, noted earlier, 'What activates impulse ... is precisely an impression capable of directly impelling an appropriate action'.[108] To put the point differently, the theory reflects the approach I am associating with the idea of 'structure', rather than 'composition'. The component parts of motivation (rational impression, assent, impulse) are conceived as functioning solely in relation to the whole motivational process. They are not understood as psychic parts of the type Galen presupposes, that is, as independent and potentially conflicting sources of motivation.[109] This point applies to the Stoic analysis of motivation generally, but emotions represent one clear expression of this general characteristic.

A second dimension of the theory is psychophysical holism, a feature of Stoic thinking which is much closer to Galen's approach.[110] Of course, given Stoic physicalism about psychology, all psychological processes are conceived as being physical, as modalities of *pneuma*.[111] But the account of emotions represents a striking

[107] For Galen's underlying assumptions, based on Platonic–Aristotelian ideas, see text to nn. 33–4 above, also 4.3 below. In fact, the Stoic analysis of motivation is often seen by modern scholars as close to Aristotle's, though the Stoic account lays a greater stress on psychological unity: see further Inwood 1985: 9–17, Long 1996: 266–75, esp. 268–9, Gill 1991 (also considering the relationship to some modern ideas).

[108] Stobaeus 2.86.17–18 (LS 53 Q(1)), LS trans., slightly modified; see further Inwood 1985: 224, whose translation brings out the point even more clearly: 'What stimulates impulse is nothing but a hormetic presentation (*phantasia hormētikē*) of what is obviously (or immediately, *autothen*) appropriate'). See also Brennan 2003: 268–9, Gill 2006: 138–9, Graver 2007: 24–8, and text to n. 101 above.

[109] On the composition–structure contrast, see text to nn. 37–9 above and Ch. 1, text to n. 40. On Galen's psychological assumptions, see 4.3 below.

[110] See 3.5 above.

[111] See Ch. 3 above, text to nn. 258–77.

instance of this view; the 'impulses' (motivational responses) involved are characterized in physical terms, for instance, as 'contraction' or 'swelling' in the control-centre. The theory thus illustrates a point made earlier about the Stoic theory, that it presents physicalism about psychology in a way that accommodates scope for the exercise for rational agency.[112] As Anthony Price puts it, the Stoic thinkers 'invite us to analyse emotion as a psychophysical union of intentionality and physiology, while emphasizing that it is psychic assent that forms the locus of the subject's responsibility for his own emotions'.[113] Galen presents these strongly physical, and sometimes bodily localized, characterizations of emotions as inconsistent with Chrysippus' view of emotions as judgements.[114] But, taken in the context of the theory as described here, the combination is fully intelligible and reflects the psychophysical, as well as psychological, holism that is characteristic of the theory. Similarly, dispositions to have one or other emotion are also described in physical terms, as brought out later.[115]

To make sense of the third aspect of Stoic thinking about emotion (the negative characterization of emotion as, for instance, the 'rejection of reason') and the idea that it constitutes what Galen calls 'defective use' (*kakōsis*) of reason, we need to take into account their ideas about the final stages of ethical development, which constitute one of the most important and controversial features of their thinking. The ideal outcome of ethical development in adult human beings is seen as being a move from increasingly rational selection of 'appropriate things' (taken to be goods) to recognizing that the only real good, which alone is worthy of choice, is virtue. This is accompanied by the understanding that the appropriate things pursued as goods in the previous stage, such as health, wealth, or social status, are of a radically lower order of value than virtue; they are—relative to virtue—'matters of indifference' (*adiaphora*), at most to be regarded as 'preferable' (*proēgmena*) rather than 'dispreferable' (*apoproēgmena*).[116] Despite this radical contrast between the type of value placed on virtue rather than other so-called goods, there

[112] See Ch. 3 above, text to nn. 297–9.

[113] Price 2005: 475; cf. Gill 2006: 248, Graver 2007: 28–34.

[114] *PHP* V.362–5, 4.1.6–14 De Lacy.

[115] See text to nn. 147–54 below.

[116] Cic. *Fin.* 3.21–2 (LS 59 D(4–6)), taken with LS, vol. 1: 368, and LS 58.

is an important, though implied, link between the earlier and final stage. Virtue is taken to consist, in part at least, in a more complete and structured version of the kind of rational selection of appropriate things that is characteristic of the earlier stage of development. However, there are at least two important points of difference. One is the recognition that what matters, ultimately, is the rational selection and not the 'appropriate things' such as health which constitute the object of selection in the previous stage. The other is that virtue consists, in a whole series of ways, in a *completely structured state*, as regards knowledge and understanding, character, actions, pattern of social relationships, and so on. In this respect, virtue (that is, the virtue of human beings) reflects the character of goodness more generally in Stoic thought, which is conceived in terms of order, structure, and rationality in various contexts too, including the natural universe or logic.[117] This dimension of ethical development is paralleled by a social aspect that builds on the other-benefiting motive that is presented as fundamental to all animals, of which the paradigmatic illustration is parental love for children. In adult humans, this motive is, in the course of development, expressed in increasingly structured and broader forms of social engagement, in which the other-benefiting motive is extended to any given human being.[118]

The Stoic theory of value and the correlated account of ethical development, though they had partial parallels in earlier thought,[119] were intensely controversial. These ideas were subjected to intense scrutiny and criticism both by Academic sceptics such as Carneades (mid-second century BC), and by Antiochus (first century BC), whose thought combines Platonic, Aristotelian, and Stoic strands. One target of criticism was the allegedly twofold system of valuation, according to which value (of different kinds) was placed both on

[117] For this interpretation of the theory, see Gill 2006: 145–66; for other readings of Cic. *Fin.* 3.20–2 (an important but problematic text) and the theory implied, see Annas 1993: ch. 5, Striker 1996: ch. 12, M. Frede 1999*b*, Brennan 2005: chs. 8–13.

[118] See LS 57 E–H, esp. F (Cic. *Fin.* 3.62–8), also LS 67. The later stages of social 'appropriation' can include (rational and structured) family and communal engagement as well as cosmopolitanism and the expression of the kinship of humankind. See further Annas 1993: 262–76, 302–11, Reydams-Schils 2002.

[119] Cf. e.g. the core thesis of Plato's *Republic*, that justice constitutes happiness (357a–358d) or Aristotle's view is virtue is done 'for its own sake' (or 'for the sake of the fine'), e.g. *EN* 2.4, 1104^{a}32.

'indifferents' and on virtue. Another was the claim that, in the case of the perfectly wise person, material and social advantages made absolutely no contribution to her happiness.[120] Also controversial was the Stoic claim that this process of ethical development was a *natural* one, even though the Stoics also acknowledged that hardly anyone—or perhaps no one at all—actually carried this process to its ideal outcome.[121] Critics asked why, if this process is natural, it is so rarely taken to its conclusion. Chrysippus, as Galen himself tells us, identified two special sources of corruption, which disrupt the completion of this process. One is the 'persuasiveness of impressions' (or 'the very nature of the things around them') and the other is 'the conversation of the majority of people' (or 'of those around us').[122] Although there is no surviving Stoic systematic analysis of this aspect of their theory, the underlying rationale seems to be this. There is a natural human tendency to continue to regard 'appropriate things' such as health as goods and not simply as 'preferable' indifferents; this type of 'impression' thus continues to be 'persuasive', though mistaken. This tendency informs the beliefs and 'conversation of the majority of people' (or those who are 'around us') and their discourse reinforces our mistaken inclinations.[123] Despite the influence of these corrupting factors, and the widespread failure to complete the process of ethical development, the Stoics believe that all human beings are constitutively capable of doing so, and remain capable throughout their lives. As they put it, 'All human beings have the starting points of virtue', that is, the innate capacity to form true conceptions of notions such as good and god.[124] Also, in the Stoic unified or holistic account of psychology, there are no irrational parts that can become so corrupted by innate character or habituation that they prevent someone from completing this developmental process at any point.[125] As brought out later, there are substantive differences

120 See LS 64; also Annas 1993: 180–7, 419–25, Striker 1996: 239–48.

121 On Antiochus' criticisms, see Gill 2006: 168–79; and on the Stoic theory, see further text to nn. 129–33 below.

122 D.L. 7.89, Gal. *PHP* V. 462, 5.5.14 De Lacy.

123 See further Gill 2006: 257–8, Graver 2007: 151–63; also Tieleman 2003*a*: 132–9, referring esp. to Calcidius' report.

124 See LS 61 L (Stob. 2.65.8, *SVF* 1.566), my trans. See also LS 60 B–F.

125 See further Gill 2006: 132–4, 137–45, Graver 2007: 151–3; also Gill 2006: 134–7 for the contrast with Platonic–Aristotelian thinking.

between this conception of ethical development and that presupposed by Galen and by much preceding Platonic–Aristotelian thinking.[126] But the Stoic conception has its own coherence and credibility, and it provides a background against which we can see the process of development as natural, and as the highest fulfilment of human nature, even though it is rarely if ever carried to its conclusion.

Stoic thinking about development provides a crucial part of the background for making sense of the third aspect of the Stoic characterization of emotions. This is a negative qualitative description of the emotion in terms such as 'runaway motion', 'excessive impulse' or 'rejection of reason'. Galen maintains that such descriptions only make sense if we assume that they refer to the operation of a non-rational part of the psyche, and that Chrysippus' use of these phrases is a sign of inconsistency—or an acknowledgement of the facts of human nature.[127] However, I think that these and other apparently puzzling features of Stoic thinking about emotions can be explained in a way that is consistent with their psychological and psychophysical holism. Stoic specification of the kind of irrationality involved in emotion, while complex in its analysis, can be seen as, in Galen's phrase, a form of 'defective use' (*kakōsis*) of reason, though not a type that Galen's own preferred framework can accommodate.[128]

As outlined earlier, ethical development, in Stoic theory, involves moving from selecting 'appropriate things', such as health, taken as good things, to recognizing that all such things are only 'matters of indifference', in comparison with virtue, which is the only real good.[129] Someone who has completed this process, that is, the wise person, experiences only a limited range of affective states, namely what the Stoics call 'good emotions' (*eupatheiai*). These are wish, caution, and joy, corresponding to three of the primary (bad) emotions of appetite, fear, and pleasure.[130] This limited emotional register goes along with the other features of complete ethical development,

[126] See 4.3 below.

[127] See e.g. Gal. *PHP* V.366–70, 4.1–18 De Lacy. See text to nn. 72–5 above.

[128] See text to nn. 74–5, 116–18 above.

[129] See text to n. 116 above.

[130] There is no equivalent for the fourth emotion, pain or distress, because the wise person is never affected by the presence of the only thing that is really bad, i.e. ethically defective character. See D.L. 7.116 (LS 65 F), Cic. *Tusc.* 4.12–14; also Brennan 1998: 34–9, Graver 2007: 51–9.

including having a fully structured and stable character as well as framework of understanding.[131] The psychological state of the non-wise person—which is that of virtually all of us—is marked in various ways by the failure to complete this developmental process. For one thing, we have a set of false or defective beliefs, in particular, the belief that things such as health, wealth, and social position are goods, instead of merely 'preferable indifferents'. Having false beliefs, by contrast with the wise person's completely stable and secure knowledge, is a general feature of the non-wise person. But the application of beliefs of this type—more precisely, the 'fresh', still powerful, application of these beliefs[132]—generates specific by-products such as 'impulse which is excessive and disobedient to the dictates of reason, or a movement of the psyche which is irrational and contrary to nature'.[133] The implications of these phrases are quite complex, as brought out shortly. But the main point is that the failure to achieve the wise person's state of internal order and emotional calm means that our state is one of internal disorder and intense and unstructured affective states.

In a number of passages from Chrysippus' *On Passions* cited by Galen, we can see an attempt to bring out and explain the combination of rationality and irrationality involved in this kind of state, and also to show how it is compatible with Stoic 'psychological holism'.

> the rational animal is by nature such as to follow reason and to act with reason as his guide. But often he moves in another way towards some things and away from some things in disobedience to reason when he is pushed too much... Therefore some people not inappropriately say that an emotion of the psyche is a movement contrary to nature, as in fear and desire and the like. For all such movements and states are disobedient to reason and reject it; accordingly, we say that such persons are moved irrationally, not in the sense of reasoning poorly, as one might speak of someone who reasons the opposite of well, but in the sense of rejecting reason.[134]

[131] See Cic. *Fin.* 3.21 (LS 59 D9(4–5)), also D.L. 7.46–8 (LS 33 B), LS 63, esp. L–M (Cic. *Tusc.* 5.40–1, 81–2).

[132] According to Galen, *PHP* V.416, 4.7.1–4 De Lacy, the word 'fresh' was Chrysippus' addition to Zeno's definition of an emotion; on its significance, see Inwood 1985: 146–55, Tieleman 2003*a*: 115–18, Graver 2007: 178–9.

[133] Stob. 2.88.8–10, LS 65 A(1), LS trans. slightly modified (=*SVF* 3.378).

[134] *PHP* V.368, 385, 4.2.10–11, p. 240.18–21, 4.4.16–17, p. 254.13–19 De Lacy, trans. De Lacy, slightly modified.

Passages of this type seem designed to convey a number of interrelated claims about the emotions of the non-wise. (1) The emotions reflect rationality in that they involve the normal cognitive processes of adult humans (or rational animals), namely assent to rational impressions. (2) They are 'irrational', partly in the sense that they depend on errors of judgement (false beliefs about what is good and how it is appropriate to react). (3) But they differ from other such errors because they involve intense affective states, such as 'expansion' and 'contraction' in the psyche, and the person concerned is not really in control of herself. Her state is that of 'runaway motion', characterized in terms of the contrast between running and walking legs.[135] This state is not conceived as that in which one part of us ('the rational part') fails to control another ('the non-rational part').[136] Rather the person as a psychological whole is reacting in an unstructured, disordered way that disables normal functioning. These further features of emotional states represent the way Chrysippus distinguishes emotions from other kinds of errors—a distinction that Galen thinks he cannot make without positing a non-rational part of the psyche. They also show how Chrysippus can consistently conceive emotion as, in Galen's phrase, a 'defective use' (*kakōsis*) of reason (and not its complete absence, *sterēsis*).[137] To put the point differently, this analysis can show how the Stoics interpret features typically associated with emotion, including intense bodily reactions of which the person concerned is strongly aware and which cause loss of self-control, in a way that is consistent with their unified account of human psychology.

In some cases, at least, for instance those of 'blind' rage, it seems likely that the phrase 'rejection of reason' represents an objective description of the emotional state, rather than a characterization of the thought-processes of the person concerned.[138] However, in other cases, it seems clear that the emotional person consciously rejects

[135] *PHP* V.369–70, 4.2.13–18 De Lacy. This image may have contributed to Posidonius' introduction of the idea of 'emotional movements', which seems also to be used to convey an idea that can be characterized as that of 'psychological (or psychophysical) inertia' (n. 86 above).

[136] Galen maintains that this is what Chrysippus' description must imply: *PHP* V.373–7, 4.2.28–44 De Lacy.

[137] See text to nn. 74–5, 116–18 above.

[138] For such states, cited by Chrysippus, see *PHP* V.414–15, 4.6.44–6 De Lacy.

reason, even while recognizing the misguided character of her action and state of mind. Chrysippus' most famous example of this phenomenon is Euripides' Medea,[139] who concludes the monologue prior to killing her own children (to take revenge on her husband for rejecting her) with these lines (*Med.* 1078–80) : 'I know that what I am about to do is bad (*kaka*), but spirit (or anger, *thumos*) is master of (or stronger than, *kreissōn*) my plans.'[140] Galen assumes that the case of Medea, like other such examples, can only be explained by reference to a part-based psychological model such as Plato's tripartite one. For him, Medea's state is only intelligible as that of someone experiencing the simultaneous pull of reason and anger and finally giving way to anger.[141] However, her case can be credibly interpreted in line with the Stoic holistic analysis of psychology.[142] Medea's decision to kill her children, like all human motives, is based on beliefs and reasoning, such as that 'taking vengeance on my husband is more beneficial than saving the lives of my children'.[143] Medea herself, in Chrysippus' view, sees the motivation involved as excessive and unnatural. Despite seeing this, she is unable, in her current emotional state, to counteract the strength of her motivational impulse (the 'running legs') based on the belief that retaliation is good and that it is appropriate for her to feel anger. In this state of mind, she (consciously) disobeys or rejects what she herself sees as the reasonable way to behave.[144] What underlies this analysis, in addition to the holistic psychological model, is the Stoic belief that, as noted earlier, 'all human beings have the starting points of virtue', and they retain these 'starting points' throughout their lives, as a constitutive feature of being a human being or rational animal.[145] The force of

[139] On Chrysippus' intense interest in this play, see D.L. 7.180, Gill 1983.

[140] *PHP* V.372, 4.2.27 (which seems to summarize Chrysippus' analysis), V.403–14, 4.6.1–43, esp. 19–23 De Lacy. It is uncertain exactly where in *On Passions*, Chrysippus' discussion of Medea was located. A link with Chrysippus' definition of passion (and his distinction between emotions and other kinds of errors) is suggested by V.370–2, 4.2.19–27 De Lacy, implying that it came in Book 1 (see Gill 1983: 139–40). But Tieleman (2003*a*: 172) suggests that it appeared in the fourth ('therapeutic' book).

[141] *PHP* V. 306–8, V.338, 3.3.13–22, 3.7.14–16 De Lacy.

[142] See refs. in n. 144 below.

[143] For this way of analysing her motivation, see Epict. *Diss.* 1.28, esp. 7–10, 28. On Epictetus' interest, following Chrysippus, in Medea, see Long 1996: 277–80, 2002: 76–7.

[144] See further Gill 2006: 255–60, esp. 259; also Gill 1983, 1996: 223–5, 227–32, 1998: 118–21.

[145] See text to n. 124 above.

this example for Chrysippus must have derived partly from this point. *Even Medea*—on the face of it, a paradigm of evil character—could see that what she was doing was 'bad' and that her emotional state constituted a kind of 'rejection of reason'. Her example thus illustrates the continuing power of the natural motive to virtue in all of us, as well as the fact that our fundamental rationality sometimes issues in appalling acts whose wrongness we can ourselves recognize.

A further feature of Stoic theory that is explained by this general line of thought is their view of the long-term disposition to have emotions of a certain kind. Galen comments on Chrysippus' idea that at least some non-wise people have quasi-dispositional states such as being 'mad on women' or 'mad on birds' or the reverse.[146] Other sources support this theme: we are told of their view that different people are 'more inclined' (*procliuiores*) to different sicknesses; they show 'irascibility' (*iracundia*), for instance, rather than just (occurrent) 'anger' (*ira*).[147] This theme, on the face of it, resembles the idea, central to Aristotle's thinking, that most people, even those who are not fully virtuous, have stable dispositional patterns (*hexeis*) as regards their character (*ēthos*).[148] However, fundamental to the Stoic version of this idea is the fact that, even if these dispositions are relatively lasting and well marked, they are inherently unstable and are often coupled with opposing inclinations. This instability is indicated in Chrysippus' comment, cited by Galen: 'We must suppose that psychic disease is most similar to a feverish physical state in which fevers and chills do not occur at regular intervals but irregularly and at random from the character (of the person) and at the incidence of small causes.'[149] This can be taken with Chrysippus' characterization of emotion, as an occurrent phenomenon as a 'flutter' (*ptoia*), and as 'moving at random'.[150] We can

[146] *PHP* V.396, 4.5.20–2 De Lacy.

[147] Cic. *Tusc.* 4.27, also 23–30. See also D.L. 7.115, Stob. 2.93.1–13 (10e), trans. Inwood and Gerson 1997: 219.

[148] Arist. *EN* 2.3–5; a particularly significant indicator of this line of thought is the distinction between (stable but defective) dispositions such as 'self-indulgence' and (unstable) 'weakness of will' (*akrasia*), *EN* 7.8. See further Gill 2006: 232–3, 321, on the influence of this idea on Plutarch.

[149] *PHP* V.435, 5.2.14, p. 298.3–7 De Lacy, trans. De Lacy, slightly modified.

[150] *PHP* V.392, 4.5.6 De Lacy, also Stob. 2.88.11–12 (=LS 65 A(2)), Plu. *Mor.* 447 A.

also take it together with the identification of a class of psychic ailments 'with weakness' (*arrōstēmata/aegrotationes*), which are sometimes interpreted as inclinations to have competing sets of emotions.[151] What underlies this idea, like the characterization of emotion as a (perhaps conscious) 'rejection of reason' is the view that human beings are constitutively capable of developing towards the recognition that virtue is the only good and also towards the complete consistency of beliefs and character that constitutes perfect wisdom.[152] Failure to develop towards wisdom results in an inherently unstable and incoherent psychological state, even if it is marked by some prevalent or quasi-dispositional tendencies. Even if someone is inclined to one or other emotion, this inclination may at any point come into conflict with another emotion or with the capacity to form a more rational understanding that lies latent in all of us.[153] Galen finds this account of psychic sickness, which is found in Posidonius as well as Chrysippus, problematic in several ways.[154]But it consistently reflects the general Stoic pattern of thinking about ethical development and its failure and the impact of this success or failure on our emotional state.

As Tieleman points out, Stoic thinking about psychic sickness, as well as other aspects of their ideas about emotions, expresses their theory of causation, as involving both the specific character of the agent and the stimulus of the specific situation, and also reflects their physicalist approach to psychology.[155] These are features of Stoic thought that are, up to a point at least, shared with Galen, and constitute aspects of their shared naturalism of approach.[156] Thus, one might have expected that Galen would show a degree of constructive interest in these ideas, as he responds positively to some other Stoic ideas.[157] In fact, of course, as brought out earlier in this section, his response is uniformly negative. Galen's own comments,

[151] Stob. 2.93.12–13, D.L. 7.115, Cic. *Tusc.* 4.23; see further Kerferd 1983: 88–93, Gill 2006: 262–3, Graver 2007: 133–45.

[152] See text to nn. 116–26 above.

[153] See further for this type of analysis Gill 2006: 261–4, also 222–4, discussing Plu. *Mor.* 446 F–447 A (=LS 65G), and 450 C–D.

[154] *PHP* V.432–6, 5.2–1–19 De Lacy; see further on this passage, 5.4 below, text to nn. 271–81.

[155] Tieleman 2003*a*: 102–14, 155–7.

[156] See text to nn. 90–3 above.

[157] See 2.3 above, text to nn. 192–201.

which are often polemical and tendentious, do not take us very far in understanding the depth or nature of his differences with Stoic thinking on this subject. But important factors include the radical holism and revisionism of the Stoic theory, illustrated in the preceding analysis of their thinking on emotions, and the contrast between these features and salient aspects of Galen's psychological assumptions. To go further in making sense of his consistently negative response to these Stoic ideas, we need to consider more fully what Galen's own assumptions are and how they are formulated in *PHP* 4–5. This is the topic pursued in the next section (4.3), before returning in the final section (4.4) to the question how profound the differences are between Galenic and Stoic thought on these aspects of psychology.

4.3 GALEN'S PSYCHOLOGICAL ASSUMPTIONS

What are the psychological assumptions that underlie Galen's critique of the Stoic theory and his attempts to isolate the Chrysippean version of this theory, considered in the first part of the preceding section? Galen does not present these assumptions in analytic or expository form in *PHP* 4–5, but they emerge especially in three sections of Book 5, on psychic parts and wholes, on ethical development, and on Plato's argument in *Republic* 4.[158] The discussion of psychic parts and wholes is considered in the next section; I examine here his reading of Plato's argument for psychic parts and his treatment of ethical development. Obviously, the main assumption Galen makes is that the psyche consists of a combination of rational and non-rational parts, or at least functions. But Galen's discussion of Plato's argument, which I take first, brings out a crucial assumption underpinning the whole critique of Stoic theory in *PHP* 4–5. This is that the psychic parts or functions are not simply different and in some sense separate but are also independent, and potentially conflicting, sources of motivation. It is this assumption that, I think,

[158] These are (1) *PHP* V.439–54, 5.2.30–3.30 De Lacy, (2) V. 459–68, 5.5.1–40 De Lacy, (3) V.479–501, 5.7.1–82 De Lacy.

underlies Galen's claim earlier in *PHP* 5 that Chrysippus is not entitled to use the notion of 'part' at all, despite the fact that Galen himself offers some relatively credible candidates for this role in Stoic theory.[159] It seems likely too that this idea lies behind his psychological thinking in *PHP* 1–3, 6, and reinforces his desire to show that each of the three relevant organs, including the liver, is the 'source' (*archē*) of a physical communication system which is in some way correlated with the relevant psychological role.[160]

Galen offers an extended discussion of Plato's argument for separate psychic parts in *Republic* 435–41 towards the end of *PHP* 5.[161] The discussion, formally at least, falls outside the critique of Stoic ideas and forms a bridge to the full-scale presentation of tripartite psychophysiology in *PHP* 6; but, as just indicated, conceptually, it is very important for the interpretation of Galenic psychology in Book 4–5 and, to some extent, for *PHP* 1–6 as a whole. Plato's argument, in outline, takes this form.[162] After asking whether the psyche has parts comparable with those in the state, Socrates states a general principle by which this question can be determined. The principle is that 'the same thing will not be willing to do or undergo opposites in the same part of itself, in relation to the same thing, at the same time.'[163] This principle of non-contrariety or conflict is then applied to the psyche.[164] Socrates distinguishes as opposites such processes as assent and dissent, desiring to take and refusing, drawing to and thrusting away. He locates appetites (*epithumiai*) within the first of these two types of process. He gives thirst as an instance of appetite, directed at drinking. He considers a case when someone is thirsty (wants to drink) but also does not want to drink. He argues that this must be understood as the simultaneous presence of 'something in their psyche ordering them to drink and something different forbidding them to drink' (439c6–7). The forbidding element is said, in such cases, to derive from reasoning; and this argument is said to establish

[159] *PHP* V.441, 443, 5.2.35–8, 44–5 De Lacy; see text to nn. 227–30 below.

[160] See further on this point, text to nn. 254–7 below.

[161] V.480–501, 5.7.1–82 De Lacy.

[162] The rest of this paragraph is based closely on Gill 2006: 307.

[163] *R.* 436b8–9, trans. Grube, rev. Reeve in Cooper 1997.

[164] For these formulations of the principle, see, respectively, Price 1995: 40–1, Annas 1981: 137.

the difference between the reasoning (*logistikon*) and appetitive (*epithumētikon*) parts of the psyche (*R.* 437b–d, 439b–d). Similarly, instances of conflict between anger or indignation (characterized as 'spirit', *thumos*) and appetite, are said to enable us to distinguish these two parts from each other. Spirit is said never to conflict with reason, although it can occur separately from it, as it does in non-human animals and human children; and on this basis it is distinguished as a third (*thumoeides*) part of the psyche (439e–441c).

How does Galen read this argument and what use does he make of it? In the first instance, what is significant is that Galen chooses this passage, rather than any other in the *Republic* or elsewhere, to display the conception of human psychology he has in view.[165] In some ways, as Galen himself allows, this passage is not ideal for his purposes. He concedes from the start that the argument does not support everything he wants to claim, namely that the psyche consists of 'parts' (*merē/moria*) with separate bodily locations as well as distinct functions. Hence, in Galenic terms, the argument is really about 'functions' or 'powers' (*dunameis*), rather than 'parts'. However, Galen argues that separate location is implied in Plato's *Republic*, as well as being presented, albeit in mythic form, in *Timaeus* 69–72. Hence, he maintains, the argument is, in effect, about 'parts' in a strong sense, even if this is not shown in *R.* 435–41.[166] Why is he so attracted by this argument? First of all, it is significant that Plato's account is presented as a logical demonstration, more so than other Platonic discussions of psychology in the *Republic* or elsewhere. Galen, clearly, thinks that this gives the passage a strong methodological grounding, one that is notably lacking, he maintains, in Chrysippus' analysis of the psyche. It is worth bearing in mind that, although Galen gives special weight to the combination of logic and empiricism in

[165] This passage most of all emphasizes the distinctness and independence of the parts; other passages focus either on the harmony and integration of the parts (e.g. in the account of the psychic virtues, 441d–443e) or on the complex forms of interplay between the three parts (in the defective psychic types of books 8–9). See further Gill 1998: 131–3, 2006: 310–11, 315–20, stressing that these latter features lend themselves to a reading in terms of a more integrated, Stoic-style picture of psychology.

[166] *PHP* V.479–81, 5.7.1–9 De Lacy, including a very strained interpretation of *R.* 435c9–d3 in V.481, 5.7.6–9 De Lacy. See further on this passage and Galen's terminology and assumptions, Tieleman 2003*a*: 26–9, 2003*b*: 141–8.

establishing the truth, he also recognizes reason or argument as an independent source of knowledge.[167]

However, the main, and obvious, reason why Galen turns to this passage is because it offers support for his central thesis that the psyche is a combination of rational and non-rational parts, and thus reinforces his opposition to the unified Stoic picture. In summing up the significance of Plato's argument, Galen spells out this message repeatedly. For instance, he says, 'Plato shows that the part (*meros*) of the psyche which desires is other than the part which rationally determines how and in what manner we seek to be filled with food when we are hungry, and with drink when we are thirsty'.[168] The concept of 'part' here, in effect, means independent source of motivation; since, as Galen stresses, this is what the argument shows. As Galen puts it: 'The irrational faculty in us draws the person who feels the need to each of the desired objects, while reason pulls in the opposite direction and checks the untimely motion. And often the conflict between the two becomes violent, thus indicating clearly that the nature of the contending faculties in us is two-fold.'[169] The damaging implication for the Stoic theory, as Galen supposes, is spelled out a little later. We can 'conclude indisputably that it is not within the province of the same faculty both to reason and to desire food or drink or sexual pleasure, a fact that somehow escaped Chrysippus and the other Stoics'.[170] The feature of Plato's argument that is most crucial for Galen's case is the separation of reason and appetite. However, Galen goes on to consider the implications of Plato's argument for the separate existence of a 'spirited' (*thumoeides*) part, including the Leontius example (*R.* 440a–b). Galen presents this argument as showing 'that the part which feels anger is other than the part which desires, that the rational part is different from both, and that the angry part never allies itself with the desiring

[167] Galen uses the term *apodeixis* ('proof') or the cognate verb repeatedly in his summary of Plato's argument, and also reiterates the point that Chrysippus fails to answer Plato's argument (e.g. *PHP* V. 490–1, 5.7.43–4 De Lacy, V.493, 5.7.51–2 De Lacy). On Galen's thinking on reason as a criterion and his critique of Stoic (Chrysippean) methodology, see Ch. 2 above, text to nn. 93–8, 135–6.

[168] *PHP* V.483, 5.7.16, p. 340.7–9 De Lacy, trans. De Lacy, slightly modified.

[169] *PHP* V.485, 5.7.22, p. 342.1–5 De Lacy, trans. De Lacy, slightly modified.

[170] *PHP* V.490, 5.7.42, p. 346.11–13 De Lacy, trans. De Lacy, slightly modified.

part'.[171] The main implication of this section of Plato's argument, as Galen recognizes, is the difference between the functions of anger and desire or appetite. The argument does not show that the spirited part constitutes an independent source of motivation from reason in the same way as appetite. The main role of spirit is to react emotionally in line with the judgements of reason, though it is none the less presented as a distinct psychological function or agency.[172] However, taken overall, Galen feels confident in finding in Plato's argument a reasoned case for the un-Stoic picture of the psyche as a combination of rational and non-rational parts that are also independent sources of motivation.

Galen does not mount a separate argument of his own for this picture of human psychology. Nor does he discuss explicitly in this context the relationship between Plato's argument and the brain-centred anatomical account he argues for in *PHP* 1–3, 6, though he clearly regards them as compatible.[173] However, his endorsement of the Platonic account, as he interprets this, does underline some of the difficulties discussed earlier in correlating his tripartite psychology with his psychophysiology. The main emphasis in the physiological side is on the idea of the three organs as sources (*archai*) of distinct, and independent, communication systems, housed in brain, arteries, and veins respectively.[174] The Platonic argument provides a psychological model that supports this picture, at least as far as reason and appetite are concerned, though spirit is presented, rather, as an emotional adjunct to reason. But the Platonic argument also lays stress, as Galen's own summary brings out, on interaction between the parts, both in the form of competing pressure between reason and appetite, and in the form of responsive reactions by spirit to reason, including opposition to appetite.[175] However, as Mansfeld

[171] *PHP* V.495, 5.7.57, p. 350.23–5 De Lacy, trans. De Lacy, slightly modified.

[172] On the normal (compliant) character of 'spirit', see *PHP* V.494–8, 5.7.53–71 De Lacy, referring to *R.* 440a–b, c–d. An exceptional indication of independence is the psychic state in which 'spirit' is corrupted and thus no longer helps reason (*R.* 441a3), a point noted in *PHP* V.499, 5.7.72 De Lacy.

[173] The linkage between them is referred to in *PHP* V.479–80, 5.7.1–4 De Lacy, and is a key theme of *PHP* 1–6; see e.g. V.454–5, 5.4.2–3 De Lacy.

[174] See Ch. 3 above, text to nn. 68–70.

[175] *PHP* V.482–3, 485, 488–90, 492, 494–6, 498–9, 5.7.12–15, 22, 36–40, 47–8, 53–63, 67–71; on Plato's argument, see text to nn. 162–4 above.

and Tieleman have pointed out, it is much more difficult to find analogues in Galen's psychophysiology for these types of interaction. Although there are some indications that the nervous system is linked with the heart and, more tenuously, with the liver, this only shows how the brain-based reason might communicate with the non-rational parts and not how communication would go in the other direction. The other side of the Platonic picture, in which appetite resists reason or spirit confronts appetite, is much more difficult to correlate with Galen's brain-centred account.[176] Also, as stressed earlier, there are major difficulties in reconciling Galen's account of the liver as a physiological organ with the idea that it also serves as the source of appetitive motivation.[177] So, even if Plato's argument meets Galen's needs in demonstrating the existence of rational and non-rational parts of the psyche, it does so in a way that underlines the tensions between his psychological and physiological accounts.

But does Plato's argument meet Galen's needs? More precisely, is it obvious that Plato's argument endorses the Galenic picture of the psyche as a complex of independent sources of motivation, by contrast with the Stoic, unified, picture? The interpretative issues are rather complex, and perhaps go beyond my immediate aim, which is to bring out how Galen supposes that Plato's argument supports his position.[178] But it is worth highlighting the fact that there is a very active debate among modern Platonic scholars about what this argument actually shows about human psychology.[179] In particular, the combination of the two ideas stressed by Galen (1) that the appetitive part is non-rational, and (2) that it is an independent source of motivation and capable of conflicting with reason, has been found problematic by some scholars. It has been suggested that, in order to be able to compete in this way, the two parts must have comparable capacities, for instance, for being goal-directed, and that this implies having beliefs about what goals are worth pursuing.

[176] See Ch. 3 above, text to nn. 72–7, 96–101.

[177] See Ch. 3 above, text to nn. 79–91 above.

[178] For a more detailed treatment of most of the points made in this paragraph, see Gill 2006: 309–21.

[179] For some recent contributions to this debate, see Lorenz 2004, Rowe 2007: 164–85, and Stalley 2007.

To put the point differently, in order to be able to *conflict* with reason, as opposed to simply reacting differently, appetite would need to have richer cognitive or rational capacities than Plato (or Galen) allows.[180] The view of psychic conflict implied in this interpretation seems to imply, rather, a Stoic-style picture of psychic division, namely that between two strands of belief (or belief-and-emotion or belief-and-desire) rather than between a rational and non-rational part.[181] An alternative line of scholarly interpretation sees the conflict described as being that between different types of motivation, namely desire for the good, that is, what is best overall, and desire for some good-independent goal. On this view also, the emphasis does not fall on the contrast between rational and non-rational functions but rather between two forms of goal-directed motivation, both of which again involve some cognitive or rational capacities.[182] This line of interpretation too could be developed in a way that is compatible with a Stoic, rather than Galenic, psychological picture. Indeed, as I have suggested elsewhere, this argument, and a number of other features of Plato's psychological thinking in the *Republic*, especially in books 8–9, can be seen as prefiguring a Stoic, unified picture, rather than a Galenic part-based one.[183] Although I do not propose to explore this idea further here, it is worth stressing that Galen's view of the argument is a selective reading, and one that favours the picture of the psyche he seeks to offer as a counterweight to the Stoic one.[184]

[180] See e.g. Annas 1981: 139–46, Price 1995: 40–57, Gill 1996: 245–60, which also discuss the relationship of the argument to the presentation of psychology elsewhere in Plato's *Republic*. See also Penner 1990: 49–61, arguing that, for the argument to be successful in proving its claims, it would need to show that both reason and appetite could act as 'executive desires'.

[181] On Stoic ideas about psychic conflict, see text to nn. 139–45 above.

[182] See e.g. Irwin 1977: 191–5, 226–33, 1995: 203–22, 243–8, Cooper 1984: 4–8, Kahn 1987: 82–91.

[183] Gill 1998: 131–7, 2006: 310–21. Whether Stoics such as Chrysippus actually *did* offer readings of Plato's accounts of psychology in the *Republic* is a matter of conjecture.

[184] Did Galen set out deliberately to counter Stoic readings of the argument? There is one passage that might indicate this. In V.486–8, 5.7.26–33 De Lacy, Galen dismisses what seem to be Stoic objections to the language used for the type of desire experienced by appetite. It is unclear whether the objection is to Plato's argument (as Galen interprets this) or simply to Platonic-style language for desire. But it is a possible indicator of debate involving Stoics about the significance of Plato's argument.

Thus, Galen's comments on Plato's argument bring out key aspects of Galen's psychological assumptions. A second revealing discussion in *PHP* 5 is Galen's treatment of ethical development, offered as correcting Chrysippus' account.[185] Although some of the ideas are presented as based on those of Posidonius (more precisely, on Platonic ideas adopted by Posidonius), the discussion is best interpreted as reflecting Galen's own views, which draw on earlier Platonic–Aristotelian thinking about development.[186] Galen's comments here, together with those in *QAM* ch. 11, are of special interest because they highlight an important contrast between two competing ways of understanding ethical development in ancient philosophy. This contrast has not been much discussed by scholars, perhaps because there are few texts before Galen that articulate the contrast clearly. But I have suggested elsewhere that this contrast forms an important strand in Hellenistic and post-Hellenistic philosophy and that it underlies the presentation of the formation and collapse of character in Plutarch's biographies and, arguably, Roman literary texts including Seneca's tragedies and Virgil's *Aeneid*.[187] We can find in Plato, especially the *Republic* and *Laws*, and Aristotle's ethical works a way of thinking about ethical development that is adopted by Plutarch and Galen among others. We can identify a contrasting approach in Stoic and Epicurean thinking; some of the salient differences are indicated in Plutarch's *On Ethical Virtue* and in Galen's treatments.[188]

The main differences between the two approaches, in broad outline, are these. In the Platonic–Aristotelian pattern, thinking about ethical development is based on the assumption that there are rational and non-rational parts of the psyche. It is also assumed that the non-rational part of the psyche needs to be habituated or 'harmonized' first as a prerequisite for the second, rational stage of development. More precisely, development is seen as depending on a combination of (the right kind of) inborn nature (*phusis*),

[185] *PHP* V.459–68, 5.5.1–40 De Lacy. [186] See further discussion below.

[187] See Gill 2006: 102–7, 131–45, 178–82, 231–3, 410–12.

[188] See Plu. *Mor.* 443 C–D, also 2 A–B, taken with Gill 2006: 231–3; on Galen, see discussion below. The view of development (as 'appropriation') offered by Antiochus and Arius Didymus represents a mixed pattern, fusing Platonic–Aristotelian and Stoic strands; see Gill 2006: 166–77.

habituation (*ethos*) in (the right kind of) upbringing, education, and social context, enabling those with (the right kind) or rational capacities (*logos*) to achieve full virtue.[189] A related feature of this pattern is the belief that, at a certain stage of adult life, character (*ēthos*) becomes either unalterable or very difficult to change, presumably because the non-rational part of the psyche has been habituated in a certain way.[190] An associated belief is that even people of relatively defective character achieve some degree of stability of character.[191]

The Stoic–Epicurean pattern differs on all these points. Although Stoic and Epicurean thinking about psychology is not identical, both theories share a unified or holistic view of psychological functions, and do not adopt the Platonic–Aristotelian contrast between rational and non-rational strands in motivation.[192] Both theories also hold that all human beings are constitutively capable of forming a true understanding of core notions such as good or god, an understanding associated in both theories with the idea of 'preconceptions' (*prolēpseis*).[193] A related belief is that, as the Stoics sometimes put it, 'all human beings have the starting points of virtue', that is, all human beings have the natural capacity to develop towards *complete* ethical excellence and happiness.[194] Although both theories recognize the influence of innate factors, the physical environment, and social factors, they do not accept that these can disable anyone permanently from progressing towards perfection. This possibility remains open

189 Versions of this pattern can be found in the two-stage educational programme of Plato's *Republic* and related ideas in Plato's *Laws*; also in Aristotle's thinking about the interplay between nature, habituation, and rational choice (see e.g. Arist. *EN* 1.3–4, esp. 1095^{b}3–8, also 1098^{a}33–^{b}4, and 10.9). See further Gill 2006: 134–6, also 1996: 272–5. Cf. Plutarch refs. in n. 188 above.

190 See Arist. *EN* 3.5, esp. 1114^{a}3–21. On Plutarch's thinking, and its background in Platonic–Aristotelian thought, see Gill 2006: 413–21.

191 This is a little noticed, but significant, feature of this line of thought; Aristotle's distinction between (stable) vice and (unstable) weakness of will is relevant to this strand of thought. See Arist. *EN* 1.13, esp. 1102^{b}13–1103^{a}10, 7.8; also Plu. *Mor.* 445 E, 446 C–D; see Gill 2006: 232–3.

192 On Epicurean thinking, see Gill 2006: 113–14, referring to the belief-based view of emotions implied in their contrast between 'natural' and 'empty' emotions and desires; on Stoic thinking on emotions, see Gill 2006: ch. 4, and 4.2 above.

193 See Gill 2006: 132–3, 180–1; also Asmis 1999: 279, M. Frede 1999*c*: 318–21.

194 See Stob. 2.65.8 (*SVF* 1.566, LS 61 L), my trans. See further Gill 2006: 131–2, 257, and text to n. 124 above.

to all human beings at any stage in their lives, a fact that underlies Stoic and Epicurean ideas about the role of therapeutic discourse, as brought out later.[195] This belief is linked with the idea that the psyche does not contain non-rational parts, which can become irreversibly shaped by habituation.[196] A related idea, maintained in a particularly strong form in Stoic thought, is that failure to achieve the highest ethical state ('wisdom') means that people are (relatively) unstable and incoherent in their psychic state and pattern of life. This degree of instability and incoherence is a lasting feature of their condition—although the possibility of progressing towards wisdom also remains permanently open.[197]

This contrast in patterns of thinking about development provides the explanatory background both for Galen's discussion in *PHP* 5,[198] and for *QAM* ch. 11. In both cases, Galen seeks to counter Stoic (Chrysippean) ideas about ethical development and to commend those associated with the Platonic–Aristotelian pattern. In *PHP* 5, he presents his views as based on those of Posidonius, who is pictured, here as elsewhere, as criticizing Chrysippean ideas and adopting Platonic ones instead. In *QAM* ch. 11, Galen speaks in his own voice, though he expresses similar views. Scholars have tended to accept the impression that Galen gives about Posidonius' thinking;[199] however, as pointed out earlier, there have been some recent strong challenges to Galen's presentation.[200] Tieleman, in particular, in a detailed examination of this section of *PHP* 5, suggests that Galen's account of Posidonius' use of Plato is highly misleading, and that Posidonius is more plausibly interpreted as highlighting links between Platonic and orthodox Stoic ideas. The main claims made in this part of *PHP* 5 express Galen's own ideas, at least his version of the Platonic–Aristotelian approach to development, supported—misleadingly—by references to Posidonius and Posidonius' readings of Plato.[201]

[195] See 5.3 below. [196] Gill 2006: 103–6, 178–82, 377–9.

[197] Gill 2006:119, 260–4, 318–20; also text to nn. 146–53 above.

[198] V.459–68, 5.5.1–40 De Lacy.

[199] *PHP* V.459–465, 5.5.1–29 De Lacy is cited as fr. 169 (V.460–4, 5.5.8–26 De Lacy is presented as LS 65 M); and V.466–8, 5.5.30–40 De Lacy is cited as fr. 31 in Edelstein–Kidd 1972/1989. [200] See text to n. 83 above.

[201] Tieleman 2003*a*: 220–42, also 136–9. See also Gill 2006: 281–90.

In *PHP* 5, as in *QAM* ch. 11, Galen rejects completely Chrysippus' ideas about ethical development. He dismisses Chrysippus' view that 'children are naturally drawn (or 'appropriated', *oikeiousthai*) to the right' (or 'fine', *kalon*), arguing that, if this were true, all corruption would necessarily be from external causes. He cites an otherwise unknown comment of Chrysippus that even children who are excellently brought up do not necessarily become good people.[202] He also refers to Chrysippus' explanation of human corruption, which is known to us from other sources, by reference to the combination of social influence ('the conversation of the majority of people') and 'the very nature of the things around them', or 'the persuasiveness of impressions'.[203] Galen criticizes these explanations without showing any sign of examining them closely. He argues that Chrysippus cannot explain why these influences have any hold on children, given his view that they are naturally drawn to what is right, rather than to vice or pleasure.[204] Galen's objections are based on his own position, outlined at the start of the section, that human beings have three natural kinds of attraction (or 'appropriation', *oikeiōsis*), to pleasure, victory, and the right. These are the natural objectives of the three parts of the psyche, the rational, spirited, and the appetitive. Children, whose faculties are non-rational, are attracted to pleasure and victory; only later, when they acquire reason, are they also attracted to the right.[205] This account of childhood development is sometimes ascribed to Posidonius, though Galen himself does not say the theory is Posidonian.[206] But, although Galen adopts the Stoic term 'appropriation', and shares with the Stoics the view that children are not yet rational, the pattern of thought is clearly Platonic or Platonic–Aristotelian. The linkage between psychic parts and forms of motivation and the idea of a two-stage developmental process, in which rational development builds on non-rational, recall the more

[202] *PHP* V.461, 5.5.10–13, esp. p. 318. 24 De Lacy, cited in the text, my trans. For the Stoic idea that human beings are naturally capable of developing towards virtue, see text to nn. 193–7 above.

[203] *PHP* V.462–3, 5.5.14–19, esp. p. 321.1–2, 17–18 De Lacy. For these causes of corruption, see also D.L. 7.89; on the Stoic explanation, see text to nn. 121–6 above.

[204] *PHP* V.462–3, 5.5.15–20 De Lacy.

[205] *PHP* V.459–60, 5.5.1–8 De Lacy.

[206] The passage is given as part of fr. 169 in Edelstein–Kidd 1972/1989, and appears as *SVF* 3.229a, as well as LS 65 M.

fully theorized accounts in Plato's *Republic* or Aristotle's ethical works.[207]

Subsequently, Galen clarifies his approach to development by referring to Posidonius' ideas, including Posidonius' use of Platonic material. The ideas to which Galen refers can plausibly be interpreted as (orthodox) Stoic ones, despite Galen's presentation. But they can also, on different assumptions, be taken as giving further content and specificity to Galen's thinking about development. Galen refers to Posidonius' interest in physical factors affecting character development, including the evidence of physiognomy and environmental factors, and he suggests that Stoics such as Chrysippus ignored such factors. It is clear, however, from *QAM*, and other sources, that Stoics such as Chrysippus are fully prepared to recognize the importance of such factors—as Galen himself acknowledges in the later work.[208] What the Stoics would not accept is that physical factors disable someone completely from making progress towards virtue. However, Posidonius' interest in such factors is taken by Galen to indicate a Platonic–Aristotelian approach, which sees inborn nature as a key determinant and limiting factor in ethical development.[209] Galen goes on to note Posidonius' interest in Plato's comments in the *Laws* about shaping the character of unborn children in the womb and about rearing them appropriately after birth. As it happens, we have independent information, from Calcidius, that the Stoics recognized the possible impact on character development of physical treatment (hot baths) immediately after birth.[210] Galen also cites

[207] *PHP* V.460, 5.5.6–8 De Lacy. On the Platonic and Aristotelian accounts, see Gill 2006: 134–6; on the theory presented in *PHP* as Galenic, see Tieleman 2003*a*: 220–2. The idea of development as appropriation had become common currency long before Galen and was adopted by the Academic thinker, Antiochus (*c.*130–*c.*68 BC), whose theory is reported in Cic. *Fin.* 5.

[208] *PHP* V.464–5, 5.5.22–7 De Lacy, esp. 5.26, denying Chrysippus' interest in such factors. Contrast Gal. *QAM* IV.783, *SM* 2.45.5–11, 21–4, cited in Ch. 3 above, text to n. 271. On Stoic (including Chrysippean) interest in physical factors affecting development, see Tieleman 2003*a*: 157–66, 190–6.

[209] *PHP* V.465, 5.5.28–9 De Lacy. For Platonic–Aristotelian ideas of a similar kind, see e.g. Pl. *R.* 485a–487a (the philosophical nature as a prerequisite for complete ethical development), Arist. *EN* 10.9, esp. 1179^{b}20–31; on Plutarch's elaboration of this approach, see Gill 2006: 415, also Duff 1999: chs. 1–3.

[210] *PHP* V.465–6, 5.5.30–2, referring to Pl. *Lg.* 789a–792e. See also Calcidius, *In Timaeum* 165–7 (*SVF* 3.228); also Tieleman 2003*a*: 132–9.

evidence suggesting that Posidonius saw these and other methods as a means of pre-rational training in preparation for rational education, which is a salient feature of the Platonic–Aristotelian pattern.[211] In fact, the Stoics, like Plato and Aristotle, saw children as not yet rational, and so they too would regard any such training practices as pre-rational in their effect. But the Stoics also believed that adulthood brings a qualitative change in psychological state, and that adult motivation is consistently informed by rationality. Hence, it is quite possible for Posidonius and other Stoics to have seen childhood training as pre-rational without supposing, as Galen does, that this represents the training of a separate non-rational part, which continues to exercise motivational force throughout adult life.[212] By ignoring this difference, Galen gives the impression that Posidonius adopted the Platonic–Aristotelian approach to ethical development that he himself holds, although this does not follow from the evidence Galen cites.

The contrast between Platonic–Aristotelian and Stoic (or Epicurean) patterns of thinking about ethical development also illuminates Galen's approach in *QAM* ch. 11, discussed in 3.5 above. Galen's stance there also reflects his adoption of the Platonic–Aristotelian position and his rejection of the Stoic one. In *QAM*, as in *PHP* 5, Galen stresses the importance of innate character and rejects the Stoic view that 'all people are naturally fitted for the acquisition of virtue, but are turned away from it by the influence of those around them'.[213] In *QAM*, Galen also places special emphasis on an idea that sometimes figures in the Platonic–Aristotelian pattern, that people can become irreversibly bad in character at some point in their lives, either through inborn nature or a combination of nature, habituation, and choice.[214] In *QAM*, Galen restates the arguments of *PHP* against the idea that corruption can be wholly attributed to external

[211] *PHP* V.466–7, 5.5.33–5; on the Posidonian language cited as not necessarily indicating a part-based psychology, see Tieleman 2003*a*: 226–7, Gill 2006: 288–9. On the Platonic–Aristotelian interest in the foundational role of pre-rational education, see e.g Pl. *R.* 400d–402a, Arist. *EN* 2.1, 10.9, 1179^{b}31–1180^{a}14.

[212] See Gill 2006: 138–44; also Inwood 1985: 72–80.

[213] *QAM* IV.816, *SM* 2.74.22–75.1, trans. Singer 1997*a*: 173; cf. text to n. 194 above.

[214] *QAM* IV.815–16, *SM* 2.73.16–74.21; trans. in Singer 1997*a*: 172–3. For this motif, see n. 190 above.

influences, arguing that this view takes no account of innate differences in character.[215] He seems also to allude to the other corrupting factor cited by Chrysippus, the 'persuasiveness of impressions', though not explicitly addressing this Stoic idea. His argument takes the form of claiming that the attractiveness of pleasure affects all of us equally and so cannot be used as an explanation why some people, but not others, become bad.[216] Much of *QAM* ch. 11 is presented as Galen's own views; but he refers in the later part of the chapter to Posidonius. His comments here are more generalized than in *PHP* 5, suggesting that he is simply drawing on his memory or earlier writings and has not looked at Posidonius' treatises again.[217] Here, Posidonius is presented as endorsing Galen's claim that inborn nature is the key factor ('there is in fact a seed of evil within us') by contrast with the 'Stoic view, that evil comes into us from outside'. Although Galen does not offer specific quotations or references, it seems that he is referring again to Posidonius' comments on the importance of body-based natural inclinations, the importance of which Galen himself underlines in this connection, characterizing them here in terms of the 'mixtures' of elements in the body, in line with his main thesis in *QAM*.[218]

What implications emerge from linking *QAM* ch. 11 with the discussion in *PHP* 5 and with the larger contrast in patterns of thinking about ethical development? *QAM* ch.11 brings out still more clearly than *PHP* 5 the fact that the views offered in both cases are, essentially, Galen's own—at least Galen's version of the Platonic–Aristotelian pattern. Although, for reasons of debate, Galen stresses in *PHP* the point that, as he claims, Posidonius also adopts these views, *QAM* shows Galen expressing them in his own voice, though still enlisting the support of Posidonius. Reference to the

[215] *QAM* IV.816–18, *SM* 2.74.21–77.1; trans. in Singer 1997*a*: 173–4; cf. nn. 202–6 above.

[216] *QAM* IV.819, *SM* 2.77.1–17; trans. in Singer 1997*a*: 174; cf. text to n. 203 above.

[217] *QAM* IV.819–21, *SM* 2.77.17–79.9; trans. in Singer 1997*a*: 174–5. On Galen's (apparent) practice in reading and using Stoic materials, see Tieleman 2003*a*: 51–8, 149 n. 44.

[218] *QAM* IV.820–1, esp. *SM* 2.78.9–10, 15–17, trans. Singer 1997*a*: 175, and 2.78.23–79.9. See text to n. 208 above, and Tieleman 2003*a*: 241–2. In fact, Stoic theory also attaches importance to these factors, as is recognized by Galen himself earlier in the work, *QAM* IV.783–4, *SM* 2.45.4–46.7.

larger framework of ancient ideas about ethical development also accentuates the extreme and problematic character of the position Galen adopts in *QAM* ch. 11. As highlighted earlier, Galen there places an exceptional stress on the importance of innate character, presented as largely body-based, or physical influences on development, while at the same time insisting that people must still be held fully responsible for their character and actions and punished, or even killed, accordingly. I suggested that Galen might have improved his argument here and reached a more consistent position overall if he had engaged more closely with Stoic thinking on this question.[219] However, Galen's approach is non-standard even within the Platonic–Aristotelian framework. For instance, in Plato, Aristotle, or Plutarch, weight is placed on all three factors (innate nature, habituation, and rational choice) and on the interplay between them. Also, the question of the relationship between innate character and responsibility is treated in a more fine-grained, and theoretically consistent way elsewhere, for instance in Aristotle, *EN* 3.5 or Plato's *Timaeus*.[220] The discussion in *PHP* 5, while not explicitly focused on the question of responsibility, recognizes the importance of a variety of factors and their interplay, especially innate nature and pre-rational habituation, and is thus more in line with the Platonic–Aristotelian tradition. Hence, comparison between the two Galenic discussions both clarifies the nature of Galen's psychological assumptions and underlines the exceptional and problematic character of Galen's stance in *QAM* ch. 11.

In this section, my aim has been to bring out more clearly the psychological framework assumed by Galen in his critique of Stoic thinking about emotions in *PHP* 4–5. Galen does not offer an independent analytic statement of this framework. His assumptions emerge by implication, through his comments on Plato's arguments for separate psychic parts and on Posidonian and Platonic thinking about ethical development. Galen's main aim, in these discussions, is to show that the Stoic theory (more specifically, Chrysippus' theory) is philosophically isolated and extreme in its belief-based conception of emotions and in its implausible or unnatural presentation of

[219] See Ch. 3 above, text to nn. 292–9.
[220] See Ch. 3 above, text to nn. 289–91.

psychological functions. This leads Galen to underline ideas about psychology that are antithetical to the Stoic (Chrysippean) approach, notably the idea of psychic parts as independent sources of motivation and the part-based analysis of ethical development. However, the Stoic psychological framework, while exceptional in its radical holism and revision of previous ideas, offers a coherent and cogent analysis of human psychology and development. Seen from this standpoint, Galen's psychological approach, in so far as this is articulated, emerges as a credible alternative to the Stoic picture—but one that by no means removes the Stoic picture from serious consideration. Indeed, in some respects, as suggested earlier, the Stoic unified approach might go well with Galen's brain-centred psychophysiology,[221] though this is not a line of thought Galen even begins to pursue in this context. The main point of difference between the Galenic and Stoic approaches to psychological functions inheres in the contrast between a part-based (or 'composition') approach and holistic (or 'structure') one; and in the next section this contrast is explored further with reference to a third important discussion in *PHP* 5.

4.4 GALEN AND STOICS ON PSYCHIC PARTS AND WHOLES

In this section, I bring to a close this exploration of the relationship between Galenic and Stoic thinking on psychological functions, especially reason and emotion. I take one of Galen's criticisms in *PHP* 5 as the starting point for an examination of key features of Stoic psychology. Galen's criticism, made in the course of discussing Stoic use of the analogy between psychic and bodily health and sickness, is that Chrysippus uses the notion of psychic 'parts' without giving any intelligible content to this idea. Galen's claim is that, because Chrysippus rejects the Platonic-style notion of psychic parts that Galen himself adopts, the Stoic thinker is not entitled to use the notion of psychic parts at all in connection with the idea of

[221] See 3.2 above.

psychic health and sickness. In responding to Galen's critique, I consider, first of all, Galen's own assumptions about psychic parts and psychic health. I then suggest that Stoic theory has, in fact, a wholly intelligible conception of psychic parts, including the kind of parts relevant to psychic health and sickness, though one that is different from that presupposed by Galen. To make sense of their approach, we need to refer, especially, to Stoic ideas about ethical development, which, as indicated already, are markedly different from Galen's,[222] and consider the implications of these ideas for the contrast between the psychic state of the wise and non-wise. This contrast illuminates a number of relevant points, including their thinking about psychic health and sickness and also about the kind of irrationality involved in emotion, a topic considered earlier.[223] On the basis of this discussion of Stoic thinking about psychic parts and psychic health and sickness, I return to the broader issues raised in 4.1 about the relationship between Galenic and Stoic thinking. The contrast between Galenic and Stoic thought on this question, and to some extent on psychological functions generally, can usefully be analysed in terms of the contrast between the two different approaches to the part–whole relationship outlined earlier, those linked with the ideas of 'composition' and 'structure'.[224] However, in other respects, Galenic and Stoic approaches are not consistently differentiated in this way. This raises the question, why their ideas are so sharply contrasted in this way on this topic, a question addressed at the end of the section.

The aspect of Galen's criticisms on which I focus is his complaint that Chrysippus uses, in connection with the idea of psychic health and sickness, a concept of psychic part to which he is not entitled. What, exactly, are the Stoic ideas that Galen criticizes on these grounds? Galen offers this example, citing Chrysippus' comments:

> Just as strength and weakness, firmness and softness, are observed in the body, and also health and disease, robustness and sickliness . . . in the same way, there are certain things in the rational psyche that exist and are named analogously to all of these . . . we do in fact say that some persons are strong

[222] See text to nn. 116–18, 129–33, 188–97 above.

[223] See text to nn. 127–53 above.

[224] See text to nn. 38–56 above.

or weak also in psyche, and firm or soft, diseased or healthy; and we speak in this way of emotion, infirmity and the like in the psyche.[225]

A fuller passage, which brings out more clearly the theory involved, is cited by Stobaeus:

They say, then, that these virtues just listed are perfect in our lives and consist in theorems (*theōrēmata*); but others supervene on them, which are no longer crafts but rather certain faculties (*dunameis*) which come about as a result of practice; for instance, health of the psyche and its soundness and strength and beauty. For just as the health of the body is a good blend of the hot and cold and wet and dry elements in the body, so too the health of the psyche is a good blend of the beliefs (*dogmata*) in the psyche. Similarly, just as strength of the body is a sufficient tension (*tonos*) in the sinews, so too the strength of the psyche is a sufficient tension in judging and acting and not doing so. Just as beauty of the body is a symmetry (*summetria*) of its limbs constituted with respect to each other and the whole, so too the beauty of the psyche is a symmetry of reason and its parts (*merē*) with respect to the whole of it and to each other.[226]

I consider later what ideas these passages imply; but, first, what are Galen's objections?

What Galen criticizes is not the idea of an analogy between psychic and bodily illness as such. His objection is to Chrysippus' use of the notion of psychic parts in this connection. He cites as especially problematic passages such as this:

Therefore by analogy the psyche will also be called beautiful or ugly in terms of the proportion (*summetria*) or disproportion of certain parts (*merē*) of such and such a kind... They are parts (*moria*) of the psyche through which its reason (*logos*) and the disposition of its reason are constituted. A psyche is beautiful or ugly by virtue of its control-centre (*hēgemonikon*) being in this or that state with respect to its own proper divisions (*merismoi*).[227]

[225] *PHP* V.438, 5.2.26–7, p. 300.2–7, 8–12 De Lacy, trans. De Lacy, slightly modified.

[226] Stob. 2.62.15–63.5 (5b4 in the summary of Stoic ethics), trans. Inwood and Gerson 1997: 205, slightly modified (=*SVF* 3.278); on this passage, see Tieleman 2003*a*: 235–6.

[227] *PHP* V.443–4, 5.2.47, 49, p. 304.10–11, 18–21 De Lacy, trans. De Lacy, slightly modified.

Galen's complaint is that Chrysippus, in such passages, uses the notion of 'parts', although his conception of psychic activity does not recognize parts—at least parts of the type Galen is looking for. Galen's paradigm for 'parts' is the Platonic tripartite psyche, as he makes clear from the start: 'These parts, on Plato's view, are the spirited, rational, and appetitive, so that the analogy of psyche to body in health and disease is preserved in every respect. When the three parts are in harmony with each and not in conflict at all, they produce psychic health, but when in disharmony and conflict (they produce disease).'[228] But, in Chrysippus' case, 'As he supposes that all emotions (or experiences, *pathē*) and diseases arise in a single part, the rational (*to logistikon*), it is not surprising that he is unable to explain what those parts are, the proper proportion (*summetria*) of which is psychic health.'[229] Galen's characterization of Stoic thinking is rather misleading here; although recognizing that Chrysippus does not adopt Plato's tripartite model, Galen describes the Stoic view in Platonic terms. Chrysippus is presented as if he only recognized one of the three Platonic parts, the rational (*logistikon*), whereas, as brought out earlier, the Stoics adopted a unified or holistic approach, in which, in adult humans, rationality informs motivation as a whole.[230] However, there is still force in Galen's question: if Stoic psychology is not centred on parts, as Plato's is, what are the 'parts' whose harmony constitutes psychic health?

There are two main types of candidate for psychic 'parts' in Stoic philosophy, both of which Galen considers and rejects. One possibility is that of the various functions, those of the senses, voice, and sexual generation, which, together with the central control-centre (*hēgemonikon*), constitute the Stoic psyche. However, Galen rejects this idea, on the ground that the 'parts' relevant to psychic health are presented by Chrysippus as functions of reason, which belongs to the control-centre, and so they cannot consist in these other psychic functions.[231] The second possibility of this type considered is that the relevant parts are the two elements of which psychic

[228] *PHP* V.441, 5.2.37–8, p. 302.10–16 De Lacy; on the conception of 'part' implied in this comment, see text to nn. 244–54 below.

[229] *PHP* V.419, 5.2.45, p. 304.3–5 De Lacy, trans. De Lacy, slightly modified; cf. V.444, 5.2.48 De Lacy.

[230] See text to nn. 98–109 above.

[231] V. 446–7, 5.3.7 De Lacy; for these psychic parts or functions in Stoic theory, see also *PHP* V.288, 3.1.11 De Lacy, and LS 53 G–H; also Ch. 3, text to nn. 38–44 above.

pneuma is composed, the hot and cold or air and fire. However, Galen also dismisses this idea rapidly, arguing that these are the core elements of matter and of bodily states. What Chrysippus has in view are parts that are analogous to bodily parts but which belong to the rational control-centre, as is implied by his analogy between psychic and physical health and sickness.[232] Galen's dismissal of this idea, like his equation of Chrysippus' control-centre with the Platonic rational part, seems a bit hasty. After all, according to Stoic thinking, the psyche is a physical entity, and Galen himself in *QAM*, in a passage noted earlier, reminds us of this fact and of the use of this idea in differentiating the quality of different psychic types: 'It has, then, become clear to you now that in the view of the Stoics the substance of the psyche comes to be according to a particular mixture of air and fire. And Chrysippus has been made intelligent because of the well-tempered mixture of these two [elements], while the sons of Hippocrates... [have been made] swinish because of the boundless heat'.[233] Tieleman underlines the relevance of Stoic psychophysicalism to this question; and, indeed, argues that the 'parts' that Chrysippus has in mind are the same as the hot and cold which are the 'parts' of physical health. In arguing for this view, Tieleman appeals to a very rich vein in Stoic thinking, one de-emphasized by Galen, at least in this section of *PHP*. This includes the psychophysicalism embodied in Stoic accounts of emotions as occurrent phenomena and also of psychic sicknesses (conceived as 'feverish' states). It also includes a broadly psychophysicalist approach in connection with thinking about treatment of health and environmental influences on character.[234] In addition, Tieleman suggests that Plato's presentation of psychic illness

[232] *PHP* V.447–8, 5.3.8–11, esp. p. 306.28–31 De Lacy. On psychic *pneuma*, see LS 47.

[233] *QAM* IV.784, *SM* 2.45.21–4 (part of *SVF* 2.787), trans. Tieleman 2003*a*: 150, slightly modified; see also the translation of Singer 1997*a*: 158. See also Ch. 3 above, text to nn. 271–7.

[234] See Tieleman 2003*a*: 148–58, referring to *QAM* (passage just cited), also citing *PHP* V. 435–6, 5.2.14–19 De Lacy (psychic illness as fever) and *PHP* V.291, 3.1.25 De Lacy (emotion as psychophysical experience). See also Tieleman 2003*a*: 161–2, on Calcidius, *In Timaeum* 165 (the influence of the midwife's bath on the character of the newly-born) and 194–5 on Cic. *De Fato* 7–9 (influence of physical environment on character).

as, essentially, body-based in *Timaeus* 86b–87b may lie behind the Stoic conception and may have influenced it.[235] I accept entirely the importance of these dimensions of Stoic theory, and consider them more fully later in connection with their ideas about bodily and psychic therapy.[236] I also think that a psychophysical analysis is implied in the Stoic conception of psychic illness, and that, whatever 'parts' Chrysippus has in mind, these must have physical correlatives, which may have been conceived in terms of modalities of *pneuma* or mixtures of hot and cold. However, I still believe that Galen is making a valid point, in emphasizing that Chrysippus speaks of an *analogy* between psychic and bodily health, and that the 'parts' involved are not, primarily at least, conceived in physical terms.[237]

The second possible meaning for 'parts', which I think more likely, is one that Galen suggests as the only remaining option, but which he sees as very weak: 'But as he was unable to say what these psychic parts are, since he placed its health and disease, beauty and ugliness in one part only, the rational part, he was compelled to twist the argument and to count the activities (*energeiai*) of the psyche as its parts'.[238] The Stobaeus passage cited earlier supports this suggestion: we are told that 'the health of the psyche is a good blend of the beliefs (*dogmata*) in the psyche' and that 'the beauty of the psyche is a symmetry of reason and its parts (*mera*)'.[239] Galen also cites Chrysippus' definition of reason as 'a collection (*athroisma*) of notions and concepts', as a possible explanation of what Chrysippus means by 'parts' of reason.[240] A more plausible suggestion along the same lines is the kind of rational processes, in adult humans, involved in generating emotions: that is, the rational impressions, assents, and impulses ('beliefs' in more conventional terms) that constitute

[235] Tieleman 2003*a*: 159–60, 188–90; on the possible influence of this passage on Stoic thought, see also Gill 2006: 200–3 (also Gill 2000).

[236] See 5.4 below; this line of thought reflects one of the kinds of 'naturalism' typical of their approach (2.3).

[237] See n. 232 above.

[238] *PHP* V.444, 5.2.48, p. 304.14–17 De Lacy, trans. De Lacy, slightly modified.

[239] See text to n. 226 above. See also Cic. *Tusc.* 4.30–1, in which psychic health is defined in terms of the harmony of 'judgements and beliefs' (*iudicia opinionesque*) (30), (*opinionum iudiciorumque*) (31). See also Engberg-Pedersen 1980: 189–91.

[240] *PHP* V.445, 5.3.1, p. 304.35 De Lacy, trans. De Lacy.

emotions and reflect psychic sickness.[241] These seem to be the kind of phenomena that Chrysippus might have in mind in saying that, 'They are parts (*moria*) of the psyche through which its reason (*logos*) and the disposition of its reason are constituted (*sunestēke*). A psyche is beautiful or ugly by virtue of its control-centre (*hēgemonikon*) being in this or that state with respect to its own proper divisions (*merismoi*).'[242] There is still a question about the sense in which these constitute psychic 'parts' or 'divisions', and why Chrysippus identifies these as parts rather than something more enduring or structural. But there are, as I suggest later, intelligible and interesting reasons underlying this phraseology, and ones that reflect certain important differences between the Stoic psychological framework and Galen's.[243]

First, however, I consider Galen's reasons for regarding these as inappropriately described as psychic 'parts'. One reason is rather straightforward, the other less so, but taken together they throw light on Galen's approach to the part–whole relationship, at least as applied to questions of psychology. The more straightforward reason is that 'parts' signify basic or core elements of an entity whereas activities are the expression of the functions of the whole entity composed in this way. This kind of distinction is implied in the contrast Galen draws between 'parts' and 'activities' with respect to a number of types of entity, including the psyche, and it is formulated more explicitly elsewhere in Galen's writings.[244] A related point made by Galen is that Chrysippus' account conflates psychic health and psychic beauty when these should be kept distinct. In the case of the body, Galen says, Chrysippus maintains the distinction correctly, in that he identifies health with the proportion (*summetria*) between elements (*stoicheia*), whereas he identifies beauty with the proportion between limbs or parts of the body (*moria*). Galen maintains that, although there are widely differing views about what constitutes elements, all doctors and philosophers regard health as the proportion of the

[241] See further text to nn. 259–60 below.

[242] *PHP* V.444, 5.2.49, p. 304. 18–21 De Lacy, trans. De Lacy, slightly modified, cited in text to n. 227 above.

[243] See text to nn. 265–7 below.

[244] *PHP* V.446–8, 5.3.3–11 De Lacy. On the distinction between faculty/part (*dunamis/meros*) and activity (*energeia*) in Galen, see Hankinson 2006: 242–3.

elements.[245] He also cites a passage from Plato's *Sophist* that is presented as showing that 'the conflict of psychic parts with each other is psychic disease, while its disordered and immoderate movements, that is, its motivated activities (*energeias kath' hormēn*), constitute its ugliness'.[246] Chrysippus, on the other hand, is criticized for confusing psychic health with psychic beauty. He fails to recognize that health and sickness consist in the proportion or disproportion of core, basic elements, whereas beauty and ugliness are expressed in the movements or activities of the entity composed of these elements, such as, in the body the movements of its limbs.[247] This constitutes the more straightforward of Galen's reasons for regarding Chrysippus' use of the notion of psychic 'parts' as inappropriate.

The second reason is less straightforward, though it is intelligible. A recurrent theme in Galen's critique of Chrysippean thinking on this subject is that 'psychic disease will be disproportion *and mutual conflict* (*stasis*) in those very same parts whose proportion was psychic health'.[248] Galen supports this idea by repeated reference to a passage of Plato's *Sophist* that defines disease as 'the destruction of what is by nature congenial as a result of some dissension (*diaphora*)'.[249] As Galen explains, the rationale for this definition of disease is that it constitutes a state in which the core components of an entity, which are naturally adapted to combine in a well-proportioned way (so creating health), come into conflict, thus producing illness.[250] This point underlies Galen's critique of Chrysippus' equation of health with beauty. Disease (in the psyche as in other cases) constitutes conflict between core components or elements, whereas ugliness constitutes disproportion at a less fundamental level, namely as a property of movements or actions of whole entities.[251] Thus, when

245 *PHP* V.450.5.3.18 De Lacy.

246 *PHP* V.451, 5.3.21, p. 310.9–12 De Lacy, trans. De Lacy, modified. The passage is Pl. *Sph.* 227d–228d, cited in full in *PHP* V.452–3, 5.3.24–30 De Lacy.

247 *PHP* V.449–51, esp. 5.3.14–16, 19–21 De Lacy.

248 *PHP* V.441, 5.2.36, p. 302.8–10 De Lacy, trans. De Lacy, slightly modified, italics added.

249 Pl. *Sph.* 228a7–8, cited in *PHP* V.441, 5.2.36, p. 302.18–19 De Lacy, trans. De Lacy.

250 *PHP* V.441–2, 5.2.39–42 De Lacy.

251 See text to n. 228 above; this is supported by reference to Pl. *Sph.* 227d–228b in *PHP* V.452–3, 5.3.24–30 De Lacy.

Galen complains that Chrysippus fails to identify psychic parts properly, he has in mind two criteria for being a psychic part. One is that of being a core component of the psyche, rather than a psychic activity. The other criterion of parts is that they generate conflict between each other if they are not combined in a well-proportioned way. Galen's exemplar, again, is the Platonic tripartite psyche, whose features he characterizes in this way: 'When the three parts are in harmony with each and not in conflict at all, they produce psychic health, but when in disharmony and conflict (they produce) disease'.[252] Galen, probably, has in mind passages such as Plato, *Republic* 443–4, in which (psychic) justice is presented as the harmonization of the three core components of the psyche, as argued in 435–41, whereas injustice is presented as the dissension or 'civil war' (*stasis*) of things naturally capable of combining.[253] In the same passage, psychic justice is seen as psychic health and the opposite. For instance, Plato's Socrates says: 'To produce health is to establish the components of the body in a natural relation of control and being controlled, one by another, while to produce disease is to establish a relation of ruling and being ruled contrary to nature', and the same point applies to psychic health and disease.[254]

What larger implications follow from Galen's criteria for psychic parts in this context? In the first instance, we can see clear links with Galen's presentation of psychic parts elsewhere in *PHP* 4–5, and in *PHP* 1–6 more generally. In taking the Platonic tripartite psyche as his paradigm, as a counterweight to the Stoic pattern, Galen gives special prominence to Plato's argument for separate psychic parts (*R.* 435–41). In particular, he underlines the idea that the psychic parts are independent, and potentially conflicting, sources of motivation.[255] Similarly, in his account of psychophysiology, Galen emphasizes the idea that the three main organs function as starting points or sources (*archai*) of the three communication systems, those of nerves, arteries, and veins. He also accentuates the idea

[252] *PHP* V.441, 5.2.38, p. 302.14–16 De Lacy, trans. De Lacy, slightly modified; see also text to n. 248 above.

[253] On Galen's reading of Pl. *R.* 435–41, see text to nn. 165–72 above.

[254] Pl. *R.* 444d3–6, trans. Grube. rev. Reeve in Cooper 1997.

[255] See text to nn. 168–72 above.

that these organs function as the base for three independent sources of psychological motivation—an idea that, I argued, is in tension with his brain-centred account of the workings of the body.[256] Galen's twofold criteria in *PHP* 5 for being psychic parts (being core components of the psychic make-up and also generating conflict if not properly combined or harmonized)[257] are thus consistent with the conception of psychic parts expressed elsewhere in *PHP* 1–6.

There is a second important implication of this discussion of psychic parts in *PHP* 5. This relates to Galen's understanding of the part–whole relationship, as implied here and elsewhere in *PHP*. Earlier, I drew a contrast between two conceptions of this relationship, defined in terms of the notions of 'composition' and 'structure', respectively. In terms of this contrast, Galen's discussion clearly reflects a 'composition' conception. One aspect of the 'composition' approach is seeing the whole as identical with its parts and defined by their combination, by contrast with seeing the whole as the primary locus of identity and content, to which the parts are subordinate. A second aspect is conceiving the parts as identifiable independently of the whole, as distinct from being identifiable only in the context of the whole. A third aspect is that the structure of the whole is constituted by the combination of parts, rather than being what the whole *is*, from which the parts gain their identity. By reference to all three criteria, Galen's approach falls into the 'composition' category. The psychic whole is defined as the combination of the psychic parts, which are independently identifiable, and which constitute the structure of the whole by their combination. The fact that the psychic parts are conceived as core components with a determinate, independently specifiable character fits in with this pattern. So does the idea that the structure of the whole depends on the effective combination or coordination of the parts, which, if not achieved, gives rise to internal strife or psychic disease. As already indicated, a similar conceptual pattern is embodied in some other important features of Galen's thinking about psychology elsewhere in *PHP*, though not in all aspects of his psychological thinking, as stressed later.

[256] See Ch. 3 above, text to nn. 69–86.

[257] See *PHP* V. 439–53, 2.30–3.30 De Lacy.

Returning to Chrysippus' thinking, what conceptions of 'parts' does he have in mind, and which approach to the part–whole relationship is implied in his ideas, that of 'composition' or 'structure?[258] One of the passages cited earlier can serve as the basis for considering this question.

Therefore by analogy the psyche will also be called beautiful or ugly in terms of the proportion (*summetria*) or disproportion of certain parts (*merē*) of such and such a kind... They are parts (*moria*) of the psyche through which its reason (*logos*) and the disposition of its reason are constituted (*sunestēke*). A psyche is beautiful or ugly by virtue of its control-centre (*hēgemonikon*) being in this or that state with respect to its own proper divisions (*merismoi*).[259]

For Galen, as just explained, the 'parts' are core components or subdivisions of the psyche and also independent (and potentially conflicting) sources of motivation. The presence of proportion or its absence depends on the kind of equilibrium or hierarchy established between those core components and sources of motivation. None of those assumptions hold good in Stoic thinking. The 'parts' designed here are, as suggested earlier, 'beliefs' (as in the Stobaeus passage cited).[260] More precisely, they are the rational impressions, assent and the associated impulses by reference to which Stoic theory explains the motivation to action in adult humans. They are not, of course, 'parts' in the Galenic sense (independent sources of motivation); these parts are causally interlocked with each other, and cannot conflict in the Platonic–Galenic manner.[261] How, then, can they give rise to the *contrasting* states of proportion and disproportion or health and sickness to which Chrysippus refers? How are these contrasting states explained by reference to the way in which the governing part (*hēgemonikon morion*) is 'in this or that state with respect to its proper divisions (*oikeious merismous*)'?

[258] The following three paragraphs are based on Gill 2007*a*: 116–17.

[259] *PHP* V.443–4, 5.2.47, 49, p. 304.10–11, 18–21 De Lacy, trans. De Lacy, slightly modified.

[260] See text to n. 226 above.

[261] See e.g. LS 33 I, 53 Q–S, 62 C; see further Brennan 2003: 260–9, Price 2005: 472–81, Graver 2007: 24–34.

In addressing this question, it is helpful to ask first the more general question whether Stoic thinking about the part–whole relationship involved here is conceived in terms of 'structure' or 'composition'. The key point of difference, as highlighted earlier, is whether the whole or the part is seen as prior in identity and intelligibility.[262] I think it is clear that, in this respect as in others, Stoic thinking embodies a strongly holistic or 'structure' approach. There are several ways in which this approach is evident in this area of Stoic thought. One, just noted, is that specific psychological activities, such as, in adult humans, forming rational impressions or giving assent, only make sense when considered as part of a causally interdependent *set or system* of such activities.[263] An associated point is that both ideal and defective psychic states are viewed from a holistic standpoint. A person is psychically well or ill, well or badly proportioned, *as a whole*, in a way that reflects his entire set of (in modern terms) beliefs and reasoning, affective responses, and psychophysical reactions. In this respect, Stoic theory gives explanatory priority to the *whole* state, and sees the component part (for instance, forming this or that rational impression) as secondary. A second relevant way in which Stoic thinking is holistic is this. The wise person's state of knowledge, character, virtue, and so on, is taken as constituting the only *complete* or fully whole or structured state; all other human states are regarded as relatively incomplete or unstructured by comparison with wisdom. Hence, proportion (or psychic health) is a property, in a strong sense, only of the wise. The condition of the non-wise, by contrast, is one of relative conflict, disorder, and disproportion. Thus, while the state of mind of the non-wise person is, in one sense, conceived as an integrated whole in so far as it constitutes a causally interconnected set of psychological activities, if judged by the standard of *complete* wholeness, it lacks proportion. In this respect, the idea of wholeness has a strong normative role in Stoic thought, though one which also bears directly on the description and analysis of, for instance, adult human psychological activities.[264]

[262] See text to n. 226 above. [263] See text to nn. 107–9 above.

[264] See further text to nn. 115–18, 129–33 above, also nn. 266–7 below.

How does this point help to explain the significance of the psychic parts or divisions (*merē/merismoi*)[265] by reference to which the control-centre (*hēgemonikon*) is well or badly proportioned? These 'parts' are, I suggest, aspects of the psychological activity of, respectively, the wise and the non-wise. In both cases, these 'parts' form an integrated whole of a certain type; but the kind of structure and its degree of internal coherence and order varies dramatically in the two cases. In the wise person, these parts reflect an internally coherent structure of beliefs or, rather, knowledge. Similarly, the wise person possesses the virtues, as an interlocked set, and these generate, in turn, qualities of the whole personality, which are characterized as 'health', 'beauty', or 'harmony'. The occurrent psychological activities of the wise person reflect this fully structured character.[266] In the non-wise person, by contrast, there are inconsistent and mutually jarring beliefs, including those that generate emotions. The emotions thus generated constitute disturbed affective and psychophysical states. Also, the longer-term states of the non-wise, though quasi-dispositional, are inherently unstable and described as 'fluctuating' or 'feverish'.[267] Chrysippus is thus, despite Galen's scepticism, fully entitled to talk about 'parts' of the overall nexus of psychological states or activities of both the wise and non-wise person. But these 'parts' can only be characterized properly when viewed, first, as aspects of an interconnected set of psychological processes, and, second, in the context of the overall state of someone who possesses or who lacks psychic proportion and health. In this pattern of thinking, the whole is primary in conception and explanation, and the parts are secondary. By contrast, in the Galenic picture, the whole psychic state depends on the equilibrium established between 'parts', which are seen as independent sources of motivation and as natural, basic units within the personality.

[265] I think these two terms are used simply as synonyms here; also Chrysippus' phrase, *hēgemonikon meros* (cf. *PHP* V.288, 3.1.10–15 De Lacy) does not signify a quasi-independent 'part' in the Platonic–Galenic sense.

[266] On the wise person's consistency and harmony see e.g. LS 31 B, 61 A, F–G, 63 F, L–M, Stob. 2.62.18–24, 63.1–5 (5b3–4); on the wise person as a norm for everyone, see LS 61 G, I(1). See further Gill 2006: 150–6, and the Stobaeus passage cited in text to n. 226 above.

[267] See text to nn. 147–54 above.

Galen's discussion of this question enables us to analyse with some precision the contrast between his psychological framework and the Stoic one. The contrast between 'composition' and 'structure' approaches to the part–whole relationship illustrated here reflects differences that are strongly marked in all aspects of the two psychological frameworks examined in this chapter. In the case of Stoicism, the holistic or 'structure' approach is one that is pervasive throughout the theory. In Galen's case, the overall position is more complex; as underlined earlier, much of Galen's thinking on a variety of subjects also exhibits a holistic approach. Hence, Galen's adoption of a strongly 'composition' approach here, and his systematic rejection of a holistic approach, requires special explanation. I considered earlier (4.1) a number of possible explanations, including, of course, the influence of the Platonic tripartite theory, in a work whose overall aim is presented as combining the ideas of Plato and Hippocrates on psychology and physiology.[268] However, the most decisive factor, as suggested earlier, is that Galen sees the Stoic unified account of psychological functions as inseparably linked with the Stoic heart-centred psychophysiology, and sees the rejection of both mistakes as crucial for his larger project in *PHP*.[269] In fact, there are several reasons for questioning this assumption, and for thinking that Stoic psychology is, in certain respects, more compatible with Galen's brain-centred anatomy than the Platonic tripartite account.[270] But this is not how Galen himself sees the matter; and in his later works of practical ethics, discussed in the next chapter, Galen retains his adoption of a part-based psychological framework. Hence, the psychology of emotion is a subject on which Galen and the Stoics are more sharply divergent than any others considered here; and in which the possibility of fruitful convergence is at its most remote. Indeed, the extent of their difference on this issue may be a crucial factor in deterring Galen from closer engagement on other questions in later works.

[268] On Galen's aims in *PHP*, see Ch. 3 above, text to nn. 13–21.

[269] See text to nn. 55–6 above.

[270] See 3.2–3 above.

5

The Therapy of Emotions

5.1 PRELIMINARIES

The previous chapter has centred on Galenic and Stoic theory regarding psychological functions, especially the relationship between reason and emotion. In this chapter, the focus shifts to the practical application of philosophy, particularly the therapy of emotions. But here too, I explore the implications of Galenic and Stoic practice for understanding their ideas about psychological functions and the relationship between psychology and the body. I also consider how far Galenic and Stoic ideas about the therapy of emotions and medical therapy were—or could have been—combined. I discuss how far their ideas, taken separately or in combination, reflect the kinds of shared naturalism that are evident in other aspects of their thought. To what extent can we say that their thinking about the therapy of emotion did form—or could have formed—part of a naturalistic picture of the self as a psychological and physical whole? A related question, explored in Chapter 6, is how far we can say that Galenic or Stoic therapy of the emotions—or any actual or potential combination of their approaches—constitutes what we would recognize, from a modern standpoint, as 'psychiatry' or 'psychotherapy'?

The core material for this topic is relatively limited. On Galen's side, the main work is a short essay, *Psychological Affections* (*Aff. Dig.*), which is coupled with another short work, *Psychological Errors* (*Pecc. Dig.*). There is also a still shorter, newly discovered, essay of a similar type, *Avoiding Distress*, and a closely related work *Character Traits*, known only from an Arabic summary. The main Stoic work is the (lost) fourth 'therapeutic' book of Chrysippus' *On Passions*, for which Galen is the main, though critical, source.[1] However, both works can be, and need to be, placed in a larger context, within Galen's works and Hellenistic-Roman thought more generally, if we are to make sense of their respective contributions to the therapy of emotions and if we are to use these works as part of the basis for answering the wide-ranging questions raised here.

I begin (5.2) by examining the main themes and objectives of Galen's *Psychological Affections*. This work reflects the Platonic–Aristotelian (part-based) approach to psychology that is evident in *PHP* 4–5 and also in *Character Traits*. However, the central aim and genre of the work reflect, to some degree at least, the Stoic approach, as expressed above all, in Chrysippus' 'therapeutic' book. How does Galen come to write an essay whose main aim is to rid the psyche of emotions and thus 'cure' it—a thoroughly Stoic aim—and how far does he transform this project to express his contrasting psychological assumptions? Part of the answer is that this genre had already been adopted by thinkers working in the Platonic–Aristotelian tradition, especially Plutarch. But questions still remain, as they do for Plutarch, about how fully an essay of this kind could be abstracted from the Stoic (or Stoic–Epicurean) psychological standpoint from which the genre derives. I also discuss the related short essay *Avoiding Distress*; this also contains a combination of Stoic-style and Platonic–Aristotelian motifs, but handled in a way that is, I think, more intellectually consistent.

I consider next the distinctive features of Chrysippus' approach to the therapy of emotions (5.3). Although the fourth ('therapeutic) book of Chrysippus' *On Passions* has been lost, we can recover its main lines from Galen's comments in *PHP* 4–5, taken with Cicero's *Tusculans* 3–4. It seems clear that Chrysippus' book constituted an important and coherent expression of the Stoic approach to this topic, and that it exercised wide and sustained influence, both within and outside Stoic intellectual circles. Its distinctive features seem to

[1] The Greek term translated *Affections* (in Galen's work) and *Passions* (in Chrysippus' work) is the same (*pathē*). The variation reflects the fact that there is no universally accepted English translation of this term. The titles used for the Galenic works discussed in this section are those adopted in Singer forthcoming.

have included both (1) strong linkage between ethical and psychological theory in its analysis of emotions and (2) a nuanced and in some ways pragmatic response to treatment of those in emotional states. The latter feature can be linked with the fine-grained analysis of cases of apparent dislocation between beliefs and emotional responses by both Chrysippus and Posidonius, which Galen reports and uses for his polemical purposes. Subsequent works of Stoic practical ethics seem to have accentuated one or other aspect of Chrysippus' approach. For instance, Epictetus and Marcus Aurelius stressed in different ways the determining impact of ethical beliefs, or the degree of one's ethical understanding, on one's emotional state.[2] Seneca's *On Anger* (*De Ira*) underlines, rather, the range of practical resources offered by Stoicism for working towards the negation of emotions, as does Cicero, in *Tusculans* 3–4 (Cicero does so from an independent, non-Stoic standpoint). The presence in Chrysippus' 'therapeutic' book of a relatively pragmatic, though still consistently Stoic, approach to the treatment of emotional states and dispositions may have promoted its influence among non-Stoics. Thus, Galen, despite his critical response to Chrysippus' programme in *PHP* 5, none the less subscribes to a broadly Stoic, or Stoic–Epicurean, project in writing his own essay on the therapy of emotions.

Subsequently (5.4), I consider broader issues raised by these Galenic and Stoic works on the therapy of the emotions. How, for instance, do these theories understand the relationship between philosophical and medical therapy? On the face of it, in each case, philosophical therapy is seen as directed at the psyche and medical therapy at the body. But do we find in either theory an attempt to combine these two kinds of therapy? This question takes on added importance in the light of the shared naturalism of the theories and the fact that both theories adopt, to some extent at least, a physicalist approach to psychology. A related question is how far the Stoic approach to the therapy of emotions—or therapy in general—reflects the holism (or 'structure-centred') approach that I have presented as characteristic of their thinking? A second question explored

[2] On Epictetus' *Discourses* and Marcus Aurelius' *Meditations*, and their strategies as works of practical ethics, see further Hadot 1995, 1998, Sellars 2003, 2007: on Marcus' approach to psychology, as essentially Stoic, see Gill 2007*b*: 176–9, 2007*c*.

is how far Galen's medical approach could have been combined with the Stoic approach to the therapy of emotions. Though the question is speculative or hypothetical, raising it enables us to examine the relationship between their thinking from a new and illuminating standpoint. The question has special interest since these methods were, arguably, the most highly developed and innovative ones in their respective fields in Hellenistic and Roman thought and practice. To what extent could they have been combined to produce what would be, in some sense, a 'naturalistic', as well as a 'whole-person', approach to therapy. The question raises rather complex issues; and the answers differ according to whether one considers the question from a Galenic or a Stoic standpoint. Galen would have been very unlikely to have accepted the viability of such a combination; in any case, he offers his own attempted combination or synthesis of medical and psychological therapy, in *QAM* , for instance. However, it is less clear that the Stoics would have had in principle any objection to this kind of combination, which opens up the conceptual possibility of the merger of these two highly developed methodologies.

5.2 GALEN ON THE THERAPY OF EMOTIONS

Before looking at Galen's contributions to this subject, *Psychological Affections* and *Avoiding Distress*, we need to take note of the broader context. Many works were written on the therapy of emotions in the Hellenistic and post-Hellenistic period. Although this genre originated from Stoic and Epicurean approaches to the emotions, it was adopted by thinkers writing from a Platonic standpoint of one type or another, including Cicero, in the *Tusculans*, and Plutarch. To make sense of the genre, and to define the distinctive features of Galen's contribution, we need to review how the idea of therapy of emotions fits in with Stoic and Epicurean thinking and what kind of challenge this idea presents for Platonic, or Platonic–Aristotelian, thought.

One of the provocative, or revisionist, claims made by Stoic and Epicurean philosophy is that emotions, as normally understood, express misguided beliefs about the nature of human happiness and constitute types of psychological sickness. In Stoicism, this results in the contrast between the *pathē* (emotions or passions) of non-wise people and the more restricted range of 'good emotions' (*eupatheiai*) of the normative wise person. Although Epicurean views on this subject are not quite so sharply defined, Epicureans also regard most emotions and desires as 'empty', reflecting erroneous ideas about happiness, by contrast with the 'natural' emotions and desires characteristic of wisdom.[3] Hence, for both schools, human happiness consists, in part, in a state of freedom from such emotions and from the inner disturbance they generate, a state conceived as *apatheia* in Stoicism, and *ataraxia* in Epicureanism.[4] In Aristotle's ethical writings, by contrast, virtue is characterized, in part, as hitting the 'mean' in feelings as well as actions, that is, as having the right type or degree of emotional reaction, which is appropriate to the specific situation and the agents involved.[5] The Platonic dialogues express a wide range of ideas about emotions, which can be seen as prefiguring both of these two approaches, the Stoic–Epicurean and the Aristotelian. On the one hand, the presentation of Plato's Socrates, in the *Symposium* or *Phaedo*, for instance, as strikingly free from normal sensual desires or emotions, such as fear of death, can be taken (and was sometimes seen in antiquity) as anticipating the Stoic or Epicurean idea that wisdom brings with it freedom from emotions and desires, as conventionally understood.[6] On the other hand, other Platonic ideas, notably the tripartite psychic theory in dialogues including the *Republic*, can be seen as suggesting that the 'harmonization' or control of our emotions and desires is an integral part of virtuous character. The latter strand in Platonic thought was often combined with versions of Aristotelian thought about emotion to construct the kind of Middle Platonic (Platonic–Aristotelian) view

[3] On Stoic thinking on passions, see Ch. 4 above, text to nn. 116–33. On Epicurean thinking on emotions, see LS 21, e.g. B(1) (*Ep. Men.* 127), I, Phld. *De Ira* 42.22–34 Indelli; see further Annas 1993: 190–5, Warren 2004, Gill 2006: 112–14, 452–3, Tsouna 2007, Armstrong 2008. For a survey of Stoic and Epicurean theories of emotions, see Gill 2010.

[4] See e.g. LS 21 A(6) (Cic. *Fin.* 1.37), B (1), 63, esp. L–M (Cic. *Tusc.* 5.40–1, 81–2).

[5] See e.g. Arist. *EN* 2.6, esp. 1106^{b}16–28 (the 'mean' in feelings and actions), *EE* 2.3. See further Annas 1993: 59–61.

[6] See e.g. *Smp.* 219b–e (imperviousness to sexual desire), *Phd.* 116d, 117d (lack of fear at death); see further on the influence of such depictions in Hellenistic thought, Gill 2006: 89–93.

we find strongly marked in post-Hellenistic thinkers including Plutarch and Galen.[7]

These contrasting ideals underlie the emergence of a recurrent issue in Hellenistic-Roman writings on the emotions: whether the ideal character-state is that of 'freedom from emotions' (*apatheia*) or 'moderation of emotions' (*metriopatheia*).[8] Although the second ideal takes its inspiration from Aristotle, combined with aspects of Platonic thought, what counts as 'Aristotelian' thought is subtly transformed for the purposes of this debate. This process is evident in Cicero's *Tusculans* and Seneca's *On Anger* (*De Ira*), as well as in analogous use of Aristotelian ideas by Plutarch. For instance, we are told that Aristotle advocates the moderation of emotions, rather than that he recommends 'hitting the mean' in emotions as well as actions, which is what we find in surviving school-texts, such as the *Nicomachean Ethics.* We hear that Aristotle's approach to the 'therapy' of emotions consists in moderating rather than extirpating emotions, although this kind of therapy is not, in fact, an important idea in Aristotle's ethical treatises.[9] We are also told that Aristotle sees anger as a necessary emotional stimulus for virtue, as distinct from the idea found in the school-texts that 'good temper' is a virtue.[10] In effect, Aristotelian (and sometimes Platonic–Aristotelian) thought has been reconceived as a counterweight to the influential Stoic (or Epicurean) approach to emotions, a process we have also seen at work in Galen's thought.[11] However, although the opposition between *apatheia* and *metriopatheia* functions as a focus of debate in post-Hellenistic thought, we sometimes find in the work of any one thinker nuanced or complex versions of this antithesis. For instance, Antiochus, an Academic (Platonic) thinker (born *c.*130 BC), whose synthesizing approach prefigures much that we associate with

[7] On this selective fusion of Platonic and Aristotelian ideas, see further Donini 1974: 63–126, Dillon 1983, Vander Waerdt 1985, Braund and Gill 1997: 5–11, Gill 2006: 230–7.

[8] See Dillon 1983, Annas 1993: 61–6.

[9] On Aristotle's use of the ideas of medicine and health in his ethical writings, which are quite different from the Hellenistic–Roman ideas about the therapy of emotions, see Nussbaum 1994: chs. 2–3.

[10] See e.g. Cic. *Tusc.* 3.22, 74, 4.39–46, Sen. *De Ira* 1.7, 8.4–5, 9, 10.4, 11.1, 12.1–3. 14.1, 17.1. See also Plu. *Mor.* 444 B–C, 449 F, 451 C–452 A. Contrast the approach in Arist. *EN* 2.6, 4.5. See further Braund and Gill 1997: 6–7, Graver 2002: xvii–xix, Gill 2006: 233–4.

[11] See Ch. 4 above, text to nn. 185–8, 218–20.

'Middle Platonism', adopts *apatheia* as a norm but deploys it in a sense that is closer to that normally given to *metriopatheia.*[12] In Plutarch's essay *On Ethical Virtue*, we find both ideals used for different conceptions of the person. The ideal of *apatheia* is used for the mind, seen as the vehicle of abstract thought and knowledge, and that of *metriopatheia* is used for the whole, complex person, in which body-based emotions need to be regulated by practical reason.[13]

The emergence of the idea of philosophy as a means of therapy of the emotions, as well as reflecting distinctively Stoic and Epicurean ideas about emotions and the ideal character-state, also reflects their thinking about ethical development. As outlined earlier, there are several salient points of contrast between Platonic–Aristotelian and Stoic–Epicurean patterns of thinking about this topic, which form an important part of the intellectual context for understanding different strands in Galen's essays, *Psychological Affections* and *Character Traits.* In the Platonic–Aristotelian pattern, ethical development depends on a combination of the right kind of inborn nature (*phusis*), habituation (*ethos*) in the right kind of family and communal context, and the development of rational agency and decision-making (*logos* or *prohairesis*). The processes and phases of ethical education are conceived in terms of a part-based psychological model; in particular, the habituation of the non-rational part or parts of the psyche is seen as a necessary preliminary to rational development. Related themes include the idea that even relatively defective character-states can be stable ones, and that, at a certain stage in adult life, character defects become unalterable even if we want to change ourselves.[14] The Stoic–Epicurean pattern differs in ways that give a special importance to the idea of philosophy as a means of psychic therapy. Any given family or social context is seen

[12] On Antiochus, see Cic. *Fin.* 5.28–32, *Ac. Pr.* 135; also Dillon 1977: 77–8, Gill 2006: 172–3. For various positions taken by Middle Platonist thinkers on this issue, see Dillon 1977: 151 (on Philo of Alexandria), 241 (Calvenus Taurus), 302 (Albinus).

[13] See Plu. *Mor.* 444 C–D, also 443 C–D; see further Babut 1969: 321–33, Gill 2006: 237–8. Contrasting Platonic ideas (see text to nn. 6–7 above) underlie Plutarch's dual ideals, which are transformed into a more elaborate normative typology in Neoplatonic thought.

[14] See Ch. 4 above, text to nn. 188–91; also Gill 2006: 134–6.

as one that is likely to propagate erroneous beliefs about happiness and the kind of (defective) emotional states that derive from these beliefs. However, all human beings are regarded as constitutively capable of developing towards complete virtue and happiness. This is partly because they are thought to have the innate capacity to form ideas ('preconceptions') of ethical ideas such as good. It is also because, in a unified or holistic psychological model, motivational patterns are seen as capable of being wholly shaped or reshaped by the development of ethical understanding. There are no non-rational psychic parts that can become incurably corrupted.[15] The idea of philosophy as a means of therapy has a natural home in this framework of ideas. Philosophy is seen as a way of promoting criticism of misguided ideas, for instance, about human happiness, implanted by family upbringing or social context. Given Stoic–Epicurean ideas about psychology and ethical development, the replacement of false with true beliefs, or, ultimately, knowledge, about the human good is seen as enabling the complete 'cure' of diseased character-states and the defective emotions to which they give rise.[16]

Although the idea of philosophy as therapy of emotions emerged as a key theme in Stoic and Epicurean philosophy and was closely linked with salient ideas in those theories, it was subsequently adopted by a number of thinkers working in other intellectual traditions, including the Platonic one, in its various versions. These thinkers sometimes made a deliberate effort to assimilate this idea to a different conceptual framework. For instance, the Academic thinker Philo of Larissa (158–84 BC) evolves a three-stage version of this idea. The medical analogy was also reinterpreted in a form that was consistent with his type of scepticism.[17] Cicero's version of Academic scepticism, indebted to thinkers such as Philo, allows the possibility of adopting positions on any one issue that seem 'probable'. In line with this position, Cicero both offers a positive appraisal of the merits of the Stoic, especially Chrysippean, conception of the idea of philosophy as therapy in *Tusculans* 3–4 and, elsewhere in this

[15] See Ch. 4 above, text to nn. 116–26, 192–7; also Gill 2006: 137–44, 180–2.

[16] See further Gill 2006: 377–91, focused on the interpretation of Epictetus, and Gill 2008*d*; also 5.3 below.

[17] The three stages were those of protreptic (encouragement), therapy, and advice; see Stob. 2.39.20–41.25, taken with Brittain 2001: ch. 6, esp. 277–80.

work, evolves an independent approach to therapy that fuses Stoic and Platonic ideals of *apatheia*.[18] Plutarch's essays in the genre of the therapy of the emotions sometimes adopt a Stoic-style approach, despite Plutarch's robust critique of Stoic psychology in *On Ethical Virtue*.[19] For instance, his essay *On Peace of Mind* (*peri euthumias*), synthesizes Democritean–Epicurean and Stoic themes alongside Platonic ones; even so, I think, it defines a relatively coherent conception of how to promote peace of mind and cure discontentment.[20] In *On Avoidance of Anger*, Plutarch adopts a uniformly negative attitude towards anger, which seems to reflect the influence of Stoic thinking on this subject.[21] The approaches of Cicero and Plutarch are especially relevant for making sense of Galen's writings on this topic. Galen's *Psychological Affections* and, to a lesser extent, *Avoiding Distress*, also exhibit a mixture of Stoic–Epicurean and Platonic–Aristotelian influences, and the latter work contains several echoes of Plutarch's *On Peace of Mind*.

Galen's main contributions to this subject are *Psychological Affections* (*Aff. Dig.*), coupled with an essay on psychological errors (*Pecc. Dig.*), and *Avoiding Distress*.[22] In Galen's late work, *My Own Books* (*Lib. Prop.*), these essays are listed among twenty-three works on ethical philosophy, most of which seem to fall into the type we would describe as 'practical ethics'.[23] Most of these Galenic writings have been lost. Apart from the essays just noted, the only other work in

[18] On Cicero's philosophical position, see Glucker 1988; on his approach in *Tusc.* see Lévy 1992: 445–94. See e.g. *Tusc.* 1.71–5, in which Plato's Socrates figures as an exemplar of *apatheia*. On Chrysippean therapy and Cicero's account of this, see 5.3 below.

[19] On this critique, see Gill 2006: 219–29.

[20] See Gill 1994: 4624–31; the core idea stressed, one shared by these different ancient theories, is that consciousness of one's own virtue, if achieved, brings peace of mind despite unfavourable circumstances.

[21] See further, Dillon 1977: 189, Becchi 1990, Kidd 1992: 171–3. On Plutarch's writings on practical ethics in general, see Van Hoof 2010.

[22] The full Latin title of *Aff. Dig.* is *De Proprium Animi Cuiuslibet Affectuum Dignotione et Curatione*, in English, *Diagnosis and Treatment of Psychological Affections* (*Psychological Affections*, in brief). For the Greek text of *Aff. Dig.*, see *CMG* V 4,1,1, *SM* 1.1–44; for translations, see Harkins and Riese 1963, Singer 1997*a*, both with notes. Singer forthcoming contains translations of *Aff. Dig.*, *Pecc. Dig.*, *Indol.*, *Mor.*, and *QAM*, with introductions and commentaries. On *Avoiding Distress*, see below.

[23] *Lib. Prop.* XIX.45–6, trans. Singer 1997*a*: 21. On Hellenistic and Roman 'practical ethics' (not an ancient term), see Foucault 1990, Gill 2003: 40–4, Sellars 2007, Van Hoof 2010; on the therapeutic strand in practical ethics, see text to nn. 204–13 below.

this group which survives (in Arabic summary) is *Character Traits*. As brought out later, there are certain clear links between the surviving works, as well as connections with *PHP* 4–5 and *QAM*, ch. 11, though there are also some important differences of emphasis. Although we cannot be certain about the chronology of these works,[24] it seems likely that the first to be written was *Avoiding Distress* (193, soon after the fire in Rome in 192 that is discussed there).[25] *Character Traits* may also belong to this period; and *Psychological Affections* must be later again, since it refers to *Character Traits*.[26] Another work on psychology that belongs to this period of Galen's work (and which also refers to *Character Traits*) is *Psychological Faculties Depend on Bodily Mixtures* (*QAM*), generally seen as being, along with *Prop. Plac.*, one of his last works.[27] It looks as though the fire at Rome in 192, and Galen's rather 'stoic' (in a non-technical sense) response to his losses in that fire, sparked off a renewed interest in the questions of ethical psychology that are discussed so intensely in *PHP* 4–5 (written in 162–6). This, in turn, seems to have led Galen to address again, in *QAM* and parts of *Prop. Plac.*, questions about mind–body relations that derived from the issues about body-based psychological functions discussed in *PHP* 1–3 and 6. So, it would appear that, after some decades centred on other topics, psychology, in various senses, comes to the forefront of Galen's concerns again in the 190s and remains there till his last writings.

Galen's most sustained essay on the therapy of emotions is *Psychological Affections* (*Aff. Dig.*), which I discuss first, followed by the

[24] The following comments are indebted to Nutton's note on *Indol.* 54 in Singer forthcoming, which provides more detailed support for the sequence outlined here.

[25] *Indol.* 54 makes negative comments about the emperor Commodus and so is unlikely to have been published before his death at the end of 192; see also Boudon-Millot 2007*b*: 76, Hankinson 2008*d*: 21–2. *Hipp. Epid.* 6.8, *CMG* V 10, 2, 2, 486.19, 495.2, 494.22, 495.5–12, combines similar themes (losses in the fire and criticism of Commodus) and seems to belong to the same period.

[26] *Mor.*, in a passage not included in Mattock 1972, cites an incident that is implicitly critical of Commodus and so is likely to have appeared after 192. See further Walzer 1962: 158 n. 2, Nutton 1999: 140 n. 2, and Hankinson 2008*d*: 21. *Aff. Dig.* ch. 6, V.27–9 refers to *Mor.*

[27] *QAM* ch. 1, IV.768 (trans. Singer 1997*a*: 150); on *QAM* and related passages from *Prop. Plac.*, see 3.5 above. See also the chronological outline of Galen's works in Singer 1997*a*: l–lii, and Hankinson 2008*d*: 21–5.

shorter *Avoiding Distress* (though, as just noted, the latter work seems to have been written first). In *Aff. Dig.*, Galen's overall strategy includes several themes that are standard in the genre of writing on the therapy of emotions, regardless of the philosophical perspective of the writer. These include the need for self-understanding, to enable us to recognize and correct our own susceptibility to emotions; the importance of using a reliable and judicious adviser to guide our self-criticism; and the need to carry out self-criticism in a consistent and sustained way.[28] A more individual feature—often cited—is Galen's specific reference to his own parents, as contrasting paradigms of good or bad behaviour, and to his father's role as a model of good character and as promoting Galen's wide-ranging education.[29] However, I focus on the indications of contrasting philosophical traditions in Galen's presentation of these ideas. As indicated, the approach seems to be a mixed or eclectic one. The basic framework and a number of motifs evoke the Stoic, or Stoic–Epicurean, standpoint. On the other hand, also present, especially in the later stages of the work, are several well-marked characteristics of the competing Platonic–Aristotelian approach. Hence, it is difficult to say, as Hankinson points out, whether Galen's normative character-state is that of *apatheia* or *metriopatheia*.[30] I review the main contrasting strands in the essay before attempting to explain this—rather surprisingly—ambiguous standpoint.

The idea that emotions are sicknesses which need to be removed or 'cured' is closely linked with the Stoic–Epicurean approach, as is the genre (therapy of the emotions) in which Galen is working here. A number of motifs throughout the essay evoke the Stoic–Epicurean connotations of the genre. Galen begins by referring, though rather critically, to an otherwise unknown work by Antonius the Epicurean on *The Control of Specific* (or *Individual*) *Emotions*.[31] He locates his work in the broader tradition of writings on the therapy of emotion, citing especially that of Chrysippus, which he discusses at length in the earlier

[28] See e.g. ch. 2 (V.3–7) (need for self-knowledge), ch. 3 (V.8–14) (role of adviser), ch. 4 (V.14–21) (importance of practice).

[29] See ch. 8 (V.41–3).

[30] Hankinson 1993: 198–204.

[31] *Aff. Dig.* ch. 1, V.1–2: Galen criticizes the work for lack of clarity about the nature of 'control' (*ephedreia*), and for failing to distinguish between errors and emotions (on the latter point, see text to nn. 45–8 below).

work *PHP* 5.[32] Subsequently, he refers, in a positive tone, to the Stoic Zeno and the Cynic Diogenes; Zeno is linked with the idea of justifying our actions to our teachers or guardians (*paidagōgoi*) and Diogenes with blunt criticism directed towards anyone (even kings).[33] The associations implied here, linking Zeno with ethical teaching or doctrines and Diogenes with plain speaking and indifference to social and political status, are rather standard ones in post-Hellenistic practical ethics. They appear, for instance, in Epictetus' *Discourses*.[34] These (predominantly) Stoic allusions are combined with phraseology implying the Stoic ideals of *apatheia* and of the extirpation of emotions. For instance, we are told early in the essay that we should identify 'all the emotions (*pathē*) that need correction', and that we should 'free ourselves' (*eleutherōsai*) or 'remove' (literally 'knock off', *ekkoptein*) the emotions of the psyche. The emotions 'which everyone recognizes' are specified as 'spirit (*thumos*), anger, fear, envy, and excessive appetite'.[35] Although the addition of 'excessive' (*sphodra*) to 'appetite' might seem to mark an Aristotelian note, the inclusion of 'spirit' (*thumos*) is striking, given its—typically positive—association with the Platonic tripartite psyche.[36] Subsequently, the wise person or god is associated with someone who has 'practised *apatheia*' throughout his life'.[37]

Other features which reinforce this Stoic tone include the idea that the expression of anger, even in its less extreme forms, is a kind of 'madness' (*mania*), a mark of subhuman (bestial) character, and 'sickness' (*nosēma*) of the psyche.[38] In the same context, a similar

[32] *Aff. Dig.* ch. 1, V.3, *SM* 1.2.13–15; cf. *PHP* V.432–45, 5.2.1–52. Galen also refers in general terms to works in this genre by Plato and Aristotle (*SM* 1.2.15–18), but, significantly, does not specify any (there are none known in this genre, which seems to have emerged in the Hellenistic era).

[33] *Aff. Dig.* ch. 3, V.12–13, *SM* 1.9.22–10.4, 10.11–17.

[34] See e.g. Epict. *Diss.* 3.3.19; see further Schofield 2003: 233–5. Diogenes is also referred to in Plutarch's essay *On Avoidance of Anger* (*Mor.* 460 E).

[35] *Aff. Dig.* chs. 2–3, V.5, 7–8, *SM* 1.3.25–6 (the passage is bracketed as textually dubious in *SM*), 1.5.16–20, 24.

[36] For Aristotle, virtue consists in hitting the 'mean' in desires, emotions, and actions and avoiding the vices of excess and deficiency (*EN* 2.6). For the 'spirited' part, see Pl. *R.* 439e–440c, and, in this work, see text to n. 50 below. Singer 1997*a*: 412–13, note on p. 103, notes the potential inconsistency of Galen's inclusion of 'spirit' among emotions to be got rid off.

[37] *Aff. Dig.* ch. 11, V.11, *SM* 1.18.12–17.

[38] *Aff. Dig.* ch. 5, V.22–4, *SM* 1.17.3–13, 1.18.7–8.

status is attached to five emotions (grief, rage, anger, appetite, and fear) that overlap at least with the four basic Stoic emotions (grief, appetite, pleasure, and fear).[39] Also, Galen's characterization of acts of blind, intense anger is strongly reminiscent of Chrysippus' description of such behaviour, as reported by Galen himself in *PHP*.[40] A further standard Stoic motif is the idea that genuine 'freedom' (*eleutheria*) is not a function of one's legal or political status but consists in freedom from emotions such as love of money or reputation.[41] Also, Galen's strategy for the progressive therapy of emotion can be analysed in terms that recall key features of Chrysippus' therapeutic method, considered later.[42] Other themes in the essay evoke, rather, the Epicurean goal of *ataraxia*, that is, 'being undisturbed'. For instance, Galen presents himself as exemplary in remaining 'undisturbed' (*anekplēktos*) by contingent disasters such as loss of possessions, provided one has the minimum needed to look after oneself.[43] A further motif that is compatible with both Stoic and Epicurean ideas about ethical development is that aiming at perfection is a project that can continue virtually throughout one's life, since self-improvement is possible even at 50 years old.[44]

However, alongside these Stoic or Epicurean motifs, the essay also contains a number of distinctively Platonic–Aristotelian themes, relating especially to the psychological model and ethical development. Taken as a whole, these themes are more prominent or fully developed than the Stoic–Epicurean ones—as one would expect, given Galen's typical standpoint. For instance, early in the work,

[39] *Aff. Dig.* ch. 24, *SM* 1.18.8–10; cf. LS 65 E (Stob. 2.90.19–91.9) (*SVF* 3.394). Cf. the five emotions cited in text to n. 35 above.

[40] *Aff. Dig.* ch. 5, V.22, *SM* 1.16.25–17.3, cf. *PHP* V.414–15, 4.6.44–5 De Lacy; see also Hankinson 1993: 200.

[41] *Aff. Dig.* ch. 10, V.53, *SM* 1.41.11–16; cf. Epict. *Diss.* 4.1, and see further Bobzien 1998: 338–44.

[42] As Hankinson 1993: 200–1 brings out, the method (as shown in *Aff. Dig.* ch. 4, V.20–1, 53–6) can be analysed as including (1) controlling the manifestation of emotion before tackling the emotion itself, and (2) waiting until the emotion has subsided before attempting treatment. On Chrysippus' therapeutic technique, see 5.3 below.

[43] *Aff. Dig.* ch. 8, V.43–4, *SM* 1.33.14–34.2, 9–15; cf. LS 21 B(1, 4), (*Ep. Men.* 127, 130), G(1), (*Sent. Vat.* 33).

[44] *Aff. Dig.* ch. 4, V.14–16, esp. *SM* 1.11.3–7. Cf. Epicur. *Ep. Men.* 122 (LS 25 A), Lucr. 3.307–22 (LS 14 D(5)); see further Gill 2006: 103–7.

Galen introduces the distinction between errors (*hamartēmata*) and emotions (*pathē*): 'I defined error as arising from false opinion, and emotion as arising from an irrational faculty in us that is not amenable to reason'.[45] This distinction is fundamental to the structure of Galen's (two-stage) project: the essay on the therapy of the emotions is coupled with one on the therapy of (intellectual or cognitive) errors.[46] As brought out earlier, Galen claims in *PHP* that Chrysippus also recognized this distinction but was unable to apply it, because of (what Galen sees as) his intellectualist theory of emotion.[47] Although Galen does not stress this point of difference here, it constitutes a potentially major contrast with Stoic (and Epicurean) techniques of therapy, which assume that emotions are shaped by mistaken beliefs, especially about the nature of human happiness.[48]

A further difference, which is consistent with the error–emotion distinction, is that Galen conceives the operation of his therapeutic techniques in terms of a part-based, and specifically tripartite, psychological theory. In chapter 6, Galen refers to his essay *Character Traits*, where he explicitly adopts the Platonic tripartite psychology that he uses as a counterweight to Stoic thinking in *PHP* 4–5. Also, following Plato, he links the distinction between the two non-rational parts of the psyche with a contrast between two methods of treatment, namely training (*paideusis*) and discipline or correction (*kolasis*), the latter being more suitable to a more 'bestial' faculty.[49] Although the point is made with some emphasis, I do not think that there is a systematic attempt to integrate the Platonic model with Galen's account of therapeutic techniques. In this chapter, as well as elsewhere, anger, for instance, is treated as one of a number

[45] *Aff. Dig.* ch. 1, V.2, *SM* 1.2.6–9, trans. Singer 1997*a*: 100, slightly modified; also ch. 3, V.7, *SM* 1.5.14–18.

[46] On the intellectual framework of the latter essay (*Pecc. Dig.*), see Donini 1988.

[47] See Ch. 4, text to nn. 72–5 above.

[48] See further on this distinction and its relevance for Galen's strategy in this essay, Hankinson 1993: 192–7; also text to nn. 68–76 below. On Stoic (belief-based) strategies, see 5.4 below.

[49] *Aff. Dig.* ch. 6, V.27–9 (also ch. 5, V.27), esp. *SM* 1.21.10–18. On Plato's tripartite theory and Galen's use of it in *PHP* 4–5, see Ch. 4 above, text to nn. 161–72. On the linkage, in Plato's *R.*, between psychological parts and forms of education, see Gill 1985*b*, 1996: 245–60, 266–87, 2006: 134–5.

of (bad) emotions, along with those (of 'lust, greed, drunkenness, or luxuriousness') that are linked with the appetitive part, rather than being seen as the distinctive property of the 'spirited' part.[50] Nor does Galen explain further how this psychological model, especially the distinction between the two non-rational parts, is correlated with different forms of therapeutic practice.[51] However, the part-based psychological model is consistent with certain other Platonic–Aristotelian themes in the essay, notably those relating to ethical development.

One well-marked feature in the essay is the Platonic–Aristotelian idea that ethical development depends on the combination of the right kind of inborn nature and habituation, enabling, in the best cases, correct use of reasoning and choice.[52] Here, as in other Galenic works on related subjects, we find stress on the idea that individual differences, relevant to ethical behaviour and attitudes, are already evident in childhood, suggesting that they are innate.[53] There is also repeated emphasis on habituation and rehearsal, a theme that is interlocked with several other, equally Platonic–Aristotelian, motifs relating to ethical development. One is the idea, strongly marked in Aristotle's ethical writings, that correct habituation over time makes virtuous action pleasurable; this is linked, as in Aristotle's theory, with the distinction between the partial virtue of 'self-control' (*enkrateia*) and the complete virtue of 'temperance' (*sōphrosunē*).[54] Another Platonic–Aristotelian theme, which figures repeatedly in Galen's essay, is that habituation can make vices unalterable over time even if the person

[50] See e.g. *Aff. Dig.* ch. 6, V.28, esp. *SM* 1.21.4–10, cited in part, trans. Singer 1997*a*: 112; also V.30–1, *SM* 1.22.25–6, 23.13–16. Contrast Pl. *R.* 439d–441c. On this point, see also Singer 1997*a*: 412–13: note on p. 103.

[51] In *Aff. Dig.* ch. 6, V.30, Galen specifically says one should use the same techniques in the case of appetites as in anger (*SM* 1.22.25–6), namely looking for a critical adviser and deliberate self-scrutiny; see also V.33–4, esp. *SM* 1.25.16–19.

[52] On this aspect of *Aff. Dig.*, and its Aristotelian inspiration, see Donini 1974: 128–32.

[53] *Aff. Dig.* ch. 7, V.38–40; for this type of emphasis, see also Pl. *R.* 485a–487a (the philosophical nature) and Arist. *EN* 10.9, esp. 1179^{b}4–32. On this theme in other Galenic works, see text to nn. 118–36 below.

[54] Galen uses the distinction to suggest that self-control is a half-way stage to complete temperance. See *Aff. Dig.* ch. 6, V.32–4, esp. *SM* 1.25.14–15, 18–25, 1.26.2–6. Cf. Arist. *EN* 1.13, 1102^{b}25–8, 2.1, 3, 7.1, 1145^{b}8–20. On ethical habituation in Aristotle (which is not necessarily a non-rational process), see Sherman 1989: ch. 5, 1997: chs. 2, 6.

concerned wants to change.[55] The idea that, if nature and upbringing provide a sound basis, rational choice and reflection can play a significant role in ethical development appears especially in connection with Galen's own self-presentation. Indeed, the most striking and distinctive feature of the whole essay, Galen's report of the influence of his father and education, is used to illustrate this point.[56]

How should we explain the presence of these contrasting Stoic–Epicurean and Platonic–Aristotelian strands in Galen's essay, especially given the intense critique of Stoic (at least, Chrysippean) psychology in *PHP* 4–5, examined in the preceding chapter? Does Galen's essay, even so, embody a coherent and intelligible—even distinctive—approach to the therapy of the emotions? The first of these questions is easier to answer than the second. It is likely that Galen's use of Stoic and Epicurean motifs and ideas reflects the substantial role of these theories in originating and developing the genre of treatises on the therapy of the emotions, outlined earlier. The presence of Platonic and Aristotelian ideas on psychology and ethical development, on the other hand, expresses Galen's typical adoption of these ideas, sometimes as a counterweight to the Stoic approach, in *PHP* 4–5, *Character Traits*, and *QAM* ch. 11. The fact that, as noted earlier, earlier thinkers writing from a Platonic standpoint (of one kind or another), also wrote in this genre, and adapted it, in various degrees, to their approach, makes Galen's project less surprising. Plutarch, for instance, prefigures in *On Ethical Virtue* Galen's critique of Stoic psychology in *PHP* 4–5; but his essay *On Avoidance of Anger* offers a markedly Stoic-style programme for the removal of anger.[57]

It is more difficult to say how far Galen's contribution to the therapy of emotions is intellectually consistent. Much depends on what kind of work we take it to be. If we assume that the aim, like that of Plutarch's essay *On Avoidance of Anger*, is essentially practical,[58] we may think that Galen combines material from different intellectual

[55] *Aff. Dig.* ch. 5, V.5–25, *SM* 1.19.10–11; ch. 6, V.29, *SM* 1.22.10–15; ch. 7, V.36, *SM* 1.7–8, ch. 10, V.52, 54, *SM* 1.41.1–3, 1.41.23–42.4. Cf. Arist. *EN* 3.5, 1114^{a}3–21; on Plato and incurable vice, see Hankinson 1993: 219–20 n. 102, referring e.g. to *Grg.*478e–479a, 525b–c, *Lg.* 731d.

[56] *Aff. Dig.* ch. 7, V.37, esp. *SM* 1.28.20–4, ch. 8, V.40–5, esp. *SM* 1.32.21–33.16.

[57] See text to nn. 19–21 above.

[58] For this interpretation of Plutarch's essay, see Kidd 1992: 169–71.

traditions in order to produce the most serviceable instrument for this objective. On this reading, the core of the essay consists in the messages conveyed about the need for self-criticism, the proper use of advisers, and the need for sustained work on managing one's emotions.[59] Galen, on this view, simply adopts strands from the main philosophical traditions on this subject, which in any case converge in some respects, without paying much attention to the potential contradictions in aims or assumptions of the different approaches. Galen's characteristically independent or eclectic standpoint in philosophy, restated in this essay, and his impatience with—what he sees as—pointless quibbling between different schools, make this a relatively plausible interpretation of the work.[60]

On the other hand, the fact that Galen has himself engaged in intellectual debate against Stoic ideas and on behalf of competing Platonic–Aristotelian ideas on topics relevant to this essay, especially in *PHP* 4–5, makes it more difficult to suppose that he simply sets aside what he himself sometimes recognizes as important points of difference. An alternative view, which takes account of his normal intellectual stance, is that he thinks the therapy of emotions can be best achieved by presupposing a Platonic–Aristotelian psychological framework and account of ethical development. The most substantial obstacle to this reading of the essay is constituted by the indications that the objective assumed is freedom from emotion or disturbance (*apatheia* or *ataraxia*), rather than moderation of emotion (*metriopatheia*).[61] However, there is no formal statement on this point; and Galen does not refer explicitly to this well-known contrast between normative character-states. It is possible that Galen is using *apatheia*, or cognate terms, in a way that implies something closer to what is normally meant by *metriopatheia*, that is, a moderate level of emotional response.[62] At the start of chapter 3, after listing the emotions

[59] See text to n. 28 above.

[60] See *Aff. Dig.* ch. 8, V.42–3, *SM* 1.32.19–33.16, coupling independence of philosophical outlook with adopting a shared stress among philosophers on self-development of virtue and the achievement of freedom from emotional disturbance (on this as the programme of Plutarch's eclectic essay *On Peace of Mind*, see Gill 1994: 4624–31). On Galen's intellectual independence or eclecticism, see Hankinson 1992.

[61] See text to nn. 30–44 (also 8–13) above.

[62] As Antiochus seems to do: see text to n. 12 above.

to be avoided, including 'excessive appetite', he adds that 'moderation (or 'measure', *metron*) is best', and both these phrases might imply an Aristotelian type of validation of moderate emotions.[63] The Aristotelian ideal of a moderate level or type of response may also be implied in his comment later in the work that 'There is no loss that has the power to cause me grief (or 'distress') (except the loss of all my possessions)'. Subsequently, this is rephrased as the idea that 'one should not be troubled by any material loss provided that what remains is adequate for the care of one's body [thus ensuring] . . . that one is not hungry, cold, or thirsty'.[64] These qualifications mark a distinction at least from the Stoic ideal, according to which the emotion of grief or distress (*lupē*) is *always* misguided, since it involves treating as good (or bad) what is only a preferable (or dispreferable) indifferent.[65] The Epicurean position on this point is rather closer to the one specified by Galen here.[66] These indications of the valuation of *metriopatheia* rather than *apatheia* are rather un-emphatic; but they may be enough at least to qualify the impression that Galen is presupposing an unequivocally Stoic-type ideal character-state, which would be in clear tension with the Platonic–Aristotelian characterization of psychology and ethical development.[67]

However, if we suppose that Galen's aim is to produce a consistently Platonic–Aristotelian approach to the therapy of emotion, another problem arises. The difficulty derives from the apparent mismatch between the methods of therapy recommended and the psychological theory put forward. The methods of therapy cited—sustained self-scrutiny, taking account of the criticisms of an adviser, adjusting your ideas about how much property you need for a good life—are highly cognitive or rational.[68] This reflects the pattern established by Stoic and Epicurean thinkers, the originators of the

[63] *Aff. Dig.* ch. 3, V.7, *SM* 1.5.20, 23; see also text to nn. 8–13 above.

[64] *Aff. Dig.* ch. 8, V.43–4, *SM* 1.33.16–17, 1.34.12–14, 15, trans. Singer 1997*a*: 120–1.

[65] See further Brennan 1998: 30–4, 2003: 269–71, Graver 2007: 35–59; also Ch. 4, text to nn. 116–33.

[66] See e.g. LS 21 G(1) (*Sent. Vat.* 33): 'The flesh's cry is not to be hungry or thirsty or cold', and the specification of natural or necessary desires as things such as 'drinking when thirsty' (LS 21 I).

[67] For some analogous suggestions about the ideal character-state that may be implied by Galen's essay, see Hankinson 1993: 203–4.

[68] See e.g. *Aff. Dig.* chs. 2–4, 8–9.

genre, who presuppose a unified psychological theory, in which emotions and desires depend on beliefs.[69] Galen, however, presents, especially in chapter 6, a very different psychological account, including two non-rational parts, one of which is presented as only capable of 'discipline' (*kolasis*) not training (*paideusis*).[70] It is not very clear how Galen's recommended therapeutic methods fit with this psychological picture. Hankinson suggests that Galen's essay implies a largely coherent combination of psychology and therapeutic method, in which judgements and emotions or desires are mutually informing and thus both capable of gradual adjustment.[71] However, I am not sure that Galen works out in any detail how to integrate his therapeutic methods with his psychological theory.

There is an instructive contrast with the works from which Galen derives his psychological assumptions, Plato's *Republic* and *Laws*, which in turn underlie Aristotle's thinking on ethical development. In the Platonic works, the part-based psychological theories are combined with educational programmes in which different phases are directed towards different faculties or parts of the psyche. In particular, in both *Republic* and *Laws*, childhood education is conducted by means (including music and gymnastics in the *Republic* and prenatal movement in the *Laws*) that are specifically directed at non-rational aspects of the psyche.[72] Galen himself brings out this linkage between psychology and methods of training in his comments in *PHP* 5 on Posidonius' response to Plato's account of early upbringing in the *Laws*.[73] Although Galen specifies clearly the kinds of non-rational psychic parts that are the target of therapeutic modification in this essay, he does not give any indication how these parts are to be modified, except by the application of rational, belief-based methods.[74] In the kind of Platonic–Aristotelian framework assumed by Galen, the only person who will reliably

[69] See further 5.3 below. [70] See text to nn. 49–51 above.

[71] Hankinson 1993: 201–3; but see also his comment, cited in n. 76 below.

[72] See Pl. *R.* 401d–402a, 411e–412a, 429e–430a, 441e–442a, 522a; *Lg.* 789a–792e, also 653a–c, 654c–d, 655d–656b, 658e–660a (and 643e–645c, 649a–650b). See further Gill 1985*b*, 1996: 245–60, 266–75, 2006: 134–6, which also draw out the links with Aristotelian thinking about ethical habituation.

[73] *PHP* V.466–7, 5.5.30–5, esp. 32 De Lacy. See further, stressing Galen's misleading presentation of Posidonius' interest in Plato, Tieleman 2003*a*: 220–6, Gill 2006: 287–9.

[74] See e.g. *Aff. Dig.* ch. 6, V.31–4, focused on the desires of the appetitive part but taking the form of rational advice for self-monitoring and aspiration towards temperance.

respond to this kind of approach is someone whose nature and habituation make him already well equipped to respond to such rational appeals.[75] Thus, it is not clear that Galen has really worked out how to integrate the different elements he is combining in this essay, especially the Stoic–Epicurean methods of therapy and the Platonic–Aristotelian psychological model.[76]

The other surviving essay on the therapy of emotions is the recently rediscovered short work, *Avoiding Distress* (*peri alupias* or *De Indolentia* (*Indol.*)), found on the same manuscript as the complete Greek text of *Prop. Plac.*[77] This treats many of the same themes as *Psychological Affections*,[78] but in a more autobiographical form; it also has a rather tauter structure and a more explicitly defined intellectual standpoint. Like Plutarch's *On Peace of Mind*, an essay which it recalls at various points, it is couched as a letter, though to an unnamed addressee.[79] The addressee is presented as wanting to know how Galen has developed the ability to respond without distress or mental pain (*alupia*) to setbacks and losses which normally upset someone profoundly. In particular, the addressee is amazed by the equanimity with which Galen has taken the destruction of many valuable possessions and, more importantly, much of his personal library and medical resources in the fire that broke out at the Temple of Peace at Rome in 192. Much of the first half of the essay spells out these losses, thus underlining the remarkable character of

[75] That is, someone such as Galen himself, as he presents himself in this essay; see text to n. 56 above. Cf. Arist. 10.9, esp. 1179^{b}4–1180^{a}5.

[76] Cf. Hankinson's comment (1993: 203) that 'Galen's account . . . seems in danger of breaking down under the combined weight of the separate phenomena (and traditions) that he is trying to integrate'.

[77] Namely, Vlatadon 14: see Boudon-Millot 2007*b*: 73–5 and Boudon-Millot and Pietrobelli 2005: 168–70; on the Greek text of *Prop. Plac.*, see Ch. 3 above, n. 215. Boudon-Millot 2007*b* provides a full text of *Indol.* (just over 14 pages) with apparatus criticus, French translation and commentary. It is subdivided into 84 numbered sections which are used for references below.

[78] These include the emphasis on the father's influence (n. 81 below), the criticism of acquisitiveness (cf. *Aff. Dig.* ch. 9, V.48–9 and *Indol.* 43, 47, 82–3), similar accounts of the minimum conditions for a happy life (see nn. 87–93 below). On the chronological relationship between the two works, see text to nn. 24 above and 97–8 below.

[79] Points of resemblance include the opening words of each work and the anecdotes on Zeno (cf. Plu. *Mor.* 467 D and *Indol.* 48) and Aristippus (cf. Plu. *Mor.* 469 C–D and *Indol.* 42); see Boudon-Millot 2007*b*: 76 and her notes on these passages.

Galen's calm response.[80] In the latter half of the essay, Galen explains the personal and intellectual basis of his equanimity in the face of misfortune. Here, as in *Psychological Affections*, he gives a prominent place to the influence of his father, or more broadly, the nature and upbringing transmitted in his family over several generations.[81] He also refers in a more generalized way to themes and sayings that figure prominently in philosophical writings on the therapy of emotions.[82] However, he also distinguishes his underlying ethical views, on the nature of the good life, from the Stoic and Epicurean ideas which shape much previous writing on this topic. He presents his own ideal as, by implication at least, a more realistic one than the Stoic–Epicurean ones. He maintains that, by these standards, he is still able to live a happy and fulfilled life in spite of these setbacks and thus that his equanimity in the face of great losses is justified.

Like *Psychological Affections*, this essay evokes both Stoic–Epicurean and Platonic–Aristotelian ideas about the therapy of emotions and the development of character. In the first half of the essay especially, the stress on the point that Galen experiences not just little distress but none at all might suggest that Galen has in view the Stoic ideal of 'absence of passion' (*apatheia*) or the Epicurean one of 'absence of disturbance' (*ataraxia*) rather than the Aristotelian-style 'moderation (or 'control') of passion'.[83] This, ethically rigorous, note is reinforced by the fact that, as Galen underlines, the losses which might have affected him most are not those of material wealth. Rather, they are those of his books, drugs, instruments, and other resources that are vital for the practice of medicine, which Galen sees as an ethical project and vocation and not simply an occupation or means of livelihood.[84] Also, in the centre of the essay, Galen identifies as the basis of his response the

[80] See *Indol.* 4–37: sections 13–30 provide valuable evidence about Galen's personal library, on which see Nutton 2009.

[81] Cf. *Indol.* 58–62 and *Aff. Dig.* ch. 8 (V.41–3); the stress on the good influence of the father (not the mother) in *Aff. Dig.* is paralleled by the good influence of successive fathers on their sons in *Indol.*

[82] See *Indol.* 40–8, 52–6, 68–77; see further references in nn. 79 above and 88 below.

[83] See *Indol.* 2–3, 11, 31, 38: on these alternative Hellenistic ideals, see text to nn. 8–13 above.

[84] See *Indol.* 4–12, 31–7; on Galen's view of medicine as an ethical project and on the demands of training oneself for this way of life, see Boudon-Millot 2009. The closest philosophical parallel for Galen's view of the value of medical resources is, in

quality of 'magnanimity' (*megalopsuchia*), which he characterizes in Stoic terms, as courageous indifference to misfortune, rather than in Aristotelian terms, as the virtuous person's attitude towards honour.[85] However, in the latter part of the essay, Galen distances himself from Stoic and Epicurean ideas about value and about emotional ideals and also underlines themes which are strongly reminiscent of the contrasting Platonic–Aristotelian approach to the development of character. Hence, the essay has connotations of both the main philosophical traditions of thought about the therapy of the emotions.

In the case of *Psychological Affections*, I suggested that Galen's amalgamation of Stoic–Epicurean and Platonic–Aristotelian motifs is a rather uneasy one. In particular, Galen fails to explain how the highly rational or cognitive methods he advocates for the therapy of emotions are compatible with the Platonic–Aristotelian psychology he adopts, in which emotions are located in a distinct, non-rational part of the psyche.[86] However, although *Avoiding Distress* also combines motifs from contrasting intellectual traditions, it does so in a way that is, I think, more internally self-consistent. This is partly because, despite the Stoic-style character of his equanimity, Galen makes it plain that this is not based on Stoic, or Epicurean, principles but on (what he presents as) a realistic assessment of the situation and a reasonable, non-doctrinaire view of what makes for a happy life.

For instance, about half-way through the essay, he comments that he was not distressed at the loss of his property 'because what was left was more than sufficient'.[87] He then explicitly distinguishes his attitude from the Stoic ideal, exemplified in a comment ascribed to Zeno, of

fact, an Aristotelian one, namely as 'external goods' which are 'instrumental' for the effective practice of virtue (Arist. *EN* 1.8, 1099^{a}31–^{b}2, see also Annas 1993: 378–84). I am not sure if Galen is aware of this concept; Moraux 1984: 792 notes Galen's limited interest in Aristotle's conception of virtue.

[85] See *Indol.* 50–1; for Stoic thinking on *megalopsuchia*, see Cic. *Off.* 1.66–7, 69 (also Dyck 1981); on the possible influence of this thinking on writings about peace of mind by Panaetius, Seneca, and Plutarch, see Gill 1994: esp. 4609–10. For the contrasting Aristotelian idea of *megalopsuchia*, see *EN* 4.3; however, *APo.* 97^{b}7–25 points to a linkage between both these ideas, which is also implied in *EN* 1124^{a}16–20, ^{b}6–9 (see further Annas 1993: 116–19).

[86] See text to nn. 68–76 above.

[87] *Indol.* 46, trans. Nutton, in Singer forthcoming. (I am grateful to Vivian Nutton for sharing with me his translation and notes prior to publication.)

equanimity at the loss of *all* one's property.[88] Later in the essay, he explicitly distances himself from the idea that one can achieve a state of character or happiness that is completely invulnerable to misfortune. He comments: 'Possibly you imagine that like some of the philosophers who promise that one will never suffer pain, I shall make the same pronouncement, since you have never seen me distressed'.[89] But then he goes on to reject both Epicurean and Stoic versions of this idea, linked with their respective ideals of freedom from distress (*ataraxia*) and passion (*apatheia*).[90] He also makes it plain that he would indeed be distressed by *some* external events. These include the complete loss of his possessions, also 'the ruination of my homeland, or a friend being punished by a tyrant'. Putting it in more general terms, he adds: 'I am keenly aware that I depend on the quality of the state of both my body and my psyche, and so I would not like anything to arise from any external cause that could destroy my health or any disaster that could overpower my psyche'.[91] This conception of happiness, attaching intrinsic value both to qualities of mind and character and of the body, and also to the well-being of friends or relatives and material goods, recalls the Platonic–Aristotelian conception offered by Antiochus, as a counter-ideal to that of Stoicism.[92] However, it is presented by Galen as a purely individual belief, and one which underlies his reaction to misfortune, including his apparently

[88] *Indol.* 48; the anecdote cited implies the Stoic idea that things other than virtue are 'matters of indifference' (LS 58). Note also the implied distancing from Socrates and Diogenes the Cynic (often used as Stoic exemplars of wisdom), who were satisfied with having little or no possessions (*Indol.* 45–6).

[89] *Indol.* 70, trans, Nutton in Singer forthcoming.

[90] 'I make light of the loss of possessions without quite being deprived of them' (here he distances himself from the Stoic ethical ideal, cf. his criticism of the Stoic Musonius Rufus in 73–4)... and of bodily pain without quite claiming to make light of Phalaris' bull', *Indol.* 71, trans. Nutton in Singer forthcoming. The Epicurean wise person is presented as able to recognize that his life is pleasant even in the bull of Phalaris, i.e. a tyrant's instrument of torture: see e.g. Cic. *Tusc.* 2.17–18, 5.31, Plu. *Mor.* 1088 B and 1090 A (also Gill 2006: 118). See also Galen's dismissal of the Epicurean ideal of freedom from distress (characterized as 'absence of trouble' (*aochlēsia*) in *Indol.* 68, and the reference to Galen's father drawing a distinction between the good and freedom from being pained or distressed (62), which seems to refer broadly to both Stoic and Epicurean ideals.

[91] *Indol.* 72, 75, trans. Nutton in Singer forthcoming.

[92] See Cic. *Fin.* 4–5, esp. 4.2, 14–15, 19–23, 5.67–75, 77–95. See also Annas 1993: 419–23, Gill 2006: 167–8, 172–3.

Stoic-style absence of distress, underlined in the first half of the essay. Although some losses would indeed cause him distress, those resulting from the fire at Rome, though very considerable, fall short of what would be needed to produce this effect.[93] In this way, Galen suggests that his reactions reflect a consistent set of ethical ideas, and ones that are explicitly different from Stoic and Epicurean norms.

In *Psychological Affections*, I raised the question of the consistency between the purely rational methods Galen advocates for the therapy of emotions and the picture of human psychology he offers, namely as a combination of distinct rational and non-rational parts. However, *Avoiding Distress* does not give rise to this question in the same way. Galen does allocate a substantial role in this essay to rational methods of controlling emotions, especially the method recommended by some philosophers of preparing for disaster by imagining it in advance.[94] But he also stresses the role of other, less rational (or at least less theoretical), factors such as innate character and family upbringing. He also implies that a precondition of the effectiveness of philosophical methods of therapy is that one has already acquired by inborn nature and upbringing the ability to make good use of such methods.[95] This is, in fact, the standard Platonic–Aristotelian (though not Stoic or Epicurean) view about ethical development, and it is compatible with the idea of division between rational and non-rational parts of the psyche, though Galen does not refer to the latter idea in this essay.[96] Hence, both in the ideal of happiness

[93] *Indol.* 38, 46–50, 65–76, 78–9.

[94] See *Indol.* 51–6, 76–9; this theme is illustrated in 52 and 77 by reference to a Euripidean fragment (814 Mette) often cited in connection with the theme of preparation for future disasters. See e.g. Cic. *Tusc.* 3.30, Plu. *Mor.* 112 D, also Gal. *PHP* V.418, 4.7.10 De Lacy referring to Posidonius. On the role of this theme in philosophical writings about peace of mind, see Gill: 1994: 4613, 4617, 4627–30.

[95] *Indol.* 51, 57–62, 65 (in connection with Galen himself), 51, 79 (in connection with the addressee). Note also 58, suggesting that Galen's father 'developed [the virtues] naturally in himself without the need for philosophical discourse' (trans. Nutton in Singer forthcoming), and 61–4, ascribing to Galen's father, and Galen himself, 'philosophical-style' ideas which are presented as personal beliefs rather than doctrines based on theories. The brief contrast between *askēsis* ('practice') and *dogmata* ('doctrines') at the start of the essay (*Indol.* 1) takes on added significance against this background; cf. the contrast between *kolasis* ('discipline') and (*paideusis*) ('training' or 'education') in *Aff. Dig.* (text to n. 49 above).

[96] See text to nn. 72–5 above.

presupposed and in the methods presented as enabling development towards this ideal, Galen's *Avoiding Distress* seems to me more intellectually self-consistent than *Psychological Affections*.

How should we explain this difference between the two works, if my analysis is correct? As noted before, *Avoiding Distress* seems to be the earlier work. It also has a more straightforward structure and tighter focus, presenting and explaining Galen's un-impassioned response to his losses in the fire at Rome in 192. Although this response, and certain other features in the essay, have a Stoic colouring, Galen's explanation is couched in his standard (Platonic–Aristotelian) psychological style, though presented as a personal opinion and without much explicit theorizing. I suggested earlier that Galen's 'stoic' reactions to his losses in the fire seem to have reactivated his previous interest in questions of ethical psychology and the therapy of emotions, which is evident in *PHP* 4–5 (written in 162–6).[97] Both *Character Traits*, which might have been written soon after *Avoiding Distress*, and *Psychological Affections* express this interest. *Psychological Affections*, in fact, seems to be an attempt to treat similar themes to *Avoiding Distress*, but in a more elaborate and theoretically informed way, based on wider reading of previous treatises on the therapy of emotions.[98] This may explain the relatively greater prominence in *Psychological Affections* of Stoic–Epicurean motifs, which are combined (rather awkwardly, I think) with the explicitly Platonic–Aristotelian psychology. The latter side of the work is based on his earlier discussion in *PHP* 4–5, reinforced by *Character Traits* (to which he refers in ch. 6, V.27–9), which might have been written after *Avoiding*

[97] See also text to nn. 24–7 above; as noted there, this view of the chronology of Galen's writings on this topic is indebted to Vivian Nutton (in Singer forthcoming). Boudon-Millot 2007*b*: 81–2 argues that *Aff. Dig.* must be the earlier work because there is no reference there to Galen's losses in the great fire at Rome of 192 (e.g. in *Aff. Dig.*, ch. 8, V.43, where such a loss would have been a relevant fact to cite). But this may have been because the loss was less recent than it was when writing *Avoiding Distress*; and in any case Galen stresses there that he was not unduly affected by this loss (see also Hankinson 2008*d*: 22 on this point).

[98] As Tieleman suggests (2003*a*: 149 n. 43, 2009: 296–7), Galen in his later years seems to have relied on his earlier reading of Chrysippus' works (esp. *On the Psyche* and *On Passions*, including the 'therapeutic book', cited extensively in *PHP* 2–5). But *Aff. Dig.* gives evidence of other reading on the therapy of emotions, including the work of Antonius the Epicurean noted by Galen (see text to nn. 31–44 above).

Distress. In short, the relative loss of conceptual coherence in *Psychological Affections*, by contrast with *Avoiding Distress*, seems to derive from an attempt at a more ambitious version of the earlier essay, but one which has not quite been worked out at the theoretical level.

So far I have focused on locating Galen's essays *Psychological Affections* and *Avoiding Distress* in the context of writings about the therapy of emotion and the competing intellectual traditions that inform this genre. How do these essays relate to other Galenic writings of a comparable kind; and does this comparison help to explain the mixed or inconsistent character of the essay? As noted earlier, most of the other works on ethics listed by Galen in *Lib. Prop.*, ch. 12, have been lost, except for the companion essay on the errors of the psyche (*Pecc. Dig.*) and a summary of *Character Traits*. However, also relevant for understanding the project of these three ethical works are *PHP* 4–5 and *QAM* ch.11.[99] In considering the relationship between these works, I am especially concerned with the question, central to this book as a whole, of Galen's relationship to Stoic theory. I review the main features of *Character Traits*, and then consider the relationship between these various works and the overall implications for understanding Galen's approach to the therapy of emotions.

Character Traits (*Peri Ēthōn*) (*De Moribus* = *Mor.*) survives in a fairly full Arabic summary of a lost, medium-length essay, in four books, supplemented by some other evidence.[100] There is a complete English translation of the Arabic summary, and limited scholarly discussion, especially two articles by Richard Walzer, whose expertise spans Arabic and Classical thought.[101] As noted earlier, it seems to belong to the same period as *Avoiding Distress*.[102] The work is more theoretical in approach than *Aff. Dig.*, though it is not very technical or analytic, to judge from the Arabic summary. The closest surviving

[99] *PHP* and *QAM* are included in *Lib. Prop.*, ch. 13 (XIX.45–6, trans. Singer 1997*a*: 21), under 'works concerning the philosophy of Plato'. But there are quite close links with *Aff. Dig.*, *Indol.*, and *Mor.* (which are listed in *Lib. Prop.*, ch. 12 under 'ethical philosophy').

[100] For Arabic text, see Kraus 1939, also Stern 1956.

[101] For translation, see Mattock 1972 (24 pages long); a revised and more complete translation by D. Davies will appear in Singer forthcoming. See also Walzer 1949, 1954, reprinted as Walzer 1962: 142–63 and 164–74. See further Kollesch and Nickel: 1994: 1398, and Singer 1992: 208–11.

[102] See n. 26 above.

parallel known to me is Plutarch's essay *On Ethical Virtue*, which is also a résumé of Platonic–Aristotelian ethical psychology that advocates a certain type of character-state. Both works also react against Stoic psychology, though this theme is more prominent in Plutarch's essay.[103] The key term in Galen's essay, *ēthos* ('trait or quality of character'), is strongly evocative of Aristotle's ethical writings, in which this term took on a special importance. But, as elsewhere in Galen, and in much Middle Platonic writing, Aristotelian and Platonic ideas are merged;[104] and the Platonic tripartite psyche provides the basic framework of the essay. After the opening account of *ēthos*, the first book centres on the traits linked with the 'spirited' part of the psyche (or 'spirited psyche', as it is presented), the second book deals with those traits linked with the appetitive psyche, the third with the training of character-traits, and the fourth with the traits associated with the rational psyche.[105]

Much of the work represents a restatement of well-known Platonic or Aristotelian ideas that figure in other Galen works considered here.[106] However, some more distinctive features emerge if we focus closely on Galen's account of *ēthos*. One important emphasis is to associate *ēthos*, more unequivocally than in Aristotle, with the

[103] On Plu. *Mor.* 440 D–452 D, see Gill 2006: 219–38, with refs. to previous discussions. Plutarch's essay combines two norms, *metriopatheia* and *apatheia* (*Mor.* 444 C–D, cf. Gill 2006: 237–8). For Galen's protreptic to 'liken yourself to god' (i.e. to realize your god-like mind rather than your embodied emotional nature'), see XIL.214–XL.217, Mattock 1972: 248–50, and Walzer 1954 (=1962: 164–74). (NB the Latin and Arabic numbers cited for *Mor.* refer to Kraus 1939, not Kühn; the work does not appear in Kühn.) The attitude implied in this protreptic is strongly dualistic, typical of much Middle Platonic thinking, but less typical of Galen, and very different from *QAM*. On 'likeness to god' as a goal in Middle Platonic philosophy, see Dillon 1977: index under 'Likeness to God' and Annas 1999: ch. 3.

[104] Again, Plutarch's essay on ethical virtue is a useful analogue: see Gill 2006: 231–4.

[105] See Walzer 1962: 145. For the idea of three psyches (rather than three parts or faculties of psyche), see XXVI.192–3, Mattock 1972: 237 (Galen makes it clear the variation in terminology is not meant to carry any special significance). For the idea that the dominant character-traits of the person concerned derive from the dominance of one or more of the psychic parts (or psyches) within them, see XXXIX. 213–14, Mattock 1972: 247–8.

[106] See e.g. the idea of internal struggle between parts as determining the overall character of the psyche (XXIX.213–14, Mattock 1972: 247–8, XLII.218–19, Mattock 1972: 250–1) (cf. Ch. 4 above, text to nn. 248–54); the idea that traits of character are ingrained by habit and may become unalterable in time, XXXI.201 (cf. text to n. 55 above).

non-rational part(s) of the psyche.[107] This point is signalled firmly from the start of the essay:

> A trait of character is a state of the psyche that induces a man to perform the actions of the psyche without consideration or precise knowledge... Philosophers have... studied traits of character, in order to discover whether they belong only to the irrational psyche or whether some part has to do with the rational psyche... Aristotle and others considered that a part of character had to do with the rational psyche, but that the greater part was located in the irrational; later philosophers claimed that the whole of character belonged to the rational psyche, and went so far as to associate with the rational psyche the accidents [i.e. *pathē*]—anger, desire, fear, love, pleasure, grief—that occur to the psyche. Observation, however, provides evidence that those people's claims are false.[108]

Although Galen's account of *ēthos* resembles other definitions of the term found in post-Hellenistic writers,[109] the usage differs from Aristotle's conception in ways indicated by Galen himself. For Aristotle, 'ethical virtue' (that is, virtue of *ēthos*) is a quality of the whole person, including both parts of the psyche, whereas intellectual virtue is that of the purely rational part of the psyche. Aristotle also stresses the interdependence of right character (*ēthos* or *hexis*) and practical reasoning, a theme not reflected in Galen's essay.[110] The last part of the passage cited from Galen's essay indicates the motivation for this new emphasis. The Aristotelian idea of *ēthos*—or at least a modified or simplified version of this—is being recruited to challenge the Stoic conception of emotions as (in Galen's account) purely rational functions, which is clearly alluded to here.[111] In other words, Galen here adopts a version of Aristotle's idea of character-traits to support this challenge, combined with the Platonic tripartite psyche,

[107] On this emphasis, see also Walzer 1962: 146–51 (he follows Galen in *PHP* 4–5 in attributing this kind of view to Posidonius).

[108] *Mor.* XXV–XXVI.191–2, trans. Mattock 1972: 236–7, 'soul' modified to 'psyche' and bracketed phrase added.

[109] See e.g. Arius Didymus: '*ēthos* is a quality of the irrational part of the psyche which is in its turn accustomed to subordinate itself to reason' (Stob. 2.38.3–4, trans. Walzer 1962: 147, slightly modified); also Plu. *Mor.* 443 C, 444 B.

[110] See e.g. Arist. *EN* 1.13, 1103^{a}3–10, 6.12, 1144^{a}6–9, 6.13, 1144^{b}30–2, 10.8, 1178^{a}10–20. See further Gill 1996: 247–50.

[111] A similar process can be seen at work in Plutarch; see further Donini 1974: 63–126, 80–1, Becchi 1978, Gill 2006: 230–4.

which was adopted for this same reason in *PHP*, a work cited in this opening passage.[112]

A number of other themes in *Mor.* reflect this presentation of *ēthē* as properties of the non-rational psyche.[113] One is the idea that character-traits are evident in non-human animals and human children, who do not possess (or have not yet acquired) rationality. This point is also made early in the essay: 'A similar indication is provided by the traits of character that we see in infants and in irrational animals; we find that some animals, such as the hare and deer, are cowardly, some, such as the lion and the dog, are brave and some, such as the fox and ape, are crafty'.[114] The idea that traits of character, which express the non-rational psyche, are manifested in human children almost from birth, is developed at some length later in the essay. Although Galen also highlights a process of development (signs of shame or shamelessness and of love of honour appear later than birth), he emphasizes that young children give early indications of whether they are inclined towards virtue or vice.[115] This theme is subsequently linked with the tripartite psyche, in the idea that natural differences in character reflect variations in the relative strength of the parts of the psyche (or the three psyches, as this is presented here). 'The difference between the various types of character is caused only by a greater or lesser degree of inclination in each of these psyches, according to the extent of its [one of the three psyches] natural strength'.[116] The cumulative effect of these features is to suggest a rather different picture of the development of character from that offered by Plato in the *Republic* or *Laws* and Aristotle's ethical works. There, the view is that the developed character of adult human beings is a product of the interplay between inborn nature, habituation in the family and community, and rational decisions made by the person

[112] *Mor.* XXVI.192–3, Mattock 1972: 237.

[113] For the view that these themes form part of a connected line of thought, see Walzer 1962: 151–61.

[114] *Mor.* XXV.191, Mattock 1972: 236. As pointed out by Walzer 1962: 152–3, this idea figures in Arist. *HA* 8.1 but does not appear in his ethical writings. In *QAM* ch. 7, IV.791–8, and *PHP* V.465, 5.5.34–7 De Lacy, the character-traits of animal species are also illustrated by reference to Aristotle and taken to show the influence of bodily make-up (mixtures of elements) on psychological states; for the significance of Aristotle's use of the term *ēthē* in this connection, see *PHP* V.465, 5.5.27, p. 322.14–17.

[115] *Mor.* XXVIII–XXX.197–9, Mattock 1972: 239–40.

[116] *Mor.* XXIX.213, Mattock 1972: 247.

herself. This Platonic–Aristotelian view is reflected elsewhere in Galen's writings as well as in other Imperial thinkers such as Plutarch.[117] It is not difficult to see what might motivate this modification or simplification of the Platonic–Aristotelian pattern. Again, the effect is to reinforce the rejection of the Stoic view that all human beings are naturally capable of developing complete virtue and that they are corrupted (in part at least) by external influences. Although this rejection of Stoic thinking on development is not made explicit in the surviving summary, it is cited as one of Galen's views in an Arabic commentator on Galen's ethical views, probably referring to this work.[118]

How do these works (*Psychological Affections*, *Avoiding Distress*, *Character Traits*) fit into Galen's thinking on ethical psychology, as far as we can tell from our remaining texts? What do they tell us about Galen's relationship with Stoic thought—the question that is my main focus in this study? There are clear links between the three works and also with *PHP* 4–5 and, to some extent, *QAM* ch. 11. One recurrent theme is that of childhood behaviour as an indication of innate qualities of character, though this theme is rather differently handled in each of the four works. Specifying the different treatment of this theme can help us to bring out the interrelationship between these Galenic writings.

Broadly speaking, all five works convey two related ideas: the Platonic–Aristotelian part-based psychological theory and the correlated account of ethical development, centred on the interrelationship of inborn nature, habituation, and rational agency or choice. But they do so in different ways and give varying degrees of prominence to these ideas. The fullest and most philosophically articulated version of these ideas is offered in the earliest of these works, *PHP* 4–5. As brought out in 4.3 above, Galen presents his thoughts about the part-based psyche through discussion of Plato's tripartite psyche in the *Republic* and frames his ideas about ethical development as a commentary on Posidonius' reading of Plato in a way that, I think, misrepresents Posidonius' position. In both cases, the ideas offered are formulated explicitly as a counterweight to orthodox Stoic psychology and thinking about ethical development. The theme of

[117] See text to nn. 52–6, 72–5, 94–6 above; also Ch. 4 above, text to nn. 185–91.

[118] Walzer 1962: 160–1, referring to Miskawaih's comments on Galen.

childhood expression of character figures in *PHP* 5 in connection with the idea that there are three natural types of 'appropriation' (*oikeiōsis*), to pleasure, victory or honour, and to virtue. The first two types of appropriation, according to Galen, are apparent among non-human animals and human children, whereas the inclination towards virtue only appears rather later, as children become more rational.[119] Two features of this passage are worth noting. One is that the theme of the expression of character in children or animals is coupled with the standard Platonic–Aristotelian idea of a two-stage developmental process, in which non-rational training provides the basis for the development of rationality and virtue.[120] The other is that this theme, like the whole discussion of ethical development in *PHP* 5, is interlocked with a rather complex intellectual debate, in which Galen pits his own version of earlier, mostly Platonic–Aristotelian, ideas against Stoic unified psychology. The debate of *PHP* 4–5 itself forms a subdivision—and, in a sense, a digression—in a larger debate between Stoic and Platonic–Galenic ideas about embodied psychology, a point whose significance in understanding Galen's framework of ideas on these topics has been considered earlier, and which I refer to again shortly.[121]

Character Traits (*Mor.*) seems, to judge from the Arabic summary, to be a summary of the main themes of *PHP* 4–5 but presented as Galen's own ideas rather than as Platonic or Posidonian ideas recruited to challenge those of Chrysippus. Traits of character (*ēthē*) are explained by reference to the interactions of the three parts of the Platonic tripartite psyche and by a modified or simplified version of the Platonic–Aristotelian account of ethical development. The emphasis is on the idea that character is a function of the non-rational part of the psyche, as indicated by the behaviour of

119 *PHP* V.459–60, 5.5.1–8 De Lacy (part of V.459–68, 5.5.1–38 De Lacy); see esp. V.460, p. 318.5–8 De Lacy on the later emergence of the appropriation to virtue. A related point is the presence, in animals (both human and non-human) of characteristics that reflect innate, body-based 'mixtures' of elements, or the effect of environmental influences on body-based temperament: *PHP* V.464–5, 5.5.22–7 De Lacy.

120 *PHP* V.466–7, 5.5.30–5 De Lacy, which combines Posidonius' interest in Plato's discussion of prenatal shaping of character and in the childhood training as a basis for adult (rational) action. On these passages, and on Galen's misleading presentation of Posidonius, see Ch. 4 above, text to nn. 208–12.

121 See 4.1 above and text to n. 144 below.

non-human animals and human children. A motif here that marks a partial difference from the treatment in *PHP* 5 is that indications of ethical virtue or vice are said to appear very early, before the development of rationality. Thus, when 'children reach their third year, they begin to show signs of shame and impudence... These signs appear in those who have not yet been disciplined by chastisement or fear [that is, they are innate features]'. The point is spelled out that 'some children tend towards virtue and some towards vice, without thought or firm judgement', as is indicated by the willingness of some children to help each other while others take pleasure in spiteful behaviour. 'In short, no accident or trait of character [*pathos* or *ēthos*] exists in the grown man unless it already exists in him as a child.'[122] This is only a partial modification of the standard Platonic–Aristotelian pattern that underlies *PHP* 4–5: Galen goes on to explain that behaviour can be altered subsequently by habituation or the exercise of judgement.[123] But the emphasis on early indications of character in children, which is signalled from the start of the summary, is striking.[124] The summary offers few indications of the specific purpose of the essay. But, although there is no longer explicit reference to competing philosophical positions, a number of phrases indicate that Galen is still motivated by the wish to counter the Stoic (as he sees it) over-rationalistic account of psychology. Indeed, the reference to manifestations of early human and animal character (*ēthos*) and the 'accidents' (*pathē*) that reflect this character—by contrast with actions that result from reasoned judgements—is designed to support this position.[125] So it seems that the debate of

[122] *Mor.* XXIX–XXX.198–9, Mattock 1972: 239–40, with added phrases in square brackets; see also the translation of these passages in Walzer 1962: 154–5.

[123] *Mor.* XXX–XXXI, 200–1, Mattock 1972: 240–1.

[124] See Walzer 1962: 151–6.

[125] This comment follows the comments about early indications of virtue and vice in children: 'It is wrong, then, to suppose that all accidents [*pathē*] happen as a result of judgement and thought... [an accident] is a brutish movement that comes about without the exercise of thought, consideration or firm judgement', *Mor.* XXX.199, Mattock 1972: 240 (additions in square brackets). See also the citation of children's and animal behaviour to support the idea that 'character' is shown in instinctive reactions, text to n.114 above (*Mor.* XXV.191, Mattock 1972: 236). Also, 'The cause of those [actions] that stem from nature or habit is a trait of character, and the cause of those that stem from thought and consideration is judgement' (*Mor.* XXXI.201, Mattock 1972: 241).

PHP 4–5 still underlies this essay, and that it motivates even the modifications from the pattern of thinking about development found in the earlier work.

In *QAM* (to take this work next),[126] there are salient differences from the other three works discussed here. The central focus is on the physical or body-based factors shaping psychological capacities and qualities, whether innate or environmental. Also, although the Platonic-style tripartite psyche figures here also,[127] the psychological functions associated with these parts play a much less important role than in *PHP* 4–5 or *Mor.* Also, as stressed earlier, Galen in this work virtually adopts a type of physicalism in psychology that places him close to Stoic thinking and at odds with Platonic psyche-dualism.[128] However, there are some lines of continuity with the thinking of the other discussions considered here, especially regarding development of character. Variations in the behaviour of young children[129] are presented early in the essay as a key indicator of the fact that 'there are innate differences in the faculties of each of the three forms or parts of the psyche'.[130] Later in the work, variations in the psychological capacities and characteristics of different kinds of animal species are taken to show that these features are based on their physiological make-up.[131] In chapter 11, Galen sums up in a more analytic way the implications of this essay for questions of character development. He argues against the possible criticism that his focus on the body-based (innate and environmental) influences on psychological quality prevents us from making well-grounded ethical judgements about character and actions. In this connection, he restates the criticism of *PHP* 4–5 against the Stoic view that all human beings are constitutively capable of developing towards

[126] *QAM* is the last of these four works to be composed; but I take it next in order to place *Aff. Dig* and *Indol.* against the background of Galen's other works on similar themes.

[127] See e.g. *QAM* ch. 2, IV 770–2, ch. 3, IV.772, ch. 4, IV.782, Singer 1997*a*: 153–4, 157.

[128] See 3.5 above.

[129] 'Some small children show great cowardice and timidity; some are insatiable and gluttonous, others quite the opposite; some are completely lacking in shame while others are modest', *QAM* ch. 2, IV.768, *SM* 2.32.17–33.3, trans. Singer 1997*a*: 150.

[130] *QAM* ch. 2, IV.768, *SM* 2.33.5–8, trans. Singer 1997*a*: 150.

[131] *QAM* ch. 7, IV.791–8, Singer 1997*a*: 161–4, referring to Arist. *PA* and *HA*. See text to n. 114 above, on *Mor.*, though the emphasis there is on the idea that these characteristics are non-rational, not that they depend on bodily mixtures.

complete virtue and that they are corrupted by social influences and pleasure. Posidonius is presented again as supporting this critique by emphasizing the innate, and thus non-rational, causes of corruption.[132] The stress on body-based (innate or environmental) influences on character is coupled with the theme that the medical art is best placed to modify or improve psychological qualities, by offering guidance on such factors as diet and exercise.[133]

As stressed earlier, the argument of *QAM* ch. 11 is non-standard, within the Platonic–Aristotelian approach, in stressing innate (or at least body-based) factors on character, at the expense of social habituation and exercise of rational agency. It is also non-standard in arguing that the question of one's degree of responsibility for the ethical quality of one's actions and character can simply be set aside in responding to wrongdoing or bad character.[134] The discussion of *PHP* 5 is more characteristic of the Platonic–Aristotelian approach in giving some recognition to the role of all three factors.[135] However, there is a partial parallel with *Character Traits* in this respect, in that this work also cites infant human and animal behaviour as an indication of character. The focus here, however, is on the idea that traits of character (*ēthē*) are functions of the non-rational part of the psyche, rather than that they are body-based and products of the mixture of elements in the body.[136] However, the strongest contrast is between *QAM* and *Aff. Dig.*, in this respect, as is brought out shortly.

If we place Galen's essays on the therapy of the emotions (*Aff. Dig.* and *Indol.*) in the context of these other works, there emerge both well-marked similarities and differences. There is an explicit reference in *Aff. Dig.* to *Character Traits*, to reinforce the point that the shaping of character must take account of the fact that two parts of our psyche are, in different ways and degrees, non-rational.[137] The essay thus signals a linkage with the Platonic-style tripartite psyche that

[132] *QAM* ch. 11, IV.814–21, Singer 1997*a*: 172–5; cf. *PHP* V.459–67, 5.5.1–35 De Lacy. See further Ch. 4 above, text to nn. 208–12.

[133] *QAM* ch. 9, IV.808, ch. 11, IV.821, Singer 1997*a*: 169, 175. On this point, see further text to nn. 305–12 below.

[134] See Ch. 3 above, text to nn. 284–92.

[135] See Ch. 4 above, text to nn.189–212.

[136] See text to nn. 122–5 above.

[137] See text to n. 49 above.

figures in all the works considered here (except *Indol.*). But *Aff. Dig.*, like *Indol.*, resembles *PHP* 5—rather than *Mor.* or *QAM*—in reflecting the normal Platonic–Aristotelian pattern of thinking about ethical development, giving full roles to social habituation and rational agency as well as innate features. Thus, although *Aff. Dig.* restates the point that figures in other works, that individual differences of character emerge even in childhood, this motif is explicitly coupled with those of the importance of habit and rational education.[138] Of course, the main difference between *Aff. Dig.* and the other discussions are the Stoic-style motifs. As well as adopting a (predominantly) Stoic–Epicurean genre, that of the therapy of emotions, Galen uses expressions that might imply the adoption of the Stoic norm of *apatheia* ('freedom from emotion'). He also focuses on cognitive and rational strategies of therapy that imply a Stoic–Epicurean unified psychological theory, according to which emotions, and changes of emotion, depend on beliefs and reasoning. I suggested earlier that the two strands in Galen's essay (the Platonic–Aristotelian psychological model and the Stoic–Epicurean motifs) do not seem to be effectively integrated.[139] In *Indol.*, by contrast, Galen's apparently Stoic-style equanimity in the face of disaster is explained, in the course of the essay, in consistently Platonic–Aristotelian terms.[140] This survey of these five Galenic ethical works helps to bring out the relatively atypical character of *Aff. Dig.* in this respect. The Stoic-style motifs in *Aff. Dig.* emerge as relatively isolated in a group of works that are dominated, though in different ways, by a Platonic–Aristotelian approach to psychology and ethical development. The contrast between these aspects of *Aff. Dig.* and *QAM*, especially chapter 11, is particularly stark. Whereas the main focus of *Aff. Dig.* is on rational strategies for the therapy of the psyche, *QAM* underlines the extent to which our character

[138] *Aff. Dig.* ch. 7, V.38–9, Singer 1997*a*: 117–18; the differences noted include early indications of ethical character (e.g. modest or shameless, cowardly or fearless) as well as other qualities. For stress on habituation and education or rational choice, see *SM* 1.28.20–4; this theme is linked with that of childhood nature in *SM* 1.29.39–30.2, 1.30.16–31.6. In *Indol.*, we find a stress on the combination of innate nature, upbringing, and rational choice (57–65, 79) but not on childhood nature. For the childhood theme in the other three works, see text to nn. 118–30 above.

[139] See text to nn. 57–76 above.

[140] See text to nn. 86–96 above.

and psychological capacities are shaped by bodily make-up, and stresses the role of the medical doctor in improving our psychic state.[141]

What explains the variations in the position adopted in these various Galenic works on related subjects; and what general picture do we form of the formation and unfolding of this line of thought? As P. N. Singer suggests, variations between Galenic works on related topics seems better explained by the project and rhetoric of the specific work rather than by a supposed development of ideas over time.[142] Although, as Hankinson has brought out in his work on many aspects of Galen's thought, there is a strong ambition to create a unified system of ideas, there is also a tendency to focus on the main thesis in any one work, sometimes to the exclusion of themes important in other contexts. The starting-point for the approach to ethical psychology that is dominant in these works seems to be the adoption of a Platonic-style conception of human psychology and ethical development which is closely linked with his critique of Stoic psychology in *PHP* 4–5. *Character Traits* seems to represent a summary of the main themes of *PHP* 4–5, presented in less analytic and rather simplified form, but with the same broad polemical contrast in view. In *Aff. Dig.*, although Galen refers explicitly to *On Characters* and thus by implication to *PHP* 4–5, there is an unacknowledged tension between the Stoic–Epicurean conceptual frame and the Platonic-style psychology that Galen injects into this frame. In *Indol.*, in partial contrast, Galen finds an autobiographical mode for presenting his approach to the therapy of emotions that brings this theme more fully into line with his recurrent (Platonic–Aristotelian) assumptions about ethical development. *QAM* has its own distinctive project and thesis. Although there is some linkage with the psychology and account of development of *PHP* 4–5 and later writings, the stress on bodily factors is more single-minded than in the other works. This focus is also markedly at odds with the Stoic-style stress on the scope for rational agency in ethical development that is present in *Aff. Dig.*

[141] On *Aff. Dig.*, see text to nn. 68–71 above, and on *QAM*, see text to nn. 127–34 above.

[142] Singer 1997*a*: xxviii–xxxvi.

A further question raised by this group of discussions is this: what is the nature and basis of Galen's commitment to the Platonic (or Platonic–Aristotelian) psychological theory and account of ethical development? On the face of it, it may appear from these works to be a matter of philosophical allegiance. But, in fact, in *Aff. Dig.* and elsewhere, Galen repudiates the idea of philosophical allegiance,[143] and the indications of Stoic-style thinking in that essay, and in other contexts, suggests that this eclectic stance reflects significant features of his practice. I argued earlier (4.1 above) that Galen's adoption of the Platonic picture of psychological functions in *PHP* 4–5 may be a by-product of his anatomically based convictions about the role of the brain as the psychological centre. I have also suggested that his adoption of the Platonic tripartite psychology may be more at odds with his anatomical picture than he supposes, and that he might have done better to adopt a theory based on the Stoic unified control-centre.[144] Whether or not these suggestions are accepted, it is clear that Galen's adoption of a brain-centred anatomical theory and his espousal of the Platonic–Aristotelian account of ethical psychology rest on grounds of different type. One is based on an independently (and highly sophisticated) method of natural inquiry;[145] the other derives simply from Galen's co-option of a theory that is consistent—as Galen supposes—with the outcomes of that natural inquiry. If this view is correct, Galen's commitment to a Platonic–Aristotelian framework of thinking about ethical psychology is a more second-hand and derivative move than his adoption of a brain-centred anatomical picture. Hence, despite the apparent firmness of Galen's convictions about the Platonic–Aristotelian framework and rejection of Stoic thinking in this group of works, the intellectual basis for these positions is less secure—and less the result of sustained independent work—than his rejection of the Stoic heart-centred psychophysiology. For related reasons, I think it is fair to say that there is less in this group of works that represents genuinely original and innovative thought than in other areas of Galenic work considered so far in this book. These and other issues relating to the different aspects of Galenic thought in this area are pursued further later in this chapter

[143] *Aff. Dig.* ch. 8, V.42; see further Hankinson 1992.

[144] See 3.3 above.

[145] See Ch. 2 above, text to nn. 92–110.

(5.4 below), as part of a more wide-ranging consideration of the relationship between approaches to medical and psychological therapy in Galen and in Stoicism.

5.3 CHRYSIPPUS ON THE THERAPY OF EMOTIONS

I now juxtapose Galen's thinking about the therapy of emotions to Stoic ideas on this subject, which form an important part of the background for Galen's essays (*Aff. Dig.* and *Indol.*). I focus on Chrysippus' (lost) fourth, 'therapeutic' book of his work *On Passions*, taken in the context of Stoic writing on this subject, including Seneca's *On Anger* (*De Ira*), the one complete surviving Stoic text on the therapy of emotions. By contrast with Galen's essay, which was a late and rather minor exercise in this genre, Chrysippus' book was a major and influential work in the development of Hellenistic and Roman thought about the therapy of emotions. It is also a work whose approach Galen criticizes in *PHP* 4–5, as part of his sustained attack on the Stoic conception of psychological functions. Hence, examining Chrysippus' therapeutic strategy, against which Galen reacts in *PHP*, can shed further light on the relationship between Galenic and Stoic psychology, which is central to my concerns in this study. This discussion also provides a significant part of the basis for comparing Galenic and Stoic thinking about physical and psychological therapy, which is the third topic of this chapter (5.4 below).

Tieleman offers a reconstruction of Chrysippus' 'therapeutic' book as part of his review of the evidence for Chrysippus' *On Passions.*[146] This reconstruction is based on correlating Galen's comments, which refer explicitly to Chrysippus' book, with Cicero's more generalized discussion of Stoic thinking in his review of approaches to the

[146] The book is sometimes referred to as the 'therapeutic book' or, less often, 'ethical book' (or the two terms are combined). Although Galen sometimes presents the book as in some sense 'written separately' from the rest (*PHP* V.493, 5.7.52, p. 348.29–31 De Lacy), he also makes it plain that it was the fourth book of *On Passions* and that it reflects its overall theoretical approach; see Tieleman 2003*a*: 140–1.

therapy of emotions in *Tusculan Disputations* (*Tusc.*) 3–4. Although it is not possible to reconstitute the contents and structure of this book in great detail, we can identify the main topics and (to a limited extent) their order together with some salient quotations.[147] A key theme, which seems to have come at the start of Chrysippus' book, is the analogy between medical (physical) and philosophical (psychological) therapy.[148] This is linked with a number of other ideas, already noted in this study: the connection between psychological health, strength, and beauty, the idea of emotion as a 'feverish' state, and of long-term emotional states as susceptibility to certain kinds of fever.[149] The Stoic (and Galenic) idea that psychological states reflect the 'mixtures' of elements in the body may have figured in this connection, as it does in Seneca's *On Anger*.[150] Other themes linked with this book include the idea of emotion as a 'rejection' of reason, as a form of psychological weakness or 'lack of tension' (*atonia*) and as a form of 'madness' or psychological blindness.[151] Chrysippus' book also offered advice that is more directly concerned with modes of therapy of the emotions. One important motif is that the timing and form of the therapy has to take account of the emotional state of the person concerned. Another point relates to the modification of the two kinds of belief involved in an emotion. A third motif is that therapy can be directed usefully even at people who do not hold (what the Stoics see as) true beliefs about ethical principles.[152]

This bare outline of themes brings out a number of significant features of the Stoic approach deployed by Chrysippus. For one thing, it bears out the point put rather negatively by Cicero: 'when Chrysippus and the Stoics discuss the emotions, they concern

[147] Tieleman 2003*a*: chs. 4, 6; also the summary of main topics and relevant sources on p. 326. See also Fillion-Lahille 1984: part 2, esp. 82–118; on Cic. *Tusc.* 3–4, see Graver 2002.

[148] See Gal. *PHP* V.437–8, 439–40, 5.2.22–4, 26–7, 31–3; also Cic. *Tusc.* 3.6, 4.23, 58. On the analogy and the physical–psychological relationship, see 5.4 below.

[149] See Gal. *PHP* V.432, 435, 440, 443, 444, 5.2.3, 14, 32–3, 47, 49 De Lacy; also Cic. *Tusc.* 4.23–31. See also Ch. 4 above, text to nn. 147–54.

[150] *PHP* V.447, 5.3.7–8 De Lacy, *QAM* IV.783–4, *SM* 2.45.5–46.7; also Sen. *Ira.* 2.19 (on the latter passage, see text to n. 221 below).

[151] *PHP* V.396, 403–6, 408–9, 414–15, 4.5.21–2, 4.6.4–9, 11, 19–20, 23–5, 34–5, 44–6 De Lacy; also Cic. *Tusc.* 4.22, 76–7.

[152] On these points, see text to nn. 176–93 below.

themselves primarily with classifications and definitions, and the part of their treatment devoted to calming the mind and freeing it from disturbance is quite short'.[153] The Epicurean Timaxagoras, apparently, was even more critical: Chrysippus in his 'therapeutic book' is grouped with those who 'only criticize [emotions] and do nothing else at all except a little bit'.[154] These comments, especially the second, are neither fair nor wholly accurate. But there is a more sympathetic way of putting the ideas expressed. The outline of themes in Chrysippus' book indicates two important general features of his approach, which are strongly reflected in our evidence for the work. One is that Chrysippus' approach to the therapy of emotions (like his view of emotions generally) is closely integrated with other aspects of his ethical theory, including his theory of value, of psychology, and of ethical development. Several of the themes just noted in connection with the 'therapeutic' book restate, or reflect, core features of Stoic thinking about emotions, as presented in the first three, theoretical books of *On Passions*.[155] This does not mean that these themes are of no practical use for therapy. On the contrary, as brought out shortly, the presentation of these ideas can in itself serve a therapeutic function—if the person to whom they are directed responds appropriately. But this point needs to be coupled with a second feature, which is associated in our sources specifically with Chrysippus, as distinct from earlier Stoic thinkers.[156] This is a practical, even sensitive, approach regarding the circumstances in which therapeutic treatment can usefully be offered, and regarding the kind of therapy that is appropriate in different cases. The second, more pragmatic,

[153] Cic. *Tusc.* 4.9, trans. Graver 2002; it is not clear that Cicero is referring to Chrysippus' 'therapeutic' book specifically, as distinct from *On Passions* or Stoic writings on emotions generally. Cicero contrasts this approach with that of followers of Aristotle who focus more on remedies.

[154] Philodemus, *Ira* 1.10–20 Indelli 1988 (cf. *SVF* 3.470); also Tieleman 2003*a*: 320 n. 69. Philodemus is a well-known (1st-cent. BC) Epicurean writer and teacher; Timaxagoras is a more obscure figure.

[155] See esp. text to n. 148 above. The analogy between medical and philosophical therapy seems to be a distinctive feature of the 'therapeutic' book, though it fits well with other aspects of Stoic thinking about emotions.

[156] This feature might be connected with the fact that, as far as I am aware, Chrysippus was the first Stoic thinker to have written a book explicitly called a 'therapeutic' one.

aspect might seem to run counter to the first, more theoretically based, one and to mark a compromise with consistency of thinking. But, in fact, both features can be seen as fitting in with Stoic thinking about emotion, and indeed about values, psychology, and development. In short—and by contrast with Galen's less coherent approach in his essay on the therapy of emotion—Chrysippus' strategy is both highly consistent and, in various ways, potentially highly effective.

I begin by discussing the first feature of Chrysippus' approach, which I take to be the core point of the Stoic strategy. The main problem raised by this feature—as shown by ancient and modern reactions—is that of seeing in what sense it represents a form of therapy at all. Let us consider the principal moves made by Chrysippus in his book, especially what seems to have been the first part of it. Crucial for the strategy is the analogy between philosophical (psychological) and medical (physical) health and therapy. In essence, what Chrysippus seems to be doing is re-describing key features of the theory presented in the first three books of *On Passions*—but doing so *in terms of* the ideas of health and sickness. Fundamental to Chrysippus' analysis of emotions, as Tieleman suggests, is the application of the causal theory also deployed in the theory of determinism. This is based on a combination of an antecedent (external) cause and a 'sustaining' cause (internal to the character of the agent). The judgement, or set of judgements, involved in an emotion reflects the combination of the way a situation 'appears' to someone at the relevant time and her underlying character.[157] Earlier books of Chrysippus' work, it would seem, explored different aspects of this analysis. Book I centred on definitions of passions as occurrent psychological events and book 2 on the kind of judgements involved (and on possible conflicts between these judgements), as well as the developmental process that produced the defective beliefs underlying emotions.[158] The fourth ('therapeutic') book seems also to have focused on the relationship between occurrent emotions, presented as outbursts of illness, and the underlying

[157] Tieleman 2003*a*: 108–13; on Stoic causal theory, see also Ch. 2 above, text to nn. 122–4.

[158] See the summary of the contents of these books in Tieleman 2003*a*: 325–6 (see also his ch. 3); the contents of book 3 are unknown.

character-state that gives rise to these outbursts. A particularly important theme, stressed especially by Cicero, is the idea that different people are disposed towards different types of passion. However, an important corollary—and a distinctive feature of the theory—is that these states are only quasi-dispositional, and that they are fundamentally unstable or 'feverish'.[159] Chrysippus seems also to have examined in some detail the pattern of behaviour and the belief-structure associated with the weakness of character or 'absence of tension' (*atonia*) that produced outbursts of psychological sickness.[160] Extreme versions of these outbursts are characterized as forms of 'madness', reflecting mental 'blindness'.[161] Thus, the idea of emotions as pathological states, expressing long-term (but unstable) psychological conditions, seems to have been worked out in the systematic and detailed way that was characteristic of Chrysippus' treatises.

These points clarify the relationship between the main contents of the therapeutic book and the analysis of *On Passions* as a whole. But the question remains: in what way does the analysis of emotion as sickness constitute a form of therapy? Cicero, as noted earlier, complains that Chrysippus concentrated too much on elaborating the idea of emotions as a form of pathology and too little on practical forms of therapy.[162] Some modern scholars are more sympathetic to the approach, characterizing it as a type of 'preventive' medicine, by contrast with the curative measures also discussed by Chrysippus. Chrysippus' focus on the fact that emotions (psychological sicknesses) express long-term, though unstable, underlying conditions, makes it especially appropriate for him to emphasize a type of therapy that is directed at shaping (relatively) lasting belief-sets and attitudes. However, the precise form of this preventive therapy has not been analysed very closely. Even scholars sympathetic to Chrysippus' approach have tended to see this side of his therapeutic method (as distinct from the more practical side) as hard to

[159] See refs. in n. 149 above, esp. Cic. *Tusc.* 4.23–31; on the incoherence, instability or 'feverishness' of these conditions, see Cic. *Tusc.* 4.29–31, Gal. *PHP* V.435, 448, 5.2.13–14, 5.3.12 De Lacy. See also Ch. 4 above, text to nn. 147–54 above, and text to nn. 272–81 below.

[160] Gal. *PHP* V.404–6, 408–9, 412, 4.6.4–9, 11, 19–20, 23–5, 34–5 De Lacy.

[161] See refs. in n. 151 above.

[162] Cic. *Tusc.* 4.23, 33.

distinguish from ethical education generally.[163] However, there are at least two ways, I think, in which we can see this aspect of Chrysippus' theory as having a therapeutic role. One function is that of *persuasive redescription*. A related function is that of *promoting understanding* of our defective state. Both functions can be seen as essential prerequisites to, and an integral part of, improving our condition and as being 'therapeutic', in this sense.

I take the function of persuasive redescription first. As just noted, the main elements of Chrysippus' analysis of emotions have already been offered in previous books of this treatise. What is distinctive in this book is the presentation of emotions and emotional (quasi-) dispositions in terms of medical pathology. This presentation underlines that emotional states are analogous to diseased bodily states, for instance, in the forms of psychological agitation, instability or 'feverishness', internal conflict, and cognitive 'blindness' that they produce. In considering the intended effect of this type of presentation, it is worth bearing in mind that the Stoic (and Epicurean) presentation of emotions as defective ran counter to most philosophical and conventional ideas in Greco-Roman Antiquity. The Platonic–Aristotelian view that emotions as such are a normal, even positive, dimension of human experience, and that only extreme emotions are to be avoided, was a much more prevalent ancient idea.[164] Hence, the presentation of emotions in general, apart from the good emotions characteristic of the wise person, as modes of psychological disease represents an important supporting argument for the Stoic view. Also, if the view is accepted, even on a provisional basis, this can serve as the starting-point of therapy. Whatever their other differences, human beings do not, in general, want to be ill; and so a genuine acceptance of the idea that emotions, as analysed by Stoic theory, are forms of illness represents an important practical move towards trying to achieve a better state. Two features of Seneca's therapeutic essay *On Anger* seem to represent analogous ways of achieving the

[163] See e.g. Inwood and Donini 1999: 711–13, Tieleman 2003*a*: 319–20. For the distinction between preventive and therapeutic medicine in this connection, see Sen. *Ira* 2.18, *Ep.* 94.13.

[164] On competing ancient views of emotion and ideal emotional states, see text to nn. 8–13 above. The prevalence of the Aristotelian, or Platonic–Aristotelian, view in antiquity is brought out by Konstan 2001, 2006, Harris 2001.

same objectives. One is the explicit challenge to the 'Aristotelian' approach to emotions, centred on the ideal of 'moderation of emotions' (in Greek terms, *metriopatheia*).[165] The other is the presentation of anger as an inherently ugly and repellent phenomenon, marked by distorted and disturbed physical appearance, and by inhumane or near-lunatic behaviour.[166] Although it is unlikely that Chrysippus' book contained precisely comparable features,[167] these dimensions of Seneca's essay seem to be ways of achieving the same type of objective as Chrysippus. This is reinforcing the Stoic analysis of emotions, conceived as defective states, by underlining the diseased character of emotions and in so doing of undermining the competing, more favourable, view of emotions associated in Seneca with Aristotle.

The idea of persuasive redescription might suggest a purely rhetorical or presentational feature. Seneca's essay is, indeed, in these and other respects, strongly rhetorical, though there is room for argument about how closely the rhetoric is informed by Stoic objectives.[168] However, in Chrysippus' book, at least, redescription is closely interlocked with another function, that of promoting understanding in the reader about the nature and roots of her psychological condition and thus of enabling a therapeutic response. In a sense, this is the aim of the whole treatise *On Passions*. The work seems to have offered a systematic analysis of the nature of the emotions, in terms of ethical psychology, including examination of puzzling and problematic psychological states, and of the means by which human beings' belief-sets are corrupted in a way that generates emotions.[169] But the fourth, 'therapeutic' book, while presupposing these ideas, also added a

[165] See e.g Sen. *Ira* 1.7, 8.4–5, 9, 10.4, 11.1, 12.1–3, 14.1, 17.1; for comparable ideas (though not stated from a committed Stoic standpoint), see Cic. *Tusc.* 3.22, 74, 4.39–46.

[166] See e.g. (distorted appearance of anger), Sen. *Ira* 1.1, 2.35–6, (repellent and near-lunatic behaviour) 3.17–21.

[167] Chrysippus seems not to have engaged in explicit arguments with earlier theories (either those being adopted or rejected) in the way that became more common in later (post-Hellenistic and Roman) philosophy; see further Gill 2006: 136–7, 212–14. I know of no evidence suggesting that Chrysippus' 'therapeutic book' contained passages of the sort cited in n. 165 above.

[168] On this point, see refs. in n. 229 below.

[169] See Tieleman's summary of the contents of books 1–2 (2003*a*: 325–6, taken with his ch. 3).

further dimension, by drawing on the medical analogy that forms a central feature of the discussion. Two aspects seem to have been especially prominent. One is the analysis of what are, in other (more Aristotelian) types of account, seen as stable dispositions or traits of character (*ēthos*), presented here as quasi-dispositional tendencies to one or other type of psychological sickness. Chrysippus recognizes the relatively lasting or recurrent quality of such features, while also stressing that they are marked by inherent instability and internal conflict.[170] The other is the use of exemplary cases of occurrent internal conflict and self-contradiction, including tragic examples such as Euripides' Medea, to demonstrate the behaviour that results from psychological and ethical 'weakness' or 'absence of tension' (*atonia*), that is, from longer term 'sickness' of character.[171] These aspects of the discussion seem designed to serve two interrelated aims. On the one hand, Chrysippus offers what is presented as a conceptually powerful explanatory framework for well-recognized features of human psychological life, both long-term and occurrent. On the other, the features identified—including prominent and well-known examples of intensely emotional responses—are offered as what one might call 'objective indicators' of the validity of the analysis being offered.[172] In other words, if we accept the account offered of Medea's paradoxical and conflicted reactions at the prospect of killing her children, we will be more likely to endorse the general form of explanation of emotions offered by Stoicism, which aims to integrate ethical, psychological, and developmental aspects.

Here too, as well as in the case of persuasive redescription, we might ask how this aspect of Chrysippus' account helps the process of therapy. But the answer is perhaps more obvious. If we can understand the roots of our own psychological behaviour—since all of us, more or less, are subject to emotions of this kind—we are likely to be more inclined, and better placed, to take action to 'cure'

[170] See refs. in n. 159 above; as noted in text to nn. 105–11 above, *ēthos*, interpreted in (broadly) Aristotelian terms, plays a prominent role in Galen's thinking on the therapy of emotions.

[171] See refs. in n. 159 above; on Chrysippus' analysis of Medea, see Gill 1983, 1996: 226–33, 1998: 121, 2006: 254–60.

[172] For a similar point, made about Plato's depiction of defective psychic types in *R.* 8–9, see Gill 2006: 318–20.

our sickness. As this comment implies, persuasive redescription and the promotion of understanding are intimately interconnected in activating the required process of self-modification. Recognizing the roots of our psychological behaviour is presented as understanding our state as being that of occurrent and long-term sickness. This kind of understanding constitutes the first stage at least in altering or 'curing' our state. In thinking about this point, it is helpful to mark a contrast with Galen's principal essay on the therapy of emotions (*Aff. Dig.*). As highlighted earlier, there is a tension between the (highly cognitive or rational) methods of therapy advocated in Galen's essay and the psychological framework assumed, which involves a combination of rational and non-rational parts.[173] In the Stoic approach represented in Chrysippus' book, there is no such tension. Stoic theory assumes both that all human beings are constitutively capable of developing towards perfect wisdom and that such development represents the modification of the personality as a whole. According to the highly unified or holistic psychological model assumed by Stoicism, changes in belief or understanding about key ethical ideas necessarily carry with them changes in motivational pattern or attitude. There is no need or scope for separate training of non-rational parts since no such parts are acknowledged.[174] Hence, the recognition of the need for psychic cure and of the roots of our sickness in itself provides the basis for self-improvement and development towards a more 'healthy' state.[175]

The holistic character of Stoic psychology, in which beliefs are seen as shaping motivation directly, is also relevant for making sense of the second main feature of the Chrysippean approach. Alongside the themes just discussed, Chrysippus also included various pieces of practical comment and advice about the therapy of emotion. This side of Chrysippus' book has aroused rather more interest among modern scholars than the other side, although it is clear from the ancient evidence that it represented a secondary aspect of his account.[176] Although, on the face of it, this aspect might seem to mark a concession or compromise of Stoic principles, closer inspection

[173] See text to nn. 67–70 above. [174] See further Gill 2006: 129–45.

[175] On this point, see also Tieleman 2003*a*: 320.

[176] See text to nn. 146–52 above.

brings out the consistency of Chrysippus' approach. His advice relates to three main points: (1) timing and preparation, (2) the two kinds of judgement involved in emotion, and (3) offering therapy to those who do not subscribe to Stoic views.

Chrysippus seems to have stressed that there is no point in offering therapeutic advice to people who are in the grip of intense passion; however, in time the passion subsides and at that stage there is more chance of them listening to reason.[177] Galen seizes on this point, maintaining that the behaviour described (correctly) by Chrysippus is only explicable on the view that the psyche is temporarily taken over by a non-rational part.[178] In fact, we know that Chrysippus did find the phenomenon of grief abating in time a puzzling one, and that he offered a rather complex explanation in belief-based terms, discussed later.[179] But, in general, Chrysippus' theory has rather rich resources for explaining why people in emotional states are not amenable to rational arguments, even though they can at other times recognize their force; indeed, in some sense they do so in the heat of emotion. In the 'therapeutic' book, for instance, Chrysippus may have cited cases of figures such as Medea acknowledging that she is not merely acting unreasonably but, as Chrysippus put it, 'rejects' or 'disobeys' reason. The Stoic analysis of emotion is designed to bring out both the intense, overwhelming affective dimension of these states at the time (even though these states are also grounded on beliefs), and the fact that all human beings have the cognitive basis for reaching a more rational view. Hence, Medea can say that 'I know that what I am doing is bad', at the same time that she recognizes that 'anger (*thumos*) masters (or 'is stronger than') my plans'. These central features of Chrysippus' theory, which underlie the examples of psychological 'weakness' such as Medea in the 'therapeutic' book, explain quite clearly why it is not useful to offer therapeutic arguments to people while they are in passionate states of this type. The same line of thought explains why therapy is usefully offered at other times: even Medea on the point of killing her children shows an awareness of the

[177] Gal. *PHP* V.422–3, 4.7.28–31 De Lacy, Cic. *Tusc.* 4.78. See also Tieleman 2003*a*: 130–1, 168.

[178] Gal. *PHP* V.424, 4.7.32–4 De Lacy.

[179] See text to nn. 194–203 below.

'badness' of her act, an awareness which could form the basis for self-modification and 'cure' under other circumstances.[180]

A related feature of Stoic advice is that of 'dwelling in advance' (*proendemein*) on future disasters, at least, what are conventionally seen as disasters, to prepare oneself to respond to these appropriately. Galen presents this as a distinctive feature of Posidonius' thinking, and one that is coupled with criticism of Chrysippus' psychological theory.[181] But Cicero, in his less polemical treatment, associates this idea with Chrysippus (as well as the Cyrenaics), and gives further detail about Chrysippus' thinking on this subject. According to Galen, Chrysippus, like earlier Stoics, characterized grief or pain (*lupē*) as a 'fresh' belief that something bad is present; Posidonius asked why, on Chrysippus' cognitive view of emotion, the freshness of the belief should make any difference.[182] Cicero records Chrysippus' explanation why fresh (unexpected) disasters have more emotional impact; this is because there is no time to appraise the magnitude of the events properly and because we blame ourselves for not preparing properly for them. Cicero's comments imply that the strategy of preparation for future disaster, attributed to the Cyrenaics, is also adopted by Chrysippus, and that the points noted form part of Chrysippus' explanation why grief fades in time.[183] Hence, Galen's attempt to present this as a point of contrast between Chrysippus' thought and Posidonius' seems to be misleading. The advice to prepare for (what are conventionally seen as) disasters seems to be part of standard Stoic therapeutic advice shared by Chrysippus and Posidonius.[184] The advice fits in with the previous point noted, advice not to attempt therapy on those in the grip of emotion, and reflects a similar concern with the timing and the normal progress of emotion. It also fits in with the general form of Stoic therapeutic advice, namely as a form of 'preventive medicine' directed at long-term states rather than responding immediately to emotional outbursts.[185]

[180] See Gal. *PHP* V.403–13, esp. 408–9, 4.6.1–38, esp. 19–22 De Lacy, also V. 368–72, esp. 372, 4.2.19–27, esp. 27 De Lacy, referring to E. *Med.* 1078–9. On Chrysippus' analysis of emotion, see 4.2 above, esp. text to nn. 134–45. For a reconstruction of the section of the 'therapeutic book' in which the discussion of Medea might have occurred, see Tieleman 2003*a*: 170–8. On the Medea example, see Gill refs. in n. 171 above; also (on Epictetus' treatment of this example), Long 1996: 278–80, 2002: 76–7.

[181] Gal. *PHP* V.416–19, 4.7.2–11 De Lacy.

[182] Gal. *PHP* V.416–17, 4.7.3–5 De Lacy.

[183] Cic. *Tusc.* 3.52 (see also 3.28–31).

[184] See Tieleman 2003*a*: 311–14.

[185] See refs. in n. 163 above.

In another, relatively well-documented feature, we can see a distinct difference of emphasis between Stoic thinkers, though one that falls within a shared theoretical framework. Cicero, reviewing types of Stoic therapy for grief, tells us that Cleanthes saw the only effective treatment as being the extirpation of the belief that death is a bad thing, while Chrysippus saw the first task as being that of removing the belief that it was right to react with grief at someone's death (*Tusc.* 3.76–7). In *Tusc.* 4.59–62, Cicero also maintains, without specific reference to the Stoic thinkers that, although it is best absolutely to convince people that, for instance, poverty or death are bad things, it is more effective in the first instance to persuade them that, even if such things are supposed to be bad, they should be borne with equanimity. One can appeal to conventional ideas such as that grieving is a mark of weakness and enduring grief a mark of strength and dignity to counteract the view that it is right to grieve.[186] This (partial) difference of emphasis between the two Stoic thinkers can be linked with a central aspect of the Stoic definition of emotion. An emotion depends on two kinds of belief, both of which the Stoics see as mistaken: that an 'indifferent' such as death is bad and that it is appropriate or right (*kathēkon*) to react accordingly, for instance, being 'contracted' with pain.[187] Whereas Cleanthes, it would seem, focused on the first type of belief, Chrysippus concentrated, initially at least, on the second.[188] It is plausible to link Chrysippus' focus with his awareness of the importance of timing and the impact of passing time. Although it is misguided to tackle people while they are still in the grip of intense emotion, when the immediate impact weakens, they may be open to considerations about the appropriateness of grief. The question whether death as such, like other 'indifferents', is a bad thing is likely to require at least a further measure of reflective calm and distance from immediate events.[189] A second advantage of

[186] For this summary of Cicero's points, see also Gill 1998: 123.

[187] See e.g. Andronicus, *On Passions* 1 (*SVF* 3.391, LS 65B), Gal. *PHP* V.366–7, 4.2.1–6 De Lacy (LS 65D), Stob. 2.90.7–18 (10b), trans. Inwood and Gerson 1997: 218. See also Ch. 4 above, text to nn. 101–4.

[188] On the linkage between these two points, the two strategies of therapy and the Stoic definitions of emotion, see further Donini 1995: 323–4, Inwood and Donini 1999: 713–14, Sorabji 2000: 175–8.

[189] The effect of the passage of time in calming grief is considered by Chrysippus in terms of his belief-based psychology; see text to nn. 194–203 below.

Chrysippus' deployment of the second type of consideration (about the appropriateness of grieving) is that it widens the circle of those at whom therapy can be applied. Whereas the first type of therapy, directed at the belief that death is bad, will only be effective if directed at those who are already wise, in a Stoic sense, or at least who hold Stoic-style ethical convictions, the second type can be applied to people with a broader range of ethical views. This point is made by Cicero (*Tusc.* 3.77, 4.60) and is also linked with Chrysippus' 'therapeutic' book by the third-century Christian writer Origen. Origen brings out the connection made earlier between the kinds of considerations used and the state of mind of the person approached. Arguments about the nature of the good are inappropriate for someone who is still severely affected by the 'inflammation' (*phlegmonē*) of emotion. Also considerations that do not depend on beliefs about the nature of the good can be usefully offered to people who hold the Aristotelian-type view that there are three kinds of good (not just ethical good) or the Epicurean view that pleasure is the good.[190] This is a further indication of the perceptive and sensitive way in which Chysipppus seems to have approached the application of the Stoic therapeutic approach.[191] However, we should not exaggerate the difference between Cleanthes and Chrysippus on this point, or suppose that Chrysippus gives up the idea that complete therapy depends on accepting the first type of belief (about the nature of good) and making this central to one's character and life. Cicero notes that this type of therapy (Cleanthes') is the only complete type, and Celsus also suggests that this is also Chrysippus' preferred method, though he also sees the value of the other one.[192] Also, as stressed earlier here, Chrysippus' core strategy is that of commending key features of Stoic

[190] Origen, *Against Celsus* (written c. AD 249), 8.51 (*SVF* 3.474, second text); text and trans. given in Tieleman 2003*a*: 166–7. For *phlegmonē*, cf. Gal. *PHP* V.422, 4.7.27 De Lacy (also Tieleman 2003*a*: 130, 168).

[191] This point is stressed by Nussbaum 1994: 318, 378, 391; see also Sorabji 2000: 2, 178–9.

[192] Cic. *Tusc.* 4.60 (end of chapter): this method is *utilior* (more useful), but not widely applicable. Origen says that Chrysippus advocates offering therapy 'preferably by means of arguments which seem sound to him [i.e. those relating to Stoic ethics] but in the second and third instance even by means of doctrines which he does not hold' (Origen ref. in n. 190 above, trans. Tieleman 2003*a*: 166). See further Tieleman 2003*a*: 166–70; also Donini 1995: 307–8.

thinking on ethics and psychology by persuasive use of the medical analogy.[193] The fact that Chrysippus also considers, in a practical and thoughtful way, how best to apply this approach does not carry with it any compromise with the Stoic theoretical framework.

I conclude this discussion of Chrysippus' therapeutic approach by considering a passage cited by Galen in which Chrysippus seeks to explain why grief reduces in time. The passage comes from Book 2 of *On Passions*, and forms part of Chrysippus' treatment of 'puzzles' (*aporiai*) there, and not from the fourth, 'therapeutic' Book.[194] However, it is worth noting here because it bears on the topics just treated (the effects of the two types of belief in shaping emotional responses and the implications for modes of therapy). Also, the passage illustrates the subtlety and explanatory power of Chrysippus' psychological thinking, in a way that sheds light on his therapeutic approach.

On the lessening of distress, the question might be asked how it occurs, whether this is because a particular opinion is altered, or with all of them persisting, and for what reason this will be so . . . I think that this kind of opinion does persist—that what is actually present is something bad—but as it grows older the contraction and, as I take it, the impulse towards the contraction,[195] lessen. It might happen that, even though this [the opinion that the event is bad][196] persists, the consequences will not correspond because a differently qualified disposition (*diathesis*) supervenes, which is not easily reasoned out.[197] So it is that people cease weeping and people weep who do not want to, when different impressions are created by different external objects, and something or nothing stands in the way. For the way grief and weeping stop is probably what happens in those cases as well: at their outset things cause greater movement . . .[198]

[193] See text to nn. 157–61 above.

[194] See Tieleman 2003*a*: 123–30 and 325.

[195] On the interpretation of this phrase, see LS, vol. 2: 413, following Inwood 1985: 149, who sees the impulse as having the content: 'here is something bad, therefore I should contract (i.e. feel distressed)'.

[196] *tautēs*, 'this': my interpretation follows Inwood 1985: 149, with his n. 94. Other possible meanings are 'the belief that one should contract' or 'the impulse' (*hormē*) just cited.

[197] Here, I follow De Lacy's reading (*dussullogiston*), p. 284.11, rather than LS. See further Tieleman 2003*a*: 125–6.

[198] Gal. *PHP* V.419–20, 4.7.13–17, p. 284.5–16 De Lacy; translation based on LS 65 O, but modified as noted in nn. 196–7 above (see also *SVF* 3.466).

Galen presents Chrysippus as quite unable to explain this phenomenon because of his unwillingness to acknowledge the role of non-rational psychic parts;[199] but the passage allows a different interpretation.[200]

What Chrysippus has in mind is not a case where the passage of time alone produces the effect—which, indeed, it could not, in Chrysippus' theory. Nor do we have an instance of what Chrysippus, like Cleanthes, would see as the only complete therapy for grief, the removal of the belief that death and other 'dispreferable indifferents' are bad things. What Chrysippus has in view is an intermediate case in which the belief that someone's death is bad persists, but in which, as I understand the passage, this does not generate the associated impulse and contraction.[201] The explanation how this can occur is given, in very compressed form, in the following lines. What happens is that 'different external objects' activate different 'impressions', which 'stand in the way' of the belief. That is, they prevent the belief from activating an impulse and contraction (and weeping). However, the belief ('that what has happened is bad') persists; and so, when 'nothing stands in the way', it activates tears, despite the fact that the people concerned 'do not want to' weep, because of the different impressions they have now formed. Both of the reactions described (weeping and not weeping) are based on beliefs, either the belief that death is bad, or the different impressions that counteract this belief.

What are the 'different impressions' that counteract the impulse to weep? In pursuing this question, it may be helpful to focus on the second kind of belief involved in an emotion, 'that it is appropriate (*kathēkon*) to react' in a given way because of the (mistaken)

[199] Gal. *PHP* V.420, 4.7.18–19 De Lacy. Galen maintains that Posidonius, by contrast, explains the phenomenon well by referring to non-rational parts (V.424–6, 4.7.36–44 De Lacy); for an alternative interpretation of Posidonius' view, see Gill 2006: 277–9.

[200] The following two paragraphs are based on parts of Gill 1998: 122–3, with modifications.

[201] The person retains the beliefs 'that death is a bad thing' and 'that what is actually present is bad' but these beliefs fail to activate the impulse whose content is 'here is something bad, therefore I should contract (feel depressed)'. For this reading, see Inwood 1985: 149–51. Posidonius (p. 284.10 De Lacy) takes 'this' to mean 'this impulse', which seems to me even more difficult to understand than 'this belief'. However, Posidonius' reading is followed by LS, vol. 2: 413, Price 1995: 164–5 taken with his n. 16, and Tieleman 2003*a*: 123 n. 130.

impression that something is good or bad.[202] This helps to bring out the possible linkage with Chrysippus' distinctive approach to therapy. In the first flush of grief, the person concerned assumes that it is appropriate to respond to death by contracting in pain. However, the passage of time allows scope for him to form different impressions, as he reflects on the situation or responds to the reflections of others. Specifically, he may become more responsive to considerations such as those cited by Cicero, which seem to illustrate Chrysippus' method. He recognizes the force of the ideas that grieving is a mark of weakness or that enduring grief is an expression of strength and dignity; and this counteracts his view that it is appropriate to grieve in this situation.[203] Hence, people in this situation 'cease to weep', as these 'different impressions' work on them. However, the belief that death is bad still remains, and so this can still sometimes produce the thought that grieving is appropriate, and thus activate weeping, even though they now 'do not want to weep' because of the altered views they have formed of what is appropriate. Interpreted in this way, the passage illuminates the nature of Chrysippus' distinctive therapeutic strategy and also brings out the explanatory effectiveness of the psychological framework associated with this strategy.

I close this section by bringing out the importance of Chrysippus' 'therapeutic' book in the context of ancient thought, and by reviewing its influence on later Stoic works, especially Seneca's *On Anger*. The analogy between physical and psychological disease and between medical doctors and philosophers seems to go back to the late fifth century BC; the idea is developed especially by Plato.[204] It is also adopted by Epicurus; as stressed earlier, the theme fits well with Epicurean (like Stoic) views about—most—emotions and ethical development.[205] Zeno, founder of Stoicism, also deploys the theme.[206] But Chrysippus seems to have been

[202] See n. 187 above. For a similar line of thought to that suggested here, see Tieleman 2003*a*: 124–5. For further suggestions, involving competing responses to 'first movements', see Sorabji 2000: 71, Tieleman 2003*a*: 127–9.

[203] See text to n. 186 above.

[204] See e.g. Democritus, DK B 31, Pl. *Chrm.* 155b–157d, *Grg.* 475d, 505c, *R.* 444c–e, *Sph.* 227c–230e, *Ti.* 86b–90d. See further Laín Entralgo 1970: 97–8, Pigeaud 1981: chs. 1, 5, Mackenzie 1981: chs. 10–11.

[205] Usener 221, *Porph. ad Marc.* 31, p. 209, 23 N: cited by Nussbaum 1994: 102. See also Nussbaum 1994: ch. 4 as a whole, and text to nn. 14–16 above.

[206] Gal. *PHP* V.439–40, 5.2.31 De Lacy.

the first to write a 'therapeutic' book, concluding his treatise *On Passions*, and to examine the medical–philosophical analogy in a sustained way, which formed part of his general systematization of Stoic theory. The significance of this work is brought out by the extensive ancient references. Among Stoics, Posidonius responds to it, as part of his full response to Chrysippus' *On Passions*,[207] and Seneca's *On Anger* was, certainly, influenced by it, although he does not cite it explicitly.[208] The Epicurean Philodemus refers to Chrysippus' approach, and Cicero discusses it extensively in his review of therapies of emotion in *Tusc.* 3–4.[209]

More broadly, Chrysippus' book seems to have acted as a major stimulus to the exploration of the medical–philosophical analogy from various philosophical perspectives. In the first century BC, for instance, Philodemus wrote a number of treatises with a therapeutic objective, for instance, *On Anger* and *On Death*.[210] About the same time, Lucretius also makes prominent use of the motif.[211] For instance, book 3 of his poem *On the Nature of the Universe* is structured as an extended work of therapy along lines similar to Chrysippus' book, integrating theoretical ideas (about the psyche–body relationship) with more practical ethical reflections about the implications of these ideas.[212] As noted earlier, the idea of philosophy as therapy is taken up in the post-Hellenistic period by other philosophical theories and reconceived, in some cases, in line with their approaches. Hence, by the first and second centuries AD, the idea of philosophy as therapy, along with the genre of the therapeutic essay, was a highly prevalent one, adopted by thinkers from different traditions including Seneca, Plutarch, and Galen, in the essays (*Aff. Dig.*, *Indol.*) discussed in the preceding section.[213] In the light of—what seems to be—the very important and influential role of Chrysippus'

[207] See e.g. Gal. *PHP* V.432–4, 5.2.2–7 De Lacy; see further Gill 2006: 278–9, n. 334. [208] See discussion below.

[209] See text to nn. 153–4, 186 above.

[210] See further Annas 1992: ch. 9, 1993: 194–5, Warren 2004: 143–53, Tsouna 2007: chs. 4, 9–10. [211] See e.g. 1. 936–50.

[212] The two sections are 3.94–829, 830–1094. Recent discussions of Lucretius' therapy for fear of death have focused on the second part; see e.g. Nussbaum 1994: ch. 6, Warren 2004: chs. 2–4. There is scope for exploring the possible influence of Chrysippus' two-part approach on Lucretius' book 3 (or on his poem more generally).

[213] See text to nn. 17–21 above. See further, on Stoic or Epicurean therapy in Hellenistic and Roman thought, Nussbaum 1994, Sorabji 2000: parts 1–2, Gill 2008*d*, and, as part of Hellenistic–Roman thought on the 'care of the self', Foucault 1990.

'therapeutic' book in the history of ancient practical ethics, Galen's extensive response to this work in *PHP* 4–5 is unsurprising. Of course, Galen's critique there forms part of his broader attack on Stoic psychology generally (as expressed in Chrysippus' *On Passions*). But Galen seems to have a particular interest in Chrysippus' use of the medical–philosophical analogy and his therapeutic approach. This interest expresses in part Galen's own concern with the relationship between medicine and philosophy, considered shortly (5.4 below). But it seems also to reflect the exceptional significance of Chrysippus' book as a powerful and influential expression of the idea of philosophy as therapy.

Charting in detail the influence of Chrysippus' book on subsequent Stoic thinking as a whole, including that in the first and second centuries AD, would be a rather large undertaking.[214] But some points can be made here, especially on Seneca's *On Anger*, which can help us to define the Stoic approach to the therapy of emotions, by contrast with the Platonic–Aristotelian approach which is (mostly) adopted by Galen. How, exactly, does Seneca's *On Anger* (*Ira*) relate to Chrysippus' book? As noted earlier, this is our only complete surviving essay on the therapy of emotions, although Seneca also wrote essays on closely related themes, and his letters, like the works of Epictetus and Marcus, draw on various genres of practical ethics.[215] In earlier scholarship, it was common to analyse works of post-Hellenistic philosophy as composites of materials drawn from earlier (lost) Hellenistic treatises; and this approach is applied to Seneca's essay by Janine Fillion-Lahille.[216] However, it is now more normal to treat works by thinkers such as Cicero, Seneca,

[214] There has been a good deal of work on Stoic therapy (see preceding note) and on Stoic practical ethics in general (see Gill 2003: 40–4, Sellars 2007). But a separate examination of this material would now be needed, in the light of Tieleman 2003*a*: chs. 4 and 6, to establish precisely the relationship of later Stoic writings to Chrysippus' 'therapeutic' book.

[215] Related works include Sen. *On Peace of Mind* (*De Tranquillitate Animi*) and *On Consistency* (*De Constantia*); on Seneca as a philosopher, see Inwood 2005; on Epictetus and Marcus and genres of practical ethics, see Sellars 2003, 2007.

[216] Fillion-Lahille 1984; her approach reflects the so-called *Quellenforschung* ('research into sources') method. However, her work was pioneering in her critique of Galen's presentation of Posidonius as an unorthodox Stoic as regards psychology; see her 153–62; also Cooper 1998, Tieleman 2003*a*: ch. 5, Gill 2006: 266–90.

and Plutarch, as independent essays, drawing autonomously on a wide range of works, many of them unknown to us, even when they are responding to earlier works of which we have some knowledge.[217] In line with this style of reading, I take Seneca's essay as responding to the main features of Chrysippus' 'therapeutic' work, but in an independent way that does not necessarily correspond to Chrysippus' work in its overall structure or specific claims. The aspects of Seneca's work that reflect the more theoretical side of Chrysippus' approach include his discussion of the nature of anger in book 2,[218] and the recurrent critique of the, relatively positive, 'Aristotelian' view of anger.[219] They also include the striking analysis of the onset of emotion in book 2 and the related discussion of 'pre-emotions'. This material has been interpreted in very different ways; but I find most plausible the view that both aspects of this discussion represent Seneca's own way of formulating orthodox Stoic ideas, which go back to Chrysippus at least.[220] Another notable feature, though one much less discussed, is Seneca's analysis of the physical basis of character, especially in terms of the four elements, which forms part of his advice about the education of children.[221] Fillion-Lahille links this material with Posidonius; but in fact, as Tieleman has stressed, such ideas form part of standard Stoic thinking. Indeed, they can probably be linked with Chrysippus' thinking, though there is no reason, I think, to connect them specifically with Chrysippus' 'therapeutic' book.[222]

[217] For this approach to Sen. *Ira*, including criticism of Fillion-Lahille, see Inwood 1993: 150–6.

[218] Sen. *Ira* 2.26–34, also 1.2.3, supplied from Lactantius, *De Ira Dei* 17.13, and reflecting a longer discussion of definitions of anger now lost. See further Cooper and Procopé 1995: 11, 19–20, Fillion-Lahille 1984: 94–7, 170–9. Chrysippus' main discussion of definitions of emotion falls in *On Passions* 1, not the 'therapeutic' book, but the latter builds on the implications of those definitions (see the summary of Chrysippus' *On Passions* in Tieleman 2003*a*: 325–6).

[219] On this view, see text to n. 10 above; also Fillion-Lahille 1984: 211–21.

[220] Sen. *Ira* 2.1–4, esp. 2.4.1. For this view, see Gill 2006: 279–81; also Inwood 1993: 164–83, Tieleman 2003*a*: 127–8, Graver 1999, 2007: 125–32; for a contrasting view, attributing more philosophical innovation to Seneca (though seeing the theory as still basically Chrysippean), Sorabji 2000: 61–3, 66–75, esp. 72–3.

[221] Sen. *Ira* 2.19.

[222] Fillion-Lahille 1984: 183–5, Tieleman 2003*a*: 148–66; see further on this point, text to nn. 245–55 below.

Other aspects of Seneca's work reflect the side of Chrysippus' theory that is concerned with the practical application of therapy. This forms an extensive part of Seneca's essay—more so than seems likely for Chrysippus' book.[223]Although there is much that we have no reason to connect with Chrysippus, some of the themes express analogous concerns. For instance, we find a comparable concern with the need for therapy to take account of the stages and normal progress of emotions such as anger.[224] Some advice is directed at avoiding the onset of anger, while other advice aims to restrain it when it has arisen.[225] Seneca also, like Chrysippus, marks the difference between long-term tendencies to anger and occurrent outbursts; and different parts of his advice are tailored to one or other aspect of our psychic life.[226] Also, the combination in Seneca's essay of strong condemnation of anger[227] and advice about how to control it may represent a reworking of Chrysippus' distinctive method of practical therapy (Cic. *Tusc.* 3.76). This method centres on deterring people from thinking that it is 'appropriate' or 'right' to feel the emotion involved—here, anger—rather than tackling the question of what should be considered good or bad as such.[228] Also, despite the explicit polemic against the 'Aristotelian' view of anger, and the allusions to Stoic ethical psychology, much of the work, especially its practical advice, seems to be directed at a wider audience and does not depend on accepting Stoic principles. Indeed, it has sometimes been suggested that some of Seneca's practical advice, and his use of striking examples of anger or its control, is not, strictly speaking, in line with Stoic thinking about ethics at all. In some cases, though not

[223] Sen. *Ira* 2.22–36, 3.5–40. On the distinctive features of Chrysippus' approach, see text to nn. 146–52 above.

[224] On this theme in Chrysippus' book, see text to nn. 177–85 above.

[225] See, respectively, Sen. *Ira* 3.5–9, 3.10.38. An interest in the stages of the onset of anger underlies the analysis of pre-emotion and the stages of the full emotion in 2.1–4.

[226] The distinction is drawn in Sen. *Ira* 1.4.1; for longer-term or preventive advice, see 2.19–24, for advice on countering the onset of anger on specific occasions, see 2.26–34. See also Cooper and Procopé 1995: 12 and 57 n. 28.

[227] e.g. by presenting the distorted physical appearance of anger (Sen. *Ira* 1.1, 2.35–6), see also 1.2, 3.1–5, and the repellent examples of 3.16–21. The polemic against the 'Aristotelian' view is also relevant (text to n. 219 above, taken with text to n. 10 above).

[228] For this suggestion, see Cooper and Procopé 1995: 10–11, referring esp. to 2.26–34.

in all, the rhetoric of Seneca's presentation of his theme runs counter to the main objective of 'extirpating' emotions such as anger.[229] If this suggestion is right, this is a feature that certainly cannot be connected with Chrysippus' book, in which the illustrative examples, such as Medea, are closely integrated with the ethical and psychological theory.[230] However, in the other respects mentioned, Seneca's approach does seem to reflect the main emphases in Chrysippus' book, though the material is handled in a quite autonomous way.

5.4 STOICS AND GALEN ON PSYCHOLOGICAL AND MEDICAL THERAPY

In this final section of this chapter, I take up broader issues raised by Galenic and Stoic approaches to therapy. This brings out lines of connection between this topic and other aspects of Galenic and Stoic thinking already explored in this study. One question is that of the relationship envisaged, in both theories, between philosophical therapy, directed at the psyche, and medical therapy, aimed at the body. Another is whether it would have been conceptually possible to combine Galen's approach to medical therapy and the Stoic approach to the therapy of emotions. The second question has a special interest because these two approaches constituted, arguably, the most powerful ancient examples of their respective types of therapy, and the combination of them—if conceptually possible—might have been, therefore, especially potent. These two questions, taken together, enable re-examination from a new standpoint of the relationship between Galenic and Stoic thinking about psychology and the body, and about reason and emotions (the topics of Chs. 3–4 above). They also allow us to ask how far Galenic and Stoic thinking about

[229] For this suggestion, see Nussbaum 1994: 431–5, in connection with 3.14–15; she questions whether the positive presentation of suppressed anger at harm to one's relatives is compatible with the Stoic view that *all* anger is defective and shows a wrong sense of value. For related concerns, see her 414–19, 435–8. See also Wilson 1997, questioning whether Seneca's intensely emotional approach to consolation in his letters is in line with Stoic principles.

[230] See text to nn. 177–80 above.

the therapy of the emotions, taken separately or in combination, reflect the kinds of shared naturalism found in other aspects of their thinking (Ch. 2). A related question is whether Stoic or Galenic thinking about therapy, or a possible combination of the two types of thinking, constitutes—or could constitute—what we might call a 'holistic' or 'whole-person' approach to therapy. This topic is pursued in 6.3 in connection with the question how this kind of ancient thinking about medical and psychological therapy relates to modern ideas and practice in this area. In particular, I ask how far the approach of either theory represents what we, from a modern standpoint, might see as 'psychiatry' or 'psychotherapy'.

I begin with the question how we should relate Stoic and Galenic thinking on the therapy of emotion to their ideas about therapy more generally. How far in either theory is there an attempt to combine or integrate the philosophical therapy of the emotions, of the type already discussed in this chapter (in 5.2–3 above), with the therapy of the body? On the face of it, both Galenic and Stoic approaches reflect a rather familiar ancient division of labour, in which medical therapy is directed at the body and philosophical therapy is intended for the psyche. But, on closer inspection, does either theory seek to bridge this dichotomy, and, if so, how effectively?

The contrast between medical therapy for the body and philosophical therapy for the mind is drawn in what seems to be a programmatic statement early in Chrysippus' 'therapeutic' book.[231] This contrast reflects earlier statements of the analogy between medicine and philosophy by thinkers such as Antiphon, Democritus, Epicurus, and, though in a rather complex form, Plato.[232] How far, in broad terms, did this contrast match the main lines of ancient thinking and practice, beginning with the medical side of the comparison? In some respects, the contrast understates the resources of medical thinking. From Hippocrates onwards, we find in medical writings recognition of the psychological dimension of human experience, though this is, typically, seen from a body-based standpoint. For instance, we find considerable interest in the idea that climate and the physical environment affect the psychological as well

[231] Gal. *PHP* V.437, 5.2.22–4 De Lacy; see further below on this passage.

[232] See refs. in n. 204 above.

as physical character of the inhabitants of a given region. There is also a well-developed tradition of explaining psychological, as well as physical, features of specific human beings in terms of their humoral constitution.[233] There was some recognition by medical authors, beginning with the Hippocratic writings, of what might be described as psychological or mental illness. We find the emergence of a typology for these types of illness and for mental states in general, both normal and defective.[234] We also find discussion of appropriate methods of treatment for the mentally disturbed.

However, there is some basis for the standard ancient contrast between medical (physical) and philosophical (psychological) therapy. For one thing, the methods of treatment falling within the competence of ancient medicine were directed primarily at the person as a body. Typically, drugs were prescribed, often with purgative functions, for acute conditions, and long-term changes in diet and regime were recommended for chronic conditions.[235] There is also evidence of the use of physical methods, including violent ones, to restrain people in states of madness or to bring them to their senses. Some doctors also used music therapy, which can be seen as a version of the Corybantic cure offered by some ancient religions. It is also clear that doctors, from an early period, also supplemented physical methods by use of dialogue. In fact, we have some quite interesting discussions on this topic, especially from a late ancient source,

[233] For reviews of these lines of thought, see Gundert 2000 and Gill 2008*a*. On Hippocratic thought on environmental influence, see Jouanna 1999: 147–8, 218–19, 226–31, and, on the humoral basis of character, see Klibansky, Panofsky and Saxl 1964 and Flashar 1966. These ideas span (what we describe as) 'medical' and 'philosophical' writings, and in any case the boundary between medicine and philosophy is a fluid one in ancient culture, as underlined in text to n. 238 below.

[234] A distinction emerges between phrenitis (an acute, delirious condition, marked by feverish hand movements and hallucination) and melancholy (a chronic condition, affecting digestion and emotions, defined by its diagnosis, an excess of black bile). See further Pigeaud 1981: 71–99, 122–33, and, on phrenitis, McDonald 2009. On mental disorder in the Hippocratic writings, explained in physical terms, see Gundert 2000: 26–31.

[235] See e.g. the treatment for *phrontis* in Hipp. *De Morbis* II, VII.108–10 Littré: 'hellebore to purge the head, then a laxative to purge the bottom. Then asses' milk, no wine, no sport or walks. Under this treatment, the illness will go away in time...' See also Pigeaud 1981: 126.

Caelius Aurelianus.[236] But the use of dialogue and other practices directed at the person as psyche seem to be external additions to the core methods of ancient medicine. The debates and controversies between the different medical schools, for which Galen is such a crucial source, centre on the most effective method of treating the body or at least the person as body.[237] We do not find a comparable set of debates about Empiricist or Methodist or Rationalist ways of treating the mind or psyche. To this extent, at least, the association of medicine with the body, rather than the psyche, is justified.

What about the other side of the contrast, the idea that ancient philosophical therapy was directed at the psyche, rather than the body? Here too, although the generalization glosses over a complex and ambiguous terrain, it has a good deal of validity. The borderline between philosophy and medicine is, in fact, extremely fluid throughout antiquity. As is clear from the ideas referred to in Galen's *QAM*, for instance, philosophers such as Plato and Aristotle are major contributors to ancient study of the human body, and Plato, in particular, offers a strikingly physicalist account of psychic illness in the *Timaeus*.[238] However, it is still generally true that the kind of method associated by Greek thinkers with the therapy of the emotions is directed at people as psychological agents, rather than as bodies. What is involved is, normally, rational or cognitive dialogue, designed to enable people to understand and modify their psychological state. This point applies to therapeutic dialogue written from various theoretical standpoints, including Epicurean, Stoic, and Platonic approaches.[239] A further feature bearing on the comparison with medical practice is that the kinds of 'illnesses' targeted in philosophical therapy were not, usually, similar in type to the psychological illnesses addressed by doctors. Philosophical therapists were not, like medical doctors, trying to treat phrenitis or melancholy; often they were not trying to cure psychological states recognized by the person concerned or by society in general as illnesses

[236] See further Pigeaud 1981: 107–12, discussing Caelius Aurelianus (5th cent. AD, though partly based on Soranus, early 2nd cent. AD) and Celsus (1st cent. AD). On Corybantic rituals, see Dodds 1951: 79–80. See also Gill 1985*a*: 309–11, 316–20.

[237] On these debates and Galen's specification of his medical approach, see Ch. 2 above, text to nn. 90–3.

[238] Pl. *Ti.* 86b–89d; see further text to n. 251 below.

[239] See 5.2–3 above.

at all. From Plato onwards, philosophical ideas about psychological illness and cure were highly revisionist, and only partly overlapped with more conventional ideas about madness, mental disorder, or even psychological distress or unease.[240] As highlighted earlier, the Stoic–Epicurean view that emotions (as normally understood) are defective or 'diseased' states was more remote from conventional thought than the Aristotelian view that only extreme emotions were to be avoided.[241] This is a further point that distinguishes the typical philosophical conception of the therapy of the emotions from normal ancient medical practice.

How far does Stoic and Galenic thinking on therapy match this broad division of labour in ancient thought, in which philosophical therapy was directed at the person as psyche and medical therapy at the person as body? Stoic therapy, to take this first, as represented in Chrysippus' 'therapeutic' book, seems, on the face of it, to fit well with this general contrast—as well as offering a clear statement of the distinction. Chrysippus' therapeutic method consists in providing an analytic framework to enable people to understand the nature and basis of their emotional state, and thus to work towards modifying this state. The person concerned is addressed as a psychological, indeed, rational agent, in principle capable of reshaping her belief-structure and the emotional responses that reflect these beliefs. The method is holistic in the sense that the person is treated as a psychological whole, in whom changes in belief and reasoning (at least about key ethical ideas) necessarily carry with them changes in motivation, desire, and emotion.[242] For similar reasons, one can see the Stoic framework as implying a 'structure', rather than 'composition', approach to psychological processes and states.[243] But the method is not—again, on the face of it—holistic in addressing the person concerned as a psychophysical whole, although, as explained earlier, Stoic theory does in general regard people as psychophysical wholes, and sees psychological states as being also physical ones.[244]

[240] For some areas of possible overlap between the two approaches, directed at what we might call 'neurosis', see Pigeaud 1981: 204–8, 506, 516–18.

[241] See n. 164 above.

[242] On the assumptions about psychology and development underlying their therapeutic method, see text to nn. 14–16 above.

[243] For this contrast, as applied to psychology, see Ch. 4 above, text to nn. 37–45.

[244] See Ch. 3 above, text to nn. 38–44, 258–77.

But is this impression correct? Tieleman, in his reconstruction of Chrysippus' 'therapeutic' book, seeks to modify the idea that Chrysippus' focus was purely psychological. He highlights a whole series of features in Stoic theory, bearing on their view of emotions or therapy, which he takes as referring to bodily states or as evoking ancient medical approaches. These features include the point just noted that the Stoics hold an explicitly physicalist position as regards psychology.[245] More specifically, he cites a passage in Galen's *QAM* which both brings out Stoic physicalism about psychology and shows that the Stoics see the mixture of elements in the body (heat and cold, dry and wet) as the basis for differences between individuals as regards intellectual ability and emotional character.[246] Tieleman suggests that this line of thought about the physical basis of psychological states is implied in Chrysippus' ideas about psychological health, beauty, and proportion, and that it helps to make sense of Stoic ideas which Galen presents as incomprehensible or inconsistent.[247] Tieleman also thinks that this line of thought may be implied in the Stoic theme that psychological illnesses (emotions) are feverish or 'fluttering', in so far as they are an unstable mixture of heat and cold.[248] Other points cited in this connection include the presentation of anger in Chrysippus' *On the Psyche* as a physical experience, that of being heated or 'inflamed' in the region of the heart.[249]

Tieleman also notes the report in Calcidius of the Stoic idea that the corruption of people's attitudes to pleasure and the good begins immediately after birth, in the midwife's bath that creates a pleasurable antidote to the sudden pain of exposure to cold air.[250] He also suggests that Chrysippus' view of emotions (psychic illnesses) as

[245] Tieleman 2003*a*: 146–8, referring to, e.g., *PHP* V.287, 3.1.10 De Lacy (*SVF* 2.885).

[246] Gal. *QAM* ch. 4, IV.783–4, *SM* 2.45.5–46.1 (*SVF* 2.787); Tieleman 2003*a*: 149–50. On this passage, see Ch. 2 above, text to nn. 218–25, Ch. 3 above, text to nn. 271–7.

[247] Tieleman 2003*a*: 147–57, referring to Gal. *PHP* V.443–4, 446–7, 5.2.47, 49, 5.3.7–10 De Lacy. On these passages, see also 4.4 above.

[248] Tieleman 2003*a*: 155–6, referring to Gal. *PHP* V.392, 435, 4.5.6 and 5.2.14 De Lacy (*SVF* 3.465, 476).

[249] Gal. *PHP* V.291, 3.1.25 De Lacy (*SVF* 2.886), also *SVF* 3.416; see Tieleman 2003*a*: 157–9.

[250] Tieleman 2003*a*: 161–2, referring to Calcid. commentary on Pl. *Ti.*, chs. 165–8 (chs. 165–7 printed as *SVF* 3.229), esp. ch. 165.

physically based is influenced by Plato's striking presentation in the *Timaeus* of psychic illnesses as products of innate bodily states.[251] The physicalist approach indicated in these features of Chrysippean thought is seen as underlying ideas that are not explicitly presented in physical terms, such as the account of the quasi-dispositional states of being inclined to one or other type of emotion (*arrōstēmata*) or the presentation of emotion as madness.[252] Tieleman also maintains that we should take more seriously than we normally do evidence relating to Stoic thought on what is regarded in ancient medical practice as regimen (*diaita*) including diet and wine-drinking.[253] He also argues that we should see Stoic thought on psychological illnesses as similar in general type to medical thought on this topic, which also presupposes a physical basis for these illnesses.[254] Similar linkages include Stoic and medical thinking on the role of environmental factors in shaping character.[255]

In general, I think Tieleman's reconstruction of Chrysippus' 'therapeutic' book, and *On Passions* in general, is highly convincing, and I have used it as the basis of my discussion. I also accept fully that the features Tieleman describes, broadly speaking, form part of Stoic thinking; and I have referred to a number of them earlier, especially in underlining the kinds of naturalism or physicalism shared by Stoicism with Galen.[256] However, I am cautious about the suggestion that they formed an integral part of Chrysippus' 'therapeutic' book in the way Tieleman proposes. I also think we need to distinguish more sharply, or at least more precisely, between the type of analysis of the physical nature and basis of psychological states, including illness, in medical writing, including Galen's, and in Stoicism.

[251] Tieleman 2003*a*: 161–2, 187–90, referring to Pl. *Ti.*, 86b1–2, b7–c3. On Pl. *Ti.* 86b–90d, and its possible influence on Stoic, as well as Galenic, thought, see Gill 2000, also 2006: 200–3.

[252] Tieleman 2003*a*: 183–7, referring to Gal. *PHP* V.396, 4.5.21–2 De Lacy (*SVF* 3.480), and Stob. 2.68.18–23 (*SVF* 3.663).

[253] Tieleman 2003*a*: 162–6, referring to passages including D.L. 7.111 (*SVF* 3.456).

[254] Tieleman 2003*a*: 191–6, referring e.g. to Hippocrates, *Morb. Sacr.*, chs. 13, 17, and *Aff.* ch. 1, which link psychological and physical phenomena.

[255] Tieleman 2003*a*: 194, linking Cic. *Fat.* chs. 7–9 (*SVF* 2.950–1) with Hippocrates, *Airs, Waters, Places* 16.1, 24.3, pp. 62.1–5, 78.17–23 Diller.

[256] See e.g. Ch. 2 above, text to nn. 197–225 and Ch. 3 above, text to nn. 258–77.

My reasons for caution centre partly on the nature of our evidence for Chrysippus' book and partly on my understanding of the kind of philosophical claims about the physical basis of psychology made in Stoicism.

As regards the reconstruction of Chrysippus' 'therapeutic' book, Tieleman acknowledges that the physicalist approach he ascribes to the Stoic account is not fully reflected in our main sources, that is, Galen *PHP* 4–5 and Cicero, *Tusc.* 3–4. However, he argues that both writers deliberately de-emphasize the physical and medical connotations of the Stoic ideas. Cicero does so because, as someone writing from a literary-philosophical standpoint, he is rather dismissive of the medical approach to psychological illness and of what he sees as unnecessary technicalities.[257] Galen also does so, though for more polemical reasons. Because he wants to present Chrysippus as failing to give real content to the medical–philosophical analogy, and to the idea of psychic health, Galen omits the physical basis for Chrysippus' thinking, and thus obscures much of the rationale of Stoic thinking on this topic.[258] In general terms, the attitudes Tieleman ascribes to these thinkers are plausible ones. Tieleman might also find some support for his view in the fact that, as noted earlier, Seneca refers to the physical basis for character in *On Anger* 2.19, in connection with the education of children in a work that seems to be at least broadly based on Chrysippus' 'therapeutic' book.[259] Features that especially recall the Stoic themes discussed by Tieleman include the ideas that mixtures of the elements (hot, cold, dry, wet) form the basis of character in animals and humans and that anger consists in the boiling of the blood around the heart.[260] Fillion-Lahille also sees these features as genuinely Stoic but ascribes them to the influence of Posidonius, rather than Chrysippus, whose ideas about childhood development are referred to by Galen.[261] In fact, however, the points

[257] Tieleman 2003*a*: 143–4, referring to Cic. *Tusc.* 4.23; also Tieleman, 304 (also 298–9) on Cicero's tendency to understate the physical aspects in his report of Stoic thinking on the emotions and their manifestations (e.g. in *Tusc.* 3.61).

[258] Tieleman 2003*a*: 147–57.

[259] On Seneca's work, see text to nn. 221–2 above.

[260] Sen. *Ira* 2.19, 1–3; cf. refs. in nn. 246 and 249 above.

[261] Fillion-Lahille 1984: 183–4, also 132–4, citing Gal. *PHP* V.464, 466–7, 5.5.22–4, 32–5 De Lacy.

cited are closer to the Chrysippean ideas to which Tieleman refers than to Posidonius' ideas, as summarized by Galen.[262] In any case, if, as Tieleman argues, there is little or no reason to see significant doctrinal difference between the two thinkers in this area, there is no special point in pinpointing the influence of Posidonius, as distinct from Chrysippus, in this respect.[263]

However, I am more inclined than Tieleman to think that Galen and Cicero *do* convey with some accuracy the main lines of Chrysippus' thinking about the nature and therapy of psychological illness.[264] My supposition is based partly on the fact that the strategy that emerges from the combination of their evidence is an inherently credible one. My view is also based on assumptions about the nature of Stoic thinking on the relationship between the psychological and physical spheres. The core idea of Chrysippus' book is, I take it, that there is an *analogy* between philosophical therapy, directed at the psyche, and medical therapy, directed at the body, and not that these types of therapy are identical or overlapping. This idea is then developed by highlighting various types of parallel between the characteristics of physical and psychological illness and also of therapy—though we are less well informed about the 'therapy' strand of the analogy.[265] One important sub-theme in the 'sickness' strand is the idea of proneness to disease (or to disease of a certain type). Although this fits in, broadly, with the medical analogy, it is also in tension with it, since these long-term states, at the psychological level, are presented as 'feverish' ones, in a way that does not

[262] Of the two passages cited earlier (text to nn. 246, 249 above) one (Gal. *PHP* V.291, 3.1.25 De Lacy) is explicitly ascribed by Galen to Chrysippus' *On the Psyche*, the other (Gal. *QAM* ch. 4, IV.783–4, *SM* 2.45.5–46.1) is presented as a summary of Stoic (not specifically Chrysippean) teaching, but is plausibly linked with Chrysippean thinking, e.g. in *On the Psyche*. (On this passage, see Tieleman 2003*a*: 149–50.)

[263] For this view, see Tieleman 2003*a*: ch. 5, and Ch. 4 above, text to nn. 82–9. Fillion-Lahille 1984: 153–63, as noted earlier, rejects Galen's presentation of Posidonius as unorthodox among Stoics in his account of emotions, but still assumes that there were some substantive differences between the theories of the two thinkers, e.g. on the physical basis of psychological development (183–4).

[264] For the main themes, see text to nn. 146–52 above, based on Tieleman's reconstruction of Chrysippus' book from the evidence of Galen and Cicero.

[265] It is not clear from our evidence how far Chrysippus or other Stoics compared in any detail the main features of their therapeutic method (both theoretical and practical) with medical practice. On the method itself, see 5.3 above.

correspond directly to medical thinking about health and sickness. Galen, reviewing this idea from a conventional medical standpoint, finds this characterization problematic and out of line with what makes sense either at the psychological or medical level. This reaction is unsurprising because, I think, the idea of feverishness stems from specific features of Stoic thinking about the nature and basis of psychological dispositions, and relies on assumptions that Galen does not share.[266] However, in this respect as well as others, we can see a plausible overall rationale in the Stoic deployment of the medical–philosophical analogy, and one that matches their theoretical understanding of the relationship between psychology and the body, as I suggest later.

I now develop some of these points in more detail, beginning with the medical–philosophy analogy. Here is Chrysippus' programmatic statement of this, as cited by Galen:

> It is not true that, whereas there is an art called medicine concerned with the diseased body, there is no art concerned with the diseased psyche, or that the latter [art] is necessarily inferior to the former in the theory and therapeutic treatment of particular cases. Therefore, just as the doctor of the body must be 'inside', as people say, the events (*pathē*) that happen to the body and the proper cure of each of these, so it belongs to the doctor of the psyche to be 'inside' both of these things in the best possible way. One might understand that this is the situation because the analogy between these things was drawn from the beginning. The parallel appropriateness with respect to these terms will also make clear to us, I believe, the similarity between the types of therapy and the analogy that both kinds of medicine have with each other.[267]

Tieleman argues that the analogy offered here implies likeness between both sides of the analogy, which depends in part on the Stoic physicalist account of psychology. In support of this view, he notes, in connection with the passage just cited that, 'whereas medicine in its ordinary sense obviously presupposes expert knowledge of the body, medicine of the soul requires knowledge of *both* body and

[266] See text to nn. 277–81 below.

[267] Gal. *PHP* V.437, 5.2.22–4, p. 298.28–38 De Lacy, trans. De Lacy, modified, partly following Tieleman 2003*a*: 144. The repeated phrase, being 'inside' implies expertise in the relevant area. The idea that the analogy was drawn 'from the beginning' implies that 'it arises *naturally* in human thought and language' (Tieleman 2003*a*: 145).

soul'.[268] He is referring especially, I think, to the second sentence cited and is interpreting 'both of these things' (*amphoterōn toutōn*) to mean 'both body and psyche'.[269] Although this is a possible reading of the phrase—and an intriguing one—I think it is more likely to mean 'both the events and the cure' as regards the psyche. In other words, here as in the other sentences cited, the focus is on the idea of *analogy* or parallelism rather than *similarity*, if this implies that there is identity between the two sides of the comparison. What Chrysippus is stressing is that, like the medical doctor, the philosopher (or a certain kind of philosopher)[270] has expertise in the pathology and treatment ('both of these things') *of the psyche* rather than that there is an expert who has mastered both of these areas (psyche and body). The fact that the remaining passages cited by Galen and outlined in more general terms by Cicero consistently explore the idea of analogy between the areas, rather than offering a unified or synthesizing treatment of both spheres, bears out this interpretation.[271]

One passage in Galen's discussion brings out clearly the point that what is at issue is analogy between two different spheres. This passage also highlights the fact that Stoic thinking about psychic illness and therapy is informed by considerations of ethical psychology rather than by medical ideas. In this passage, Galen reacts critically to comments made by Chrysippus and Posidonius about the physical analogue of psychic illness. Chrysippus' comment is this: 'We must suppose that psychic disease is most similar to a feverish physical state in which fevers and chills do not occur at regular intervals but irregularly and at random from the condition (*diathesis*) (of the person) concerned and at the occurrence of small causes.'[272] Chrysippus' description is meant to apply to the state of inferior (non-wise) people in general, that is, virtually all of us.[273] Galen objects

[268] Tieleman 2003*a*: 147, see also 146–7.

[269] Gal. *PHP* V.437, 5.2.24, p. 298.34 De Lacy.

[270] That Chrysippus' 'doctor of the psyche' is a (Stoic) philosopher is clear from the parallel passage in Cic. *Tusc.* 3.6; see also text to nn. 204–6 above on the idea of philosophy as therapy for the psyche.

[271] See e.g. Gal. *PHP* V.438–9, 443–4, 5.2.26–9, 5.2.47, 49 De Lacy; Cic. *Tusc.* 3.6, 4.23, 30–1. For this way of reading these passages, see also Engberg-Pedersen 1990: 187–91.

[272] Gal. *PHP* V.435, 5.2.14, p. 298.3–8 De Lacy, trans. De Lacy, modified.

[273] This is clear from Gal. *PHP* V.432, 5.2.3–4 De Lacy.

that Chrysippus' analogy is inappropriate because it fails to find the proper equivalents for physical health and sickness. A better analogue, he argues, would be people suffering from recurrent, but periodic, fevers. Such people are healthy between fevers but intermittently affected by disease.[274] Galen is also—unusually—critical of Posidonius on this subject, even though Posidonius is explicitly modifying Chrysippus' view. Posidonius' comment is this:

> Therefore psychic disease does not resemble, as Chrysippus had supposed, the diseased condition of the body, which makes it liable to fall into irregular, non-periodic fevers. Rather, psychic disease resembles either physical health with a proneness to disease or [physical] disease itself. Physical disease is a state that is already diseased, but what Chrysippus calls disease resembles rather a proneness to fever.[275]

Galen welcomes Posidonius' criticism of Chrysippus, which, at first sight, prefigures Galen's own critique. But he objects to Posidonius' alternative view, which compares psychic disease to physical health, though combined with a proneness to disease, *or* to physical disease. Posidonius' comment is presented as failing to mark the proper boundaries between (physical) health and disease. Galen himself proposes as an alternative to both the Stoic formulations a fivefold analogy between psychic and physical states. On the psycho-ethical side, the schema runs from the fully virtuous to those in an intense emotional state, and on the physical side from those who are immune to disease to those who are actually diseased. Chrysippus' category of those who are liable to disease from small causes is allocated to Galen's level three (ethically middle-level people, *metrioi*).[276]

Several relevant points emerge from this discussion. It is clear that, both for Galen and the Stoic thinkers, what is at issue is how to understand the analogy between psychological health and illness and physical states, rather than how to achieve a combination or synthesis of the two areas. Also noteworthy is the fact that both Chrysippus and Posidonius use the categories of physical health and sickness in a way that is, as Galen maintains, strained or unusual. This reflects the

[274] Gal. *PHP* V.435–6, 5.2.13–19 De Lacy.
[275] Gal. *PHP* V.433–4, 5.2.7, p. 296.11–17 De Lacy, trans. De Lacy, modified.
[276] Gal. *PHP* V.434–5, 5.2.8–12 De Lacy.

fact that their attention is focused on a psychological or ethical idea, and that the medical analogy is essentially a way of conveying this idea. The idea, one of the central paradoxes of Stoic thought, is that anyone falling below the level of perfect wisdom—that is, virtually all of us—lacks complete stability or coherence. The crucial contrast, then, for Stoic ethics, is between the ideal wise person and the non-wise, rather than a more fine-grained set of distinctions.[277] Hence, Chrysippus stresses the randomness and irregularity of our (non-wise) 'feverish' state. Galen, using the concept of 'fever' in a more conventional medical way, points out that fevers are punctuated by periods of health; but this idea does not match the Stoic view that only the wise person has psychic health and is not subject to 'fevers'. Posidonius nuances this account, preferring the analogue of physical health with a proneness to disease, rather than Chrysippus' proneness to fever, or of physical disease. The basis for Posidonius' revision of Chrysippus' idea is not self-evident; but what is clear—as Galen points out—is that Posidonius' readiness to equate physical health (with a proneness to disease) with illness is out of line with normal medical thinking. Posidonius' use of the analogy, like Chrysippus', is clearly shaped by ethical concerns. His overall aim, again, is to underline the gap between wisdom (perfect psychic health) and folly, an idea that can be conveyed by comparing folly equally with (certain kinds of) health or with sickness.[278] In fact, at the level of ethical psychology, Galen does not share Stoic views on this topic. As is clear from works such as *Character Traits*, Galen holds the Platonic–Aristotelian view that non-perfect people have stable character-traits (*ēthē*).[279] This assumption may underlie his attempt in this passage to restate the Stoic contrast between psychic health and illness in the form of a more finely graded set of ethical states, including that of 'intermediate' (*metrioi*) people who are healthy

[277] For this idea, see e.g. D.L. 7.127 (LS 61 I(1)), LS 61 S–U (Plu. *Mor.* 75 C, 1062 B, 1063 A–B). On the implications for their ideas about psychological stability, see Gill 2006: 94–5, 221, 223, 254, 261–4 (on quasi-dispositional states), 318.

[278] See text to nn. 274–6 above.

[279] See text to nn. 107–12 above. This point is implied by the Aristotelian idea that self-indulgence (*akolasia*), by contrast with 'weakness of will' (*akrasia*), constitutes a relatively stable dispositional trait. See e.g. Arist. *EN* 7.8; also Gill 2006: 95 (contrasted with the Stoic idea in 93–4).

(though not perfectly robust), and not subject to fevers.[280] However, more evident is his belief that the Stoic deployment of the medical analogy conflicts with standard medical uses of the categories of health and sickness.[281]

These passages, which set out and explore the medical analogy, point to a rather different picture of the significance of the analogy from that suggested by Tieleman.[282] It is worth placing this issue in a rather larger perspective, that of the philosophical implications of Stoic theory on the psyche–body relationship. In modern terms, I take it, the Stoic theory might be classified as non-reductive token-identity physicalism (or materialism) as regards psychology. The Stoics see specific psychological events, as well as general types of psychological experience, as having a physical dimension or correlative. But they do not think that this entails that accounts of psychological experience (or of their causation) should be reduced to accounts of physical events.[283] This general principle bears on the question of how to interpret Chrysippus' idea of psychic health (and beauty and proportion), discussed in the previous chapter (4.4 above). My view is that this idea should be interpreted in terms of ethical psychology, as referring to the state of mind and character of the normative wise person, by contrast with that of non-wise people.[284] Tieleman, by, contrast, has proposed that 'proportion', in

[280] Gal. *PHP* V.434, 5.2.9 De Lacy. Galen's typology recalls the graded typology in Arist. 7.1, for instance (temperance, self-control, weakness of will, self-indulgence); however, Galen adopts for this purpose some Stoic assumptions, e.g. the ideal of perfect virtue/health and the idea that emotional states are necessarily diseased. On Aristotle's typology and the contrast with the starker Stoic wise–folly distinction, see Gill 2006: 95–6. On the point that the Stoic distinction does not prevent them from having a coherent theory of ethical progress, see Inwood and Donini 1999: 724–31.

[281] For Galen's, more conventional, medical thinking on the nature of health and sickness, see e.g. *Art of Medicine* (*Ars Med.*), I.307–18, chs. 1–4, trans. Singer 1997*a*: 345–51.

[282] See text to nn. 245–55 above.

[283] For this kind of terminology, as applied to ancient theories, see e.g. Irwin 1991: 57. The question of reductionism has been debated most intensively in relation to Epicurus; see e.g. O'Keefe 2005: ch. 4, but is also potentially relevant to Stoicism. On Stoic psychology and physicalism, see e.g. Long 1996: ch. 10, 1999: 562–72, and Ch. 3 above, text to nn. 258–301. Stoic physicalism on psychological events is qualified by their claim that *lekta* (the intelligible content of thoughts) are non-material; on *lekta*, see LS 27, 33.

[284] See 4.4 above esp text to nn. 258–67.

this case, refers to the idea of a well-harmonized 'mixture' of elements (hot, cold, dry, wet).[285] I accept fully that, in line with Stoic physicalism about psychology, psychic proportion or beauty must have a physical dimension or correlative. But this does not mean that all accounts of psychological states or the causation of such states must be translated (or 'reduced') to physical accounts. I think that the Stoic analysis of psychic health and sickness is conceived primarily in terms of ethical psychology; this applies especially to the key ideas informing the analysis, including the contrast between normative wisdom and folly. The physical dimension is present in principle, and may sometimes come to the forefront of attention; but it is not, I think, primary, nor is it as prominent in this area of their theory as Tieleman maintains.

There is one further aspect of Stoic theory that needs to be noted here, if we are to make sense of their thinking about therapy and the psyche–body relationship. As stressed in 3.5 above, the Stoics combine physicalism about psychology, and determinism, with the belief that human beings are rational agents, who are responsible for their actions and, in principle, for the shaping of their character. A key relevant feature of their thinking in this area is the distinction between internal and external causes; adult humans, as rational agents, operate as 'internal' causes differently from human children or non-human animals.[286]This point bears on the present topic in two main ways. Although, as Tieleman underlines, the Stoics regard innate physical temperament ('mixtures' of elements) and environmental influences as factors bearing on the formation of character,[287] they also believe that all human beings as such are constitutionally capable of developing towards complete wisdom. This belief is made credible by reference to their thinking about the innate capacity of human beings to form ethical ideas and by their unified view of human psychology, according to which changes of belief necessarily bring with them changes in motivation and affective states. This framework of ideas, like comparable Epicurean ideas, underlies their view that therapeutic argument can help anyone, in principle,

[285] Tieleman 2003*a*: 145–57; see also text to nn. 246–7 above.

[286] See Ch. 3 above, text to nn. 297–9.

[287] See Tieleman 2003*a*: 160–2, 194.

to reshape their belief-sets and to make progress towards perfection.[288] Hence, Stoic theory *both* recognizes the role of physical factors in shaping animal and human character, as Tieleman points out, *and* presents adult humans as capable of ethical development through such means as responding to philosophical therapy.[289] The quasi-medical role of the latter process is conceived, as I have argued, in terms of ethical psychology, despite the implicit physicalism of Stoic theory.

I now raise the same type of question in relation to Galenic thought and practice. To what extent does Galenic therapy match the typical ancient pattern, in which medical therapy is directed at the person as body and philosophical therapy at the person as psyche? In Galen's case, the situation is complicated by the fact that Galen is a contributor to both types of therapy. Galen was not simply one of the foremost doctors in the Roman Empire in his day but also the author of important works on medical therapy, which refer to many aspects of his vast collection of writings on every aspect of medicine.[290] He also wrote a number of works of (largely practical) ethics, including the essays on the therapy of the errors and passions of the psyche and *Avoiding Distress*. In a late work, *On My Own Opinions* (*Prop. Plac.*), while disowning expertise in speculative theory about the nature of the psyche, Galen presents (practically oriented) ethical philosophy and medically grounded study of the psyche as falling within his areas of expertise.[291] Although Galen is unusual in contributing to both types of therapy, his work in both areas generally reflects the typical ancient pattern, in which medical therapy is directed at the body and philosophical therapy at the psyche. In so far as his medical therapy rests on ideas about the

[288] See text to nn. 18–20 above, and Ch. 4 above, text to nn. 116–33. See also Gill 2006: 132–45, 178–84, 378–9; and Gill 2008*d*: 364–7.

[289] Hence, the emphasis on the physical basis of character as regards human children, in Sen. *Ira* 2.19, is compatible with Stoic belief about the potential efficacy of rational or cognitive therapy in adults; see also Sen. *Ira* 2.20, for a brief attempt to combine the two aspects of Stoic theory (though still related to childhood, i.e. pre-rational, development).

[290] The main works are *On the Therapeutic Method* (*MM*) and *Therapeutics to Glaucon* (*MMG*); see also *Lib. Prop.* ch. 4, XIX.30–1, and van der Eijk 2008.

[291] *Prop. Plac.* 8.3–4, p. 82.9–84.6 Nutton, 14.5, 114.5–116.4 Nutton; see also Nutton 1999: 169, 211; see also *PHP* V.794, 9.9.8–9 De Lacy.

psyche as well as the body, psychological features are viewed as aspects or functions of physical ones. In the essays on errors and emotions (*Pecc.* and *Aff. Dig.*), by contrast, Galen adopts the standard philosophical approach and addresses the person as psychological agent. Although there are some cases of partial cross-over or convergence, considered shortly, this division largely holds good in Galen's works. There is also no obvious attempt, on Galen's part, to offer a theoretical overview, indicating how these two aspects of therapy are, or could be, integrated.

I review the main distinctive features of Galen's approach to medical therapy before considering more fully the contrasting strands (medical or philosophical) in his thinking about psychic illness and treatment. As Philip van der Eijk brings out, Galen's approach to therapy, as to other aspects of medicine, is marked by the application of logic, comprehensiveness, and systematicity, rather than by the evolution of any special new method.[292] Galen presents his medical method as a considered synthesis of key aspects of the Empirical and Dogmatic (or Rationalist) methods. Central to Galen's method was the combination of theoretical understanding of the branches of knowledge relevant to the human body with observation-based application to specific cases. This combination was supported, at the theoretical level, by Galen's thinking on causation and on the interpretation of 'indications' or 'signs' of health or sickness in specific patients.[293] This method was applied to the three traditional subdivisions of ancient therapeutics, namely dietetics, pharmacology, and surgery; therapy was also understood as a combination of diagnostic, pathology, and treatment. As well as offering a systematic account of these various aspects of therapy, Galen also brought out the linkage between theoretical or research-based study and effective application of these methods. For instance, especially relevant for dietetics and pharmacology was analysis of the material composition of the body, conceived by Galen in terms of mixture of elements and the humours derived from these mixtures. Galen's extensive, and partly innovative, work on anatomy, and on the roles of the three

[292] See van der Eijk 2008: 283–6, 300.

[293] See Ch. 2 above, text to nn. 91–101, 111–24; also Hankinson 1991*c*: xxvi–xxxiv, Nutton 2004: ch. 16.

major organs in the body, informed many aspects of medical practice, especially surgery. In illustrating the effective use of the combination of logic or systematic method and empirical observation, I referred earlier to Galen's work in establishing the role of the brain and the central nervous system. Analogously, in the therapeutic sphere, Galen deployed this combination of methods in, for instance, exceptionally precise measurement of different kinds of pulse and in highly developed methods of venesection (cutting of veins).[294]

As this outline may suggest, Galen's medical therapy, like that of ancient medicine generally, was directed primarily at the body. Although he sometimes reports anecdotes that show some psychological acumen in dealing with people,[295] Galen does not develop a separate area of medical therapeutics directed at the person as psyche. He does, like other ancient doctors, recognize the existence of various types of mental or psychological illness and try to cure them. But he does so through the application of standard medical methods, using types of pathology and treatment that are largely body-based. Thus, for instance, Galen regards phrenitis, and some other mental disorders, primarily as malfunctions of the brain. Melancholy, on the other hand, is treated as a humoral disorder. Treatment for such states, as in the case of many physical illnesses centres on dietetics (*diaita* or regimen, which is broadly understood).[296] As some recent discussions have stressed, Galen thus deploys two kinds of language for psychological states (*pathē tēs psuchēs*). One is medical language, in which conditions such as phrenitis or melancholy are regarded as broadly similar to physical illnesses and treated accordingly. Another is the psychological and ethical language deployed in essays such as *Psychological Affections*, *Avoiding Distress*, and *Character Traits*. Here, Galen talks in terms of emotions, virtues, and vices; he uses the discourse of philosophical approaches to ethical psychology. In *Aff. Dig.*, as noted earlier, Galen sometimes adopts the Stoic–Epicurean

[294] On this combination of theory-based analysis and precise observation, see van der Eijk 2008: 294–7, and Ch. 2 above, text to nn. 91–4, 101–19.

[295] An often cited case is Galen's recognition from an agitated pulse (at the name 'Pylades') that a slave-woman being treated for an unknown ailment is suffering from love-sickness: *Praen.* X.630–5 K, noted by Ballester 1988: 139, Singer 1997*a*: xxi.

[296] See Pigeaud 1988; also 1981: 32–70 on Galen viewed in the context of this type of ancient medical thinking.

view of emotions as sicknesses of the psyche that need to be cured.[297] But, in this essay, the methods of treatment envisaged are purely psychological, and indeed rational or cognitive. Galen makes no attempt to draw on his own medical typology or therapy for this purpose; the generic or conceptual boundaries between the two areas are kept largely intact.[298]

However, there are at least two contexts in which Galen brings the two kinds of discourse closer together. In both cases, he does so from a medical standpoint; also, in both cases, what is at issue is 'hygienic' (general care for one's health) rather than therapy (medical treatment in response to an illness), more narrowly understood.[299] In *The Art of Medicine* (*Ars Med.*), a late or perhaps post-Galenic work, Galen identifies six factors which necessarily affect health: 'the surrounding air, motion and rest of the body as a whole or of its individual parts, sleep and waking, substances [such as food and drink] taken, and psychological events (or 'emotions', *pathē*)'.[300] Galen comments further on the last item: 'Obviously one must refrain from excess of all emotions of the psyche: anger, grief, pride, fear, envy, and worry; for these will change the constitution of the body.'[301] As Luis Garcia Ballester points out, a similar line of thought is also explored in one of Galen's commentaries on Hippocrates, *Epidemics* VI. Galen is commenting on a passage in which the Hippocratic text offers a similar list of factors affecting health, including 'state of mind' (*gnōmē*).[302] Two features of Galen's comments on this list are of interest here. One is the breadth with which he understands the items. For instance, 'diet' or regime (*diaita*) includes factors such as social and leisure activities as well as food and drink; while 'living conditions' include all aspects of material life. The second is his exploration of the significance of state of mind. Galen has in view cases where someone's psychological state (for instance, an obsession

[297] See text to nn. 31–44 above.

[298] See Ballester 1988, Singer 1992: ch. 5, esp. 276–7, 295–6.

[299] On Galen's approach to this area of medicine, see van der Eijk 2008: 297–300.

[300] Gal. *Ars Med.* I.367; trans. Singer 1997*a*: 374, modified. This set of items became codified as the 'six non-natural things' in the Galenic medical tradition. On *Ars Med.*, see Kollesch 1988.

[301] Gal. *Ars Med.* I.371, trans. Singer 1997*a*: 376, slightly modified.

[302] The six items are diet, living conditions, effort, sleep, sexual relations, and state of mind; Hippocrates, *Epidemics* VI, V.352 Littré; see Ballester 1988: 148.

or *idée fixe*) is undermining her health. He stresses that, in such cases, physical health can only be improved if the doctor helps the person concerned to alter her state of mind, presumably through dialogue (though this is not specified).[303] In these passages, Galen recognizes the role of state of mind and emotions as factors affecting physical health and disease. He also presents it as part of the work of the doctor to help the patient modify her state of mind, though he does not explore how this is to be achieved. This could be by the kind of use of dialogue discussed in other medical writings, for instance, by Caelius Aurelianus[304] or by the kind of psychological therapy Galen himself offers in *Aff. Dig* or *Indol.* But this potential linkage between the two aspects of Galen's therapeutic work is not explored further.

The other context where Galen juxtaposes the two kinds of approach is *QAM*. Here, in effect, Galen maintains that the medical approach to psychological states can replace the philosophical. As he puts it, early in the essay: 'we derive a good bodily mixture from our food and drink and other daily activities, and this mixture is the basis on which we then build the virtue of the psyche'.[305] Towards the end of the work, the radical implications of Galen's thesis are stated in clearer and more polemical form:

> So it would be wise of my opponents—those who are unhappy at the idea that nourishment has the power to make people more temperate, self-indulgent, or self-restrained, brave or cowardly, soft and gentle or violent and quarrelsome—to come to me even now and receive instruction. They would derive enormous benefit from this in their command of ethical philosophy; and the improvement in their intellectual faculties, too, would have an effect on their virtue, as they acquired greater powers of understanding and memory. Apart from food and drink, I would teach them about winds and mixtures in the surrounding air, and places, instructing them which to select and which to avoid.[306]

[303] *On Hippocrates' 'Epidemics'* (*Hipp. Epid.*) VI (*CMG* 10.2.2), XVIIA.484.7–33, 485.17–19, 22–5, 487.18–23. See further Ballester 1988: 147–52, Singer 1992: 297–9.

[304] See Pigeaud 1981: 109–12.

[305] Gal. *QAM* IV.768, ch. 1, *SM* 2.32.9–11, trans. Singer 1997*a*: 150, slightly modified.

[306] *QAM* IV.807–8, ch. 9, *SM* 2.67.2–16, trans. Singer 1997*a*: 169, slightly modified.

This sweeping and uncompromising tone is maintained in ch. 11 of the essay, already discussed in this study. Here, Galen defends his central claim (that the faculties of the psyche depend on the mixtures of elements in the body) against the possible criticism that it is in conflict with moral principles. Galen maintains that, even if ethical character depends on factors we cannot control, it is still appropriate to blame and punish wrongdoers. He also argues against the Stoic view that all human beings are constitutively capable of ethical development, which he presents as amounting to the claim that all corruption comes from external causes.[307]

Whereas the two types of therapy (philosophical and medical) are normally kept firmly apart in Galen's work, here they are, in a sense, strongly juxtaposed. But Galen brings them together only to replace one kind of therapy (the philosophical) with the other (the medical). The suggestion seems to be that medical therapy—more precisely, 'hygiene' or regime—can take care of the psyche as well as the body, and produce virtue as well as physical health. This is coupled, in ch. 11, with the abrupt rejection of ethical reservations about this suggestion and the rejection of one (Stoic) alternative account of ethical development. The core of this line of thought, at least as regards therapy, is the—wholly reasonable—suggestion that regime or 'hygiene' can help people to improve their general state of being, and thus enable them to use their intellectual and ethical capacities to the full. An idea of this kind is implied in the passages just cited (from *Ars Med.* and Galen's commentary on Hippocrates), though Galen there also recognizes the reverse process, that state of mind affects bodily condition.[308] Galen's stance in *QAM*, if taken literally, would invalidate the kind of therapeutic discourse he himself offers in *Aff. Dig.*, which presupposes that rational or cognitive therapy can play a significant role in improving someone's psychological state.[309] It also runs counter, as noted earlier, to the Platonic–Aristotelian view of ethical development, which gives roles to social habituation, and reasoned choice as well as inborn nature, a view whose validity

[307] *QAM* IV.814–22, ch. 11, *SM* 2.73.3–79.24, trans. Singer 1997*a*: 172–6. See further Ch. 3 above, text to nn. 280–92; and text to nn. 131–3 above.

[308] See text to nn. 299–303 above.

[309] See text to n. 139 above: also text to nn. 28–76 (esp. 67–70) above.

Galen himself sometimes presupposes.[310] Why Galen adopts in *QAM* such an extreme and problematic position on the relationship between medical and philosophical therapy is unclear. In general, his intellectual target in *QAM* seems to be a dualist version of Platonism;[311] but he could attack that view without presenting medical therapy as, in effect, an alternative to *all* forms of philosophical therapy or, indeed, all philosophical writings designed to promote ethical development. Some recent discussions suggest that Galen sees *QAM* as a kind of manifesto for medical therapy;[312] and this might explain his exaggerated account of the scope of medical treatment. In any case, the position of *QAM* is exceptional within his work. The more typical pattern is that medical and philosophical approaches to therapy follow different pathways with a limited amount of convergence, especially in the sphere of 'hygiene'.

I close this discussion of Galenic and Stoic therapy by considering whether their main respective contributions to this area could have been coherently combined, and, if so, from what standpoint. What kind of combination is at issue? What I have in mind is a combination of Galenic medical therapy and Stoic therapy of the emotions, as expressed especially in Chrysippus' 'therapeutic' book. I select this combination because each of the two examples can be presented, with some plausibility, as the most important ancient contribution to these types of therapy. I stressed earlier that Stoic therapy of the emotions, especially as represented in Chrysippus' 'therapeutic' book, seems to be both pioneering and highly influential in subsequent thought and practice.[313] Indeed, Galen's main essay in this area (*Aff. Dig.*) shows Stoic influence, although this is—rather awkwardly—combined with a Platonic–Aristotelian pattern of thinking about ethical psychology and development.[314] However, by comparison with the Stoic, and especially Chrysippean, approach to the therapy of the emotions, Galen's contribution is a relatively minor and derivative one, interesting though it is for the present inquiry. The second-hand character of Galen's thinking emerges in part from the awkward combination of different intellectual strands just noted.

[310] See text to nn. 134–6 above.

[311] See Ch. 3 above, text to nn. 238–40.

[312] See Donini 2008: 199–202, and Jouanna 2009: 196–205.

[313] See text to nn. 207–13 above.

[314] See text to nn. 28–56 above.

Galen is writing here as the inheritor of various traditions of philosophical writing, in particular, Stoic–Epicurean writing on the therapy of emotion and Platonic–Aristotelian ethical psychology. But he is not sufficiently in command of his material to produce a new or illuminating synthesis, nor does the work give scope for any of Galen's special strengths in methodology. In fact, the companion essay on *Psychological Errors* (*Pecc. Dig.*) is, arguably, more cogent, in displaying Galen's undoubted skills in methodical classification in the analysis of intellectual mistakes and defects.[315]

The situation is quite different as regards Galen's contribution to medical therapy. In appraising his role in the development of ancient techniques of therapy, and still more his application of these techniques, we are almost entirely dependent on Galen's own massive output. Since Galen writes on this subject as a thoroughly engaged, and often combative and polemical, participant in debate as well as a self-interested practitioner, his accounts cannot be treated as if they constituted a detached historical record.[316] However, even when this is taken into account, it does seem likely that Galen was not only an outstanding practising doctor in his own day but also one who raised the analysis and systematization of medical therapy to a new level. In particular, the integration of theoretical knowledge, sometimes based on independent research, with observation-based application in specific cases emerges as an outstandingly well-conceived medical method by ancient or indeed any standards. The fact that the intense debates between different medical schools that Galen describes came to an end after his lifetime is usually taken as an indication of Galen's success in establishing his technique as a normative one.[317]

If we allow, then, that Galenic medical therapy and Stoic therapy of the emotions were the outstanding ancient examples of their kind, could they have been coherently combined? The question, though hypothetical (like some analogous questions raised earlier),[318] is

[315] See further Donini 1988.

[316] On the difficulties of reconstructing a credible picture of the Methodist school from Galen's remorselessly critical accounts, see Tecusan 2004: 7–21.

[317] See further van der Eijk 2008, esp. 300, also Nutton 2004: ch. 16.

[318] See 3.2–3 above (on the possible combination of Stoic psychology and Galen's brain-centred anatomy), and 3.5 above, text to nn. 252–310 (on the possible combination of Galenic and Stoic thought on physicalism and agency).

potentially revealing for making sense of the relationship between these two theories. Although the topic has quite complex implications, the answer to this question is, I think, relatively straightforward. From the Stoic standpoint, this combination would have been quite unproblematic, or indeed desirable. From Galen's standpoint, however, the combination would have been much more unacceptable. What is the basis for this conclusion and what explains the difference of attitude?

In considering the Stoic therapeutic strategy earlier in this section, I outlined Tieleman's proposal that their approach combines psychological and physical or medical dimensions.[319] I am sceptical about this idea, as regards the reconstruction of the content and theoretical stance of Chrysippus' 'therapeutic' book. However, I accept that it is very likely that their theory as a whole embraces the interest in the physical aspects of psychology that Tieleman identifies and that their concerns overlap with those of contemporary medicine. This holds good, for instance, for their interest in regime, and its impact on the proper management of one's life, and also in the influence of inbuilt temperamental factors on character development.[320] In general, although the Stoics did not conduct independent research into, for instance, anatomy, they seem to have been quite ready to draw on what seemed to be the best available work, by thinkers such as Praxagoras.[321] Also, their physicalist approach to psychology is quite compatible with recognition of the importance of medical study of the body and correlated therapeutic methods. I suggested earlier that, if the Stoics had been made aware of Galen's powerful arguments for locating the ruling part of the psyche in the brain, there is no obvious reason why they should not have accepted these arguments.[322] The same principle applies to Galenic medical therapy. If they had recognized that Galen's approach to medical therapy constituted the best-grounded version in ancient medicine, I can see no reason in principle why they would not have adopted it. They would not, on my view, have attempted to integrate it with their approach to

[319] See text to nn. 245–55 above. [320] See refs. in nn. 253–4 above.

[321] See Ch. 3 above, text to nn. 32, 36.

[322] See 3.2 above, text to nn. 53–4. As suggested there, the fact that Galen's brain-centred picture fits well with the Stoic psychological theory, based on a unitary 'control-centre', makes it more reasonable for the Stoics to have embraced Galen's picture.

the therapy of emotions, which seems to be conceived in purely psychological terms.[323] But, in so far as their approach accommodates a concern with the proper care of the body and with the impact of the physical state on well-being and activity, I see no reason why they should not have adopted Galenic medical methods. It is true that Stoic ethical principles have a bearing on the status they would have given to medical practice. They would have seen medicine as designed to achieve what is, in their terms, only a 'preferred indifferent', rather than a good. But their ethical principles also recognize the 'selection' of preferred indifferents as a valid element in a good life; and, in so far as medical therapy works to this end, they could have seen this as a worthwhile practice.[324] Hence, from their point of view, the combination of Galenic-style medical therapy with—at least, alongside—their own psychological therapy seems fully acceptable.

From Galen's standpoint, however, the combination is much more problematic. The fact that he himself writes two essays on the therapy of the emotions, and that he adopts, at least in one of them (*Aff. Dig.*), a number of Stoic (or Stoic–Epicurean) assumptions and themes might seem to suggest that this combination might be acceptable to him. But this is misleading. When Galen turns his attention in this essay to the question of the kind of ethical psychology and account of development that he sees as valid, he introduces Platonic–Aristotelian ideas that are at odds with the Stoic aspects of his essay.[325] He does, in fact, explicitly disagree with Stoic assumptions and seems not to be aware of the fact that Stoic-style therapy is informed by highly determinate assumptions about psychology and development. However, if he were aware of the linkage between Stoic therapy and Stoic psychology, he would, undoubtedly, repudiate the idea that he could adopt Stoic-style therapy of the emotions alongside his own medical therapy. As brought out in Chapter 4, Galen's rejection of Stoic ethical psychology and theory of development in *PHP* 4–5 is comprehensive and sustained. Galen is also highly critical of Chrysippus' use of the analogy between physical and psychological

[323] See my response to Tieleman's view, text to nn. 256–66 above.

[324] See further LS 58.

[325] See text to nn. 45–56. Also in *Indol.* the psychological and ethical assumptions are uniformly Platonic–Aristotelian in spite of the apparently Stoic-style commendation of 'absence of distress' in the first half of the essay: see 5.2 above, text to nn. 86–96.

illness and between medical and philosophical therapy. His criticism is based both on rejection of the Stoic psychological theory and also of the way that the Stoics use the analogy between psychological and physical illness.[326] Given all this, it seems clear that Galen himself would regard as quite unacceptable the combination of his own medical therapy with the Stoic therapy of the emotions.

How should we explain this contrast between Stoic and Galenic attitudes, as I interpret them, towards the possible combination of these two types of therapy? In one way, the explanation is quite straightforward, since it simply follows from points already discussed, for instance, Galen's antagonism towards Stoic unified psychology, which is implied in their approach to emotional therapy. However, it is also worth considering how far the Stoic and Galenic responses reflect larger similarities and differences explored elsewhere in this book, relating to naturalism or holism. I have suggested earlier that the Stoics share with Galen a 'naturalistic' approach in several senses. For one thing, both theories reject Platonic-style psyche–body dualism, and see both psyche and body as integrated aspects of human beings as natural entities. For another, they both adopt what I called 'high naturalism', combining a 'biological', rather than mechanical, picture of living entities and a teleological view of natural organisms.[327] The hypothesis that the Stoics could consistently adopt the Galenic approach to medical therapy—as well as his anatomically based findings on the role of the brain and nervous system[328]—reflects their shared naturalism in these respects. From Galen's standpoint, in fact, there are close links between the key elements in his 'high naturalism' and salient features of his therapeutic method. Other aspects of this therapy that mark closeness to Stoic thought include the deployment of a Stoic-style causal framework to inform diagnosis and treatment.[329] Our evidence for Stoic views on medicine is too limited to gauge whether their medical thinking also embraces these aspects.[330] But we can at least say that

326 See 4.2 above, and text to nn. 271–6 above.

327 See 2.3 above, and Ch. 3 above, text to nn. 187–9 (on the embryo).

328 See further 3.2 above, esp. text to nn. 53–4.

329 See text to n. 293 above, also Ch. 2 above, text to nn. 122–4.

330 For some suggestions, see Tieleman 2003*a*: 190–6 (more broadly, his ch. 4 as a whole).

an implication of shared Galenic and Stoic 'high naturalism' is that the Stoics too could consistently have adopted many of the main features of Galenic therapy, as expressing their shared view of human beings as teleologically shaped, unified complexes of natural faculties.

The question of holism raises more complex implications for this question. There are several relevant aspects of holism: psychological holism, psychophysical holism, and also holism as regards different branches of knowledge. All three aspects bear in different ways on the question how far Galenic medical and Stoic emotional therapy could coherently be combined. One point on which Galenic and Stoic approaches to the therapy of emotions diverge is that Galen introduces into this topic a non-holistic, part-based, psychological model and correlated account of ethical development. This is at odds with the Stoic unified or holistic psychological theory, and correlated picture of development, linked with the Stoic conception of emotional therapy and implied in the framework that Galen himself partly adopts.[331] I suggested in Chapter 4 that, as regards ethical psychology at least, we could see a major contrast between the two theories, which could be analysed in terms of the contrast between a 'structure' (holistic) and 'composition' (non-holistic) conception of the part–whole relationship.[332] That contrast has a bearing on this question also. The points of difference between Galenic and Stoic thinking on the therapy of emotion reflect in part this broader divergence of outlook.

However, another kind of holism is also relevant. To make full sense of Stoic thinking on the psychology of emotions or on ethical development, we need to refer to the contrast between the state of mind of the normative wise person and all non-wise people. This contrast, while seen as absolute and unqualified, is also taken to provide a normative framework that applies to (non-perfect) human beings.[333] This contrast underlies, for instance, the distinction between emotions (as normally understood) and 'good emotions' (*eupatheiai*), and the Stoic assumption that all human beings are constitutively capable of developing

[331] See text to nn. 28–76, also text to nn. 14–16 on the Stoic pattern.

[332] See Ch. 4 above, text to nn. 37–46.

[333] On the question how these (seemingly conflicting) aspects of Stoic thinking are combined, see Inwood and Donini 1999: 724–35.

towards perfect wisdom.[334] It also underlies the Stoic view that the psychological state of non-wise people is inherently unstable and internally conflicted, by contrast with the stability and internal consistency of the wise person.[335] These features of Stoic thinking form part of a set of radical, seemingly paradoxical claims that, I have suggested elsewhere, seem to be strongly influenced by Socrates, as the Stoics understand this figure and his ideas.[336] This aspect of Stoic theory expresses 'holism' in another sense. This is their view that the three main branches of knowledge (ethics, physics, and logic) constitute, in principle at least, an integrated set or system.[337] The aspects of Stoic thinking noted earlier reflect the assumption that questions of psychology (which fall, in part, at least under 'physics') and ethical questions are intimately interconnected. For the Stoics, the proper understanding of the nature of emotions and of natural development (or of the therapy of emotions) depends on integrating thinking about psychological processes and functions with that on ethical norms and principles.[338] This is a type of 'holism' that has far-reaching implications for the understanding of Stoic thinking in general and for its relationship with Galen.

On the face of it, this feature marks a sharp difference with Galen's outlook. But, in his case too, as noted earlier, there is an aspiration towards establishing a unified framework of knowledge, at least as regards all aspects of knowledge bearing on medicine.[339] Also, there are certain points in his arguments with the Stoics where he too highlights close links between psychological and ethical questions. For instance, in *PHP*, he clearly sees a linkage between the question whether or not the psyche is unified or part-based with the question whether virtue is one or many.[340] Also, in the Platonic arguments about the relationship between reason and other parts (which Galen takes as providing a framework for his psychological theory), normative and psychological considerations are integrally linked, though

[334] See 4.2 above, text to nn. 116–33. [335] See 4.2 above, text to nn. 146–54.

[336] See Gill 2006: 74–100.

[337] On this idea, see LS 26 A–E; also Gill 2006: 160–2, 199–200, Annas 2007.

[338] The linkage between Stoic conceptions of psyche and physics is clear in LS 53. On the linkage between ethics, physics, and logic in Stoic psychology, see Ch. 4 above, text to nn. 36–7, and Gill 2005: 454–5. [339] See Ch. 4 above, text to nn. 48–50.

[340] *PHP* V.589–600, 7.1.8–3.1 De Lacy; on the place of the topic of virtue in the structure of *PHP* see De Lacy 2005: 50.

Galen himself does not explicitly register this linkage.[341] How far this marks a general difference between the two theories could, obviously, be explored further. However, I think it is apparent that Stoic holism in this respect is one of the factors that make for difference between the two approaches. For instance, I noted earlier that Stoic ideas about psychic illness as 'feverish' and fluctuating reflect their view of the contrast between the (unstable and incoherent) psychological state of non-wise people and that of the normative wise person. Galen does not recognize this link; his criticism of their thinking is based on what he sees as a misuse of the medical categories of sickness and health.[342] But their difference on this point reflects a larger feature of Stoic ethical psychology (its integration of ethical and psychological ideas) that, I think, may well underlie the more obvious points of disagreement between Galen and Stoicism.

The final kind of holism considered here is psychophysical holism. On this point, the Stoics and Galen come very close, although Galen stops short of formally adopting a position that the Stoics make an integral part of their theory. Both theories see human beings as, fundamentally, natural embodied entities, a point which underlies their shared readiness, as suggested earlier, to adopt medical therapy alongside emotional therapy.[343] However, this raises a further question: how far in either theory we can find a move towards a 'holistic' medical viewpoint, in the sense of one that seeks to *integrate* physical and psychological aspects of therapy. What should count as 'holistic' therapy is itself a complex and contested question in modern thought.[344] But we can mark a difference, I think, between holism that begins with the body and that which begins from the mind (although both approaches, if they are holistic, assume that these starting-points can finally be integrated in a single whole). In general, the attitude to therapy I have ascribed to both theories is not fully

[341] On Galen's use of Plato's arguments in *R.* 435–41, see *PHP* V.480–502, 5.7.1–82 De Lacy, also Ch. 4 above, text to nn. 161–72. The linkage between ethical and psychological ideas is brought out clearly in the interpretations of Plato's arguments in Cooper 1984, Kahn 1987, and Irwin 1977: 191–5, 226–33, 1995: 203–22, 245–8. On 'reason' as an inherently normative idea in Plato, Aristotle, and Stoicism, at least, see M. Frede 1995: 5–17.

[342] See text to nn. 272–6 above.

[343] See text to nn. 319–24, and Ch. 3 above, text to nn. 252–79.

[344] See further Ch. 6 below, text to n. 68.

holistic in this respect. Both theories see the validity of *both* medical (body-based) *and* philosophical (psychological) therapy, of different types, but do not attempt to integrate these methods fully. I noted earlier some points where Galenic medical therapy does seek to incorporate reference to psychological factors, especially in *QAM*.[345] This could be seen as a kind of holistic approach; but, if so, it is one in which psychological factors are subsumed under physical ones or explained in physical terms, rather than one in which a distinct or overarching framework is evolved to cover both areas. Analogously, although the Stoics conceive human beings as psychophysical as well as psychological wholes (a point stressed by Tieleman), their philosophical therapy addresses them essentially as psychological agents.[346] In this respect, although both theories have the resources for conceiving a form of 'holistic' medical therapy, directed to people as psychophysical as well as psychological wholes, they do not in practice formulate or apply this method.

345 See text to nn. 305–12 above.

346 See 5.3 above, esp. text to nn. 256–66, also 4.4 above.

6

Galen and Stoicism: Paradoxes Revisited and Modern Parallels

6.1 PRELIMINARIES

In this chapter, I revisit the paradoxes that arise in this relationship highlighted in the first chapter, and re-examine them on the basis of the intervening discussion. In particular, I explore further the question raised in Chapter 1, why Galen does not go further than he does in developing his relationship with Stoicism, in spite of the fact that the two theories have a good deal in common, which can be characterized as aspects of a shared 'naturalism'. In doing so, I refer to some modern parallels with the ancient ideas treated here. I use the modern parallels to spell out more clearly what a combination of Galenic and Stoic ideas might have looked like.

I begin by restating the paradox from which this inquiry started, referring to relevant preceding sections of the book. The main common element in Galenic and Stoic thought is constituted by the approach described earlier as 'high naturalism' (2.3). Broadly put, this represents a combination of a design-centred and a 'biological' view of the natural world, by contrast with world-views that present nature as the outcome of fortuitous and mechanical processes. There are also aspects of Stoic thinking that contribute to Galen's distinctive methodology for medicine and for natural inquiry, especially as regards logic and the theory of causation (2.2). These common features constitute a basis for intellectual engagement that is at least as solid as the basis that exists between Galen and some other ancient philosophical thinkers, notably Plato and Aristotle, with which he did develop very close bonds. In fact, as highlighted earlier, there are certain points, in addition to those already noted, where Galenic and Stoic thought come very close—in spite of significant differences and disagreements in those same areas. Galen comes close to Stoicism, especially in *QAM* and *Prop. Plac.*, in that he—nearly—adopts an explicitly physicalist account of psychology (3.5). Also, his account of embryonic development in *Foet. Form.* reflects several features shared with Stoicism, including the features linked with 'high naturalism' (3.4). A different kind of shared feature is Galen's adoption in *Aff. Dig.* of the 'therapeutic' approach to emotions, pioneered especially by Stoics such as Chrysippus, along with some Stoic-style ideas regarding the aims of such therapy (5.2).

These areas of (near-) convergence between Galen and Stoicism are significant ones. But there are other, more important, types of convergence that do *not* occur. The most notable is the linkage, that can be seen as conceptually possible, between Galen's brain-centred anatomy and the Stoic unified account of psychology, centred on the idea of the 'control-centre' (*hēgemonikon*). More precisely, one can see how the Stoic account, based on a combination of the 'control-centre' and 'nature' (*phusis*), might have fitted Galen's brain-centred picture better than the tripartite psychophysiology he adopts from Plato (3.2–3). A second possible point of convergence is the combination of physicalism as regards psychology and an account of human beings as rational and responsible agents. This is a further Stoic feature that, I think, Galen could usefully have adopted in *QAM* and elsewhere, but which he does not (3.5). In the area of therapy, I have suggested that a combination of Galenic medical therapy and the Stoic therapy of the emotions could have been an exceptionally powerful combination, and one that was possible from the Stoic standpoint, though not from Galen's perspective (5.4). The psychology of emotion is a major area of disagreement between Galen and Stoicism. However, even on this point, I have asked how far such disagreement is inevitable, in the light of Galen's other intellectual commitments. It is not self-evident that Galen's brain-centred psychophysiology, a crucial outcome of his methodology of natural inquiry, requires—or is, indeed, consistent with—the radical division between reason and emotion that Galen adopts from Plato. One can argue that this brain-centred picture would have fitted as well, or better, with the Stoic view that reason and emotions are functions of a single psychological centre[1] These areas of potential convergence, taken with those of actual or near agreement, add up to an impressive body of ideas. This set of ideas can be contrasted, in many respects, with the non-naturalistic, dualistic theories of psychology developed in first- and second-century Platonism, in the work of thinkers such as Plutarch.

How should we explain Galen's failure to build on these areas of potential agreement in the construction of a set of ideas that is, arguably, more powerful than either of the two theories can offer on its own? Earlier (4.1), I outlined various possible lines of explanation. These include the contrast between medical and philosophical approaches and the significance of intellectual affiliation or allegiance. A further possible factor is the contrast between a holistic (or 'structure') and non-holistic or part-based (or 'composition') approach. The latter difference is especially prominent in Galen's response to the Stoic psychology of emotion, and seems to be the main factor determining Galen's attitude there, which is more uniformly negative even than his response to Stoic thinking about psychophysiology (4.2–4). However, I have also pointed out that the contrast between holistic and part-based approaches does not apply uniformly to all aspects of the Galen–Stoicism relationship, and so this factor may not, on its own, explain Galen's negative attitude to Stoic psychology. It may be better to see Galen's response as a secondary consequence of his disagreement with the Stoics regarding the location of the ruling part of the psyche. Galen—perhaps unnecessarily—sees the two issues as closely linked. He therefore feels impelled to undermine Stoic thinking on emotions, or, more broadly, on psychological functions, as part of a sustained critique of Stoic heart-centred psychophysiology. Although the contrast between Galen's part-based ('composition') picture of psychology and the Stoic unified ('structure') view is very marked, this difference, on its own, might not explain Galen's comprehensively negative response to Stoic psychology.

In this chapter, I take this line of inquiry forward in two main ways. I analyse in more abstract terms the type of psychological ideas that would have resulted from a combination of Stoic and Galenic

[1] See 4.1 above, esp. text to nn. 25–7.

thinking. I do so by referring to modern ideas that exhibit a comparable type of combination. This reinforces the point (which has been made already in the ancient context) that such combinations are by no means conceptually absurd or impossible. There are three main topics on which I develop this line of thought. One is the combination of a brain-centred psychophysiology and the idea of a unitary psychological centre, that is, the kind of combination envisaged in 3.2–3. Another is the combination of a brain-centred anatomy (combined with a unitary psychological centre) and a cognitive or belief-based account of emotions.[2] These topics are both discussed in 6.2, where I argue that we can find modern equivalents for both these combinations. This fact, by itself, helps to counteract Galen's negative view of the Stoic side of these combinations and to demonstrate that these combinations are psychologically credible and coherent. The third topic, examined in 6.3, is the combination posited in 5.4 of a Galenic-style (body-based) approach to medical therapy and a Stoic-style approach to the therapy of emotions. Although we can find modern analogues for both these ancient approaches (to some extent at least), it is less clear that we can find a modern equivalent for the combination of them. However, exploring this possibility is an illuminating way of analysing ancient and modern views on the interface between bodily and psychological therapy, which is a complex and often controversial area in both ancient and modern contexts.

6.2 GALENIC–STOIC PSYCHOLOGY AND MODERN PARALLELS

In this section, I consider further the implications of combining Galen's brain-centred psychophysiology with key features of Stoic psychology. On the Stoic side, there are three aspects that could usefully be considered here. They are conceptually distinguishable,

[2] This represents the combination of the synthesis of Stoic and Galenic ideas posited in 3.2–3 and the Stoic theory of emotions (or psychological functions more generally) discussed in 4.2.

though they are closely integrated in Stoic theory itself. One is the idea of the 'control-centre' (*hēgemonikon*) as a unified locus and director of all psychological functions, by contrast with the Platonic–Galenic idea of three separate and independent psychological centres. Another aspect is the unified or holistic view of psychological functions, in which emotions and desires are seen as based on beliefs. A third aspect derives from the integration of psychological with ethical ideas, which forms part of Stoic holism about the branches of philosophy. The consequences of this integration include the radical distinction between the 'good emotions' (*eupatheiai*) of the wise person and the emotions of non-wise people and the correlated idea that the state of non-wise people is one of psychological instability and incoherence (or 'feverish' sickness).[3] As brought out earlier in the book, all three aspects contribute to the kind of Stoic ideas about psychology, and about the therapy of emotions, to which Galen reacts, in different ways. Galen responds explicitly, and mostly negatively, to the first two aspects. He does not respond explicitly to the third aspect, and may not recognize its significance, though it seems sometimes to underlie his sense of bafflement or frustration with Stoic ideas, for instance, as regards their ideas about 'feverish' psychic illness.[4] However, all three aspects are potentially relevant to the question of the conceptual outcome of the combination of Galenic ideas about the brain and of Stoic psychology.

I first draw out more fully the nature of these possible combinations of Galenic and Stoic ideas by considering some modern parallels. I am especially concerned with modern parallels for the combination of the Galenic brain and the first two Stoic ideas just noted; finding a modern analogue for the third is more difficult. My aim in considering modern parallels is partly to flesh out a set of ideas that is, of course, purely hypothetical in the ancient context, since neither Galen nor the post-Galenic Stoics actually did explore this combination. It is also to bring out what I see as the conceptual coherence and credibility of this combination of ideas, and thus to

[3] See further Ch. 4 above, text to nn. 127–54.

[4] See Ch. 5 above, text to nn. 272–6. This aspect of Stoic thought also underlies their ideas about ethical development, in ways that may help to explain Galen's negative response to these ideas (Ch. 4 above, text to nn. 116–33).

counteract Galen's typically negative view of the Stoic theories involved. In correlating ancient and modern thinking in this way, I am not assuming that modern ideas are necessarily correct or true and that ancient ones can be shown to be valid or invalid in so far as they approximate to their modern analogues. To assume this would be to ignore all sorts of relevant differences between the types of argument used to support or undermine intellectual positions in the two contexts. However, in so far as modern ideas are ours, they have an obvious interest, and they also form part of the framework from which we approach ancient thinking. Also, in this instance and others, modern parallels or contrasts can highlight the conceptual credibility of options not pursued in the ancient setting.

The first combination considered is that of Galen's conception of the brain and the Stoic idea of the unitary 'control-centre' (*hēgemonikon*). More precisely, it is the combination of Galen's view that the brain (not the heart) is the seat of the part of the psyche and the Stoic view that there is a single psychological centre, and not three such centres. More precisely again, the combination envisaged is that of Galen's picture of the brain as exercising its directive functions through a system of nerves and the Stoic picture of the 'control-centre' as the focus of seven functions radiating through the body.[5] This combination can be taken alongside the Stoic idea, which has partial parallels in Galen's thought too, that certain organic or automatic processes in the body, such as growth or nutrition, are carried forward by 'nature' (*phusis*), rather than the control-centre. Earlier in the book (3.2–3), I considered in some detail the suggestion that this combination was possible, in terms of the thought-world of the period, and that, for each theory, it would have been preferable to the view actually adopted. For Galen, the main advantage would have been greater consistency with the findings of his anatomically based investigations. The Stoic unitary control-centre matches those findings better, I argued, than Galen's three-centre system, with independent sources of motivation located in brain, heart, and liver. Galen has considerable difficulties in explaining, in terms of his own physiology, in what sense the heart and the liver function as

[5] On these seven functions, in addition to the distinctive functions of the 'control-centre' on its own, see Aëtius 4.21–4 (=LS 53 H, *SVF* 2.836).

psychological as well as physiological centres.[6] A further problem is that of combining the three-centre system with those aspects of Galen's thinking that reflect or resemble the Stoic idea of (organic or automatic) 'natural' functions, distinct from those directed by the brain.[7] On the Stoic side, I think, the relocation of the control-centre in the brain involves no substantial alteration to their main theory, provided that the brain is seen as the centre of a unified psycho-physiological system, The main advantage for the Stoics of adopting the Galenic view is that this is grounded on a more secure methodology of natural inquiry than they themselves developed, though one whose combination of logical argument and empiricism is in line with their thinking. Although they did not themselves engage in independent anatomical research, they seem to have tried to base their theory on convincing work by other thinkers, such as Praxagoras. So there is an advantage in adopting what is, arguably, the most well-grounded ancient account of the location of the control-centre, namely Galen's account of the brain and nervous system.[8]

I have made this argument in terms of what is conceptually credible in ancient terms, more precisely, in relation to the ideas and methodology of the two theories concerned. However, if we broaden the framework of reference to include modern thinking, the conclusion seems still more clear-cut. Of course, within the modern context, there are a number of potentially relevant branches of inquiry, including scientific study of the brain, psychology, understood as a scientific discipline, and the philosophy of mind.[9] But I focus, in the first instance, on the findings of scientific brain research, particularly as presented in two well-known recent books on emotions and the brain, by Antonio Damasio (1994) and Joseph LeDoux (1998).[10] What is clear is that the kind of combination being considered here

[6] See Ch. 3 above, text to nn. 71–91. [7] See Ch 3 above, text to nn. 92–115.

[8] See Ch. 3 above, text to nn. 29–36, 53–4; also 2.2 above, on Galenic methodology and Stoic contributions towards this methodology.

[9] There are interesting questions that could be raised (though not here) about how far this set of disciplines corresponds to the ancient forms of inquiry (medical and philosophical) that bear on psychology. On relevant issues in the modern philosophy of mind, see discussion below.

[10] The potential relevance of these studies to the Galen–Stoic debate on emotion is highlighted in Sorabji 2000: 144–52. Both modern studies include extensive discussion of earlier scientific work on the brain.

(a Galenic-type brain and a Stoic-style unitary psychological centre), is, more or less, the standard modern picture. There is no serious debate about the fact that the brain is the sole locus of psychological functions—even if these functions are closely integrated with processes that go on elsewhere in the body.[11] The idea, for which Galen argued so passionately in *PHP* 1–6, that there are three independent psychological centres and sources of motivation, located in three separate parts of the body, finds no equivalent in modern thought. Also, the brain is seen, in Stoic fashion, as a unified system or set of subsystems (though more needs to be said about this shortly). As in the Galenic picture, the brain is understood as operating through a unified system of nerves. The idea, which forms an integral part of Stoic thought, and, less explicitly of Galenic thought, that the control-centre coexists with 'nature' (automatic or organic processes such as those of growth and nutrition), also figures in modern thinking. Some at least of these processes are now allocated to the autonomic nervous system, that is, 'the "vegetative" part of the nervous system, which controls the involuntary activity of, for example, our gastrointestinal tract, heart, and blood vessels'.[12] Thus, the combination of ideas, which, in the ancient scheme of options, would have seemed bizarre and implausible,[13] has come to seem indisputable in modern medical science.

Although the preceding outline of modern thought is, I think, tenable, there are some complications that need to be noted. The question how far we should think in terms of a single psychological centre or a number of centres, that is, in terms of wholes or parts (the issue that divides Galen and Stoicism so sharply), does, to some extent, also reappear in modern scientific thought on the brain. Attempts at localizing specific psychological functions in different parts of the brain have been made since at least the eighteenth century.[14] Two key regions are the limbic system and the cerebral

[11] On the integration of emotions with bodily processes more generally (not just in the brain), see Damasio 1994: ch. 8, also Colombetti 2007, 2008.

[12] Blakemore and Jennett 2001: 116.

[13] On these ancient schemes, their influence, and the exceptional character of the option of one psychological centre and one location, see Tieleman 2003*a*: 34–9, and 61–88.

[14] Franz Joseph Gall is an important figure (late 1700s) in this respect; see Damasio 1994: 14–17, LeDoux 1998: 74–6.

cortex, generally taken to be the oldest and newest parts of the brain in evolutionary history. A recent handbook offers this summary of functions:

> The limbic system is involved in vital cyclical activity—including appetites and sexual cycles, and emotions such as fear, anger, and aggression—and in all-important short-term memory...The cerebral cortex...is responsible for the initiation of movements, and for interpreting input from all our sensory systems, as well as for integrating motor and sensory activity necessary for speech and other cognitive functions.[15]

This subdivision of functions in different parts of the brain might seem to reproduce in another version the Galenic–Platonic contrast between reason and, at least, one non-rational psychic part. However, this impression is misleading for two main reasons. For one thing, these two regions, and the functions with which they are associated, are seen as subdivisions or subsystems of a single integrated system or structure. As in the Stoic account, and unlike the Galenic one, there is great stress on interconnections and lines of communication within and between these subdivisions.[16] For another thing, these areas of the brain and their functions are not seen as independent, and potentially competing, sources of motivation in the way that Galen conceives his three centres. The picture is, rather, one in which emotions, for instance, or motivation to action, involve coordinated responses in both these sectors and possibly other parts of the brain and the rest of the body. Hence, the 'parts' involved are more like those assumed in the Stoic account of the psyche than in the Galenic picture.[17]

Within this broad framework of modern scientific thinking about the brain and its functions, there is scope for variation between different approaches about how far stress should fall on the role of subdivisions or on interconnections between sectors. For instance, in

[15] Blakemore and Jennett 2001: 116.

[16] On the complexity of internal brain communication, see Damasio 1994: 92–3. On intra-psychic communication in Stoicism (and Pl. *Ti.* 69–71), see LS 53 B(5–9), G(6–9), Ch. 3 above, text to nn. 38–44, and on its relative absence in Galen, see Ch. 3 above, text to nn. 72–4.

[17] On Stoic psychic 'parts' (i.e. subdivisions of the work of the control-centre), see LS 65 G, H, K; on the issue of the place of psychic parts in their thought-system, see 4.4 above.

two recent studies on the brain and emotions, LeDoux stresses the role of one subsystem in activating fear, while Damasio underlines the interconnection of different subsystems in producing fear and other emotions. These differences of emphasis reflect, in part at least, different programmes of research. LeDoux's work has centred on the role of the amygdala, part of the limbic system, especially in connection with conditioned fear in rats, though the work has implications for human emotions.[18] One of his themes is the idea that there are two routes in the production of fear, one involving the amygdala alone and one involving both the amygdala and the cortical region. The first route is more rapid and is purely instinctual and unconscious; the second is slower and involves consciousness. LeDoux explains the existence of the two routes in evolutionary terms. The more rapid, amygdala-based, route has played a crucial role in the survival mechanisms of animals. It persists in higher mammals, including human beings, alongside the more developed, but slower, route involving consciousness.[19] Damasio's work, on the other hand, has centred on cases where damage in one region of the brain has led to emotional deficiencies that also disable some rational functions.[20] This has led him to stress the idea that emotions depend on coordinated activity in both main sectors of the brain. In particular, he stresses that emotional responses, whether originating from the limbic or cortical sector or a combination of the two, may be indispensable for effective decision-making and ethically responsible behaviour.[21] More broadly, he emphasizes the idea that normal psychological activity involves multiple lines of communication in various directions across all sectors of the brain and, indeed, other parts of the body.[22]

At first glance, the differences between these two theories might lead one to suppose that we have an analogous contrast to the

[18] LeDoux 1998: ch. 6. [19] LeDoux 1998: 161–78.

[20] On brain damage in Phineas Gage (a 19th-cent. case) and modern examples, see Damasio 1994: chs. 1–4. The damage examined has been mainly in the prefrontal cortex, but this has consequences for the activation of emotion by the brain operating in a coordinated way.

[21] See e.g. Damasio 1994: xvi–xix, 83–4, 128, 139–40, 143–5, 180–3.

[22] See e.g. Damasio 1994: xxvi–xxvii, 92–3, 225–6.

approaches of Galen and Stoicism, stressing, on the one hand, a more part-based and, on the other, a more holistic picture of emotion and other psychological functions. However, this would be a misleading conclusion. Both thinkers refer positively to each other's work and present themselves as engaged in complementary programmes of research. More importantly, both thinkers conceive emotions in human beings as, normally, a coordinated, multi-level response involving different sectors of the brain and other bodily reactions. Also, both researchers accommodate the findings of the other in their overall analyses of emotion, though these are made from rather different standpoints. For instance, Damasio characterizes LeDoux's two routes for emotion, involving the amygdala alone or the amygdala and the cortex, as primary and secondary emotions.[23] He also introduces the idea of 'somatic markers', that is, intuitive emotional responses ('gut feelings'), which are primarily housed in the cortex even though they also involve other bodily reactions.[24] LeDoux also describes normal human emotions as complex reactions involving, as in Damasio's account, coordinated activity in different brain-sectors and bodily responses. However, he also stresses the activation of response in the amydala as the primary and indispensable element in the arousal of fear.[25] These analyses share the general modern picture of the brain outlined earlier, in which different sectors of the brain are seen as operating, in normal cases, as subdivisions or subsystems of an integrated whole, rather than as independent and competing sources of motivation.[26] This picture, as suggested earlier, is closer to the Stoic than the Galenic one. The modern view, as illustrated by these theories, thus serves to indicate, in contemporary form, the possible outcome of the combination of a Galenic-type

[23] Damasio 1994: 131–9, referring to the work of LeDoux and others on the amygdala in 133–4.

[24] Damasio 1994: 173–5, also 180–3 on the sector of the brain most likely to house these markers, the prefrontal cortices.

[25] LeDoux 1998: 296–9, also 284–5 on the amygdala as the more active partner in inter-communication with the cortex.

[26] See also, stressing integration and interconnection between sectors or functions of the brain, Lewis and Todd 2007 and Pessoa 2008, both discussing the relationship between cognition and emotion. I owe these references to my Exeter colleague in Philosophy, Giovanna Colombetti.

brain and nervous system with the Stoic idea of a unitary psychological centre.

I now consider modern parallels for a second combination of ideas, namely that of the Galenic brain and the Stoic unified or holistic account of psychological processes, especially their view of emotions as belief-based or informed by rationality. This aspect of Stoic thinking is related to their belief in a single psychological centre, rather than multiple centres, but it is not simply identical with that belief.[27] In the ancient context, the basis for this combination of ideas is less substantial than that of the Galenic brain and Stoic unitary control-centre. I highlighted earlier certain features of Galen's work and of earlier medical thought that indicate that emotions as well as reasoning is located in the brain.[28] But, in general, Galen's rejection of the Stoic conception of emotions is even more comprehensively negative than his critique of their heart-centred psychophysiology.[29] I have suggested that Galen's rejection is based in part on his misunderstanding of the nature of the Stoic theory of emotions. Their theory is a unified or holistic one, seeing emotions as informed by beliefs and reasoning, rather than the purely intellectualistic one that Galen supposes.[30] This point would not necessarily alter Galen's view, since he also rejects the Stoic idea of a unitary psychological centre. But this makes a difference when we transpose the issue to the modern intellectual context and think about the possibility of combining the modern scientific picture of the brain and a Stoic-style theory of the emotions.

In modern thought, the most obvious parallel for the Stoic theory is what is usually called the 'cognitive' theory of the emotions, by contrast with the theory that emotions involve an irreducibly non-cognitive element. The Stoic psychological theory is relatively exceptional in the ancient context,[31] and is sometimes seen by modern scholars as

[27] An alternative view—*not* the Stoic one—would have been that we have a single (bodily based) psychological centre which houses wholly distinct and independent functions.

[28] See Ch. 4 above, text to nn. 25–7.

[29] See 4.1, text to nn. 19–20 and 4.2 above.

[30] See Ch. 4 above, text to nn. 90–115.

[31] However, there are close similarities with Epicurean thought on emotions, as well as links with aspects of Platonic and Aristotelian theory; see further Gill 2006: ch. 2, and 2010.

extreme and implausible. So it is useful to note that cognitive theories of emotion form a well-developed strand in modern thinking, although there are also non-cognitive theories that are closer to the part-based (Platonic–Aristotelian) approach presupposed by Plutarch or Galen.[32] In fact, one recent cognitive theory of emotions, that of Martha Nussbaum (2001), is explicitly presented as a revival and adaptation of the Stoic approach. Her starting-point is the idea 'that emotions always involve thought of an object combined with thought of that object's salience or importance; in that sense, they always involve appraisal or evaluation'. By 'cognition', as she explains, she means nothing more than being 'concerned with receiving and processing information', rather than more elaborate mental processes such as calculation or reflexive self-awareness.[33] Her theory is also presented as 'cognitive-evaluative', since emotions are seen as part of goal-directed behaviour directed at securing one's good (broadly put, one's happiness).[34] In the course of her book, Nussbaum incorporates into her theory a number of dimensions that go well beyond the boundaries of Stoic thinking. But the core of her 'cognitive-evaluative' theory of emotions is, credibly, presented as a contemporary version of key features of the Stoic account.[35]

Nussbaum's theory is formulated, broadly speaking, in terms of the philosophy of mind; but her discussion takes account of a wide range of other disciplines, including recent research on emotions and the brain. She notes, in fact, the studies by LeDoux and Damasio discussed here, presenting them as 'non-reductive' accounts of the relation between physiology and psychology. More positively, she finds in both treatments, especially Damasio's, support for her analysis of emotions as modes of appraisal and as closely bound up with goal-directed activity. She sees their research programmes as

[32] For examples of both strands, see Nussbaum 2001: 22–7; for surveys of modern theories of emotions (including cognitive and non-cognitive types), see Rorty 1980 and Goldie 2010.

[33] Nussbaum 2001: 23.

[34] Nussbaum 2001: 23, also 4, on the three main ideas in her theory: 'cognitive appraisal or evaluation', 'one's flourishing or one's important goals and projects', 'the salience of external objects as elements in one's own scheme of goals' (italics deleted).

[35] See Nussbaum 2001: 3–6, 11–12, highlighting her departures from Stoic thought. On comparable features of Stoic thought on emotion, see Brennan 1998: 22–39, 2003: 265–74, Graver 2007: 24–59.

designed to illustrate by reference to the operation of sectors of the brain the functions of appraisal and evaluative response, in animals as well as humans, which she sees as fundamental for the nature of emotions.[36] This seems to be a credible reading of the implications of their theories. For instance, LeDoux's account of the two possible routes for fear, through the amygdala alone or through the amygdala and cortex, reflects a view of fear as part of a mode of appraisal ensuring defence from danger and thus survival. His analysis also expresses a picture of the brain as the outcome of evolutionary development that expresses the long-term results of such emotion-guided searches for survival and other objectives.[37] In Damasio's theory, emotional reactions (including 'somatic markers') play a key role in enabling people to make the decisions by which they shape their lives and relate to other people.[38] Obviously, much more could be said about the interface between cognitive theories of emotion and contemporary brain research. But these observations are enough to show that in the modern context the kind of combination being considered here, the combination of a Galenic-type view of the brain as the psychological centre and a Stoic-style view of emotions, is a clear conceptual possibility.

Can we establish more precise correlations between contemporary thought and the Galen–Stoicism debate in this respect? Richard Sorabji suggests some highly specific points of connection. Athough he sees Damasio's research as supporting a (Stoic-style) cognitive view of emotions, he presents at least one aspect of LeDoux's work as supporting a more Galenic, non-cognitive, account. LeDoux's demonstration that fear can sometimes be activated through the amygdala alone, without the operation of the cortex, and thus the cognitive functions associated with this region, is taken by Sorabji to be damaging for the Stoic theory. Sorabji suggests that this aspect of LeDoux's work supports the competing view, ascribed by Galen to Posidonius, that emotions are at least sometimes, in adult humans, activated by non-cognitive processes.[39] As indicated earlier, I think

36 Nussbaum 2001: 114–19, also 106–7 on Lazarus 1991.

37 LeDoux 1998: chs. 5–6, esp. 161–78.

38 See n. 21 above; also n. 41 below on 'somatic markers'.

39 Sorabji 2000: 144–50; see also his chs. 6–8 on Posidonius' criticisms of Chrysippus' account of emotions and emotional conflicts, as presented by Galen.

Galen's reports of Posidonius are highly misleading and that they need very close critical examination before they can be accepted as evidence.[40] But Sorabji's comments raise from another standpoint the question whether we can, in fact, find in these modern theories support for the idea of the combination of ideas I am considering, that is, contemporary brain research and Stoic-style cognitive accounts of emotion.

I think that some of the points noted earlier about the research of LeDoux and Damasio offer the basis for somewhat different conclusions about the implications for Stoic theory and modern research from those offered by Sorabji. In both these modern studies, we can find two different levels of emotion. In LeDoux's book, we find the distinction between the two alternative routes of fear. LeDoux also offers an account of emotions, such as fear, as complex, partly cognitive, processes, while presenting the amygdala-based response as the core, indispensable element. Analogously, Damasio distinguishes primary and secondary emotions, based on criteria similar to those of LeDoux's two routes. He also identifies what he calls somatic markers, which represent intuitive emotional reactions; though involving cortical (and in some sense cognitive) responses, these do not constitute the conscious appraisals that form part of more full-blown emotions.[41] The distinction between these two levels seems to me to correspond rather closely to a contrast drawn in Stoic thinking between 'pre-emotions' (*propatheiai*) and 'emotions' (*pathē*) in the full sense. Pre-emotions are affective responses to situations, such as an involuntary shudder in danger, which can be characterized either in physical or psychological terms. But they lack key elements of emotions, as conceived in Stoicism. Notably they lack the element of belief (in Stoic terms, the assent to rational impressions) 'that it is appropriate to react' in a given way, which is seen as triggering the physiological and psychological responses characteristic of emotions in the full sense. Although our fullest evidence for Stoic pre-emotions is rather late (in Seneca's *On Anger*), recent work suggests that the idea may go back much earlier, and that it is

[40] See Ch. 4, text to nn. 82–9. See also Tieleman 2003*a*: ch. 5 and Gill 2006: 266–90. [41] See text to nn. 23–5 above.

consistent with orthodox Stoic thinking on the nature of emotion.[42] If we can accept the analogy between these two levels of affective response in Stoic theory and in these modern studies of brain research, the ancient and modern theories may seem to offer a similar overall picture. In both the ancient and the modern theories, both levels of emotion involve cognition, or at least the transmission of information, and an evaluative reaction. But the first level is basic or instinctive whereas the second is conscious or fully articulated, with corresponding differences at the physiological level.

However, in spite of the resemblance noted, this aspect of Stoic thinking brings out a point on which Stoic thinking and modern thinking of this type diverge. Although there is, as noted, some evidence for the idea of pre-emotions, the overwhelming weight in Stoic theory falls on emotions in the full sense, and on the way that certain kinds of beliefs generate specific types of psychological and physiological reactions. This fact, in turn, reflects a further, more general, point, the close integration of psychological with ethical thought, which expresses, in turn, the holistic integration of the different branches of knowledge in Stoic theory. Emotions are important in part because, unlike instinctive pre-emotions, they are ethical actions, reflecting the underlying belief-structure of adult humans as agents or rational animals.[43] They also reflect the state of ethical development of the person concerned—more precisely, their failure to complete development towards the state of mind and character in which (defective) emotions are replaced by 'good emotions', a development that all human beings are fundamentally capable of making. Associated ideas are that the emotional state of defective non-wise people, that is, virtually all of us, is one of 'feverish' instability and incoherence by contrast with the stability and coherence of which we are all capable.[44] This set of ideas finds no clear equivalent, as far as I am aware, in modern thinking either about the cognitive nature of emotions or about emotions and brain research. On the contrary, in the scientific theories noted and for

[42] See Sen. *Ira* 2.1–4, Gel. 19.1.171–8 (LS 65 Y); also Graver 1999, 2007: 85–108, 125–32, Gill 2006: 279–81.

[43] These points are brought out clearly in Inwood 1985: ch. 5, Brennan 1998, 2003: 269–79.

[44] See Ch. 4 above, text to nn. 146–54.

Nussbaum too, instinctive or intuitive reactions are as important as fully formed emotions in shaping the goal-directed behaviour of animals, including humans.[45] For Damasio, for instance, 'somatic markers' (intuitive pre-emotions) play a vital role in enabling human beings to make the decisions by which they shape their lives.[46] This difference does not mean that ethical and normative considerations are entirely absent from the modern theories. Nussbaum's theory of emotions (like the Stoic one) is 'cognitive-evaluative';[47] and the scientific theories also presuppose that emotions constitute forms of (more or less conscious) evaluative appraisal and in this sense at least are ethical responses. However, the ethical or normative dimension in these modern theories is not developed in the same way as in Stoic thought, for instance, as regards the radical distinction between the wise and non-wise person, and does not lead to a view of emotions as generally misguided.[48] Whether or not there are equivalents in modern theory of any type for these features of Stoic thought is a further and more complex question;[49] but the differences noted mark the limits of the analogy between Stoic and modern theory of brain research and cognitive emotions.

I have suggested that we can find modern analogues for the combination of Galen's view that the control-centre is housed in the brain and a Stoic (unitary) conception of how that control-centre works. We can also find at least partial parallels for the idea that the unitary psychological centre is the home of cognitive (belief-based) emotions, though differences between modern and Stoic thought emerge which reflect different ways of understanding the ethical or normative status of emotions. What implications do these points have for reflecting on Galen's rejection of these aspects of Stoic

[45] Note Nussbaum's minimal requirements for the notion of 'cognitive' (i.e. transmitting information) (2001: 23), also her p. 5 on her difference from the Stoics in recognizing emotions in animals.

[46] Damasio 1994: 173–83.

[47] Nussbaum 2001: 23 (also 4).

[48] Nussbaum 2001: 11–12 explicitly distinguishes her position from Stoicism in this respect. She characterizes her implied normative framework as that of 'a liberal brand of Aristotelianism or... a flexible virtue-oriented type of Kantianism' (12).

[49] Becker 1998 offers a vigorous modern restatement and defence of Stoic ethics and, to some extent, psychology; but his account is not linked with brain research or physiology.

thought and thus for his failure to construct the kind of conceptual combinations outlined here? In one, rather straightforward, way, these points are irrelevant to Galen's thinking, since he could have had no knowledge of them. However, in another way, the existence of these combinations in modern thought can be seen as having implications for Galen's thought. Earlier (3.2–3), I argued that the first type of combination considered, that of Galen's idea of the brain and the Stoic control-centre, was a conceptual possibility for both ancient theories, in terms of their categories. Also, I argued, the combination of the idea of a unitary (brain-based) control centre and 'nature', as conceived in Stoic thought, would have avoided a number of tensions and awkward features or gaps in his own theory. A powerful consideration for Galen against adopting the Stoic view was the fact that his own position was based on a cogent method of natural inquiry (what I called his logico-empirical method), whereas the Stoic position was based on what he saw as a defective method.[50] If Galen had been convinced that the Stoic picture of a unitary control-centre could also be based on a powerful method of natural inquiry, presumably, his response would have been very different. My suggestion is that modern brain research offers what Galen would have seen as arguments based on sound methodology for supposing that the Stoic picture, or at least a picture much closer to this than to Galen's three-centre theory, is a valid one. My supposition is that, confronted with these arguments, Galen too would have adopted a unitary model that would have rendered his own account more consistent and cogent.[51]

A possible objection to this suggestion is that Galen's adherence to Platonic ideas would have rendered impossible the adoption of a unitary account of the control-centre. It might also be thought that allegiance to Plato's part-based psychology would also make it unthinkable for him to have accepted the second combination of ideas discussed here, the combination of brain-centred psychophysiology and a cognitive or belief-based theory of emotions. It is certainly true that Galen allocates a special status to Plato as a philosophical

[50] See Ch. 2 above, text to nn. 92–110, 135–40.

[51] On the relationship between Galen and modern scientific method, see Ch. 2 above, text to nn. 104–10.

influence, and that the union of Platonic and 'Hippocratic' (medical) ideas is fundamental to the project of *PHP.* On the other hand, as pointed out earlier, Galen is an explicitly independent thinker without fixed allegiances and with his own distinctive medico-philosophical projects. His version of 'Platonic' (and also of 'Hippocratic') ideas is often highly selective and shaped by his own objectives.[52] Particularly in some later works, including *Foet. Form.*, *QAM*, and *Prop. Plac.*, Galen is capable of taking a detached or even critical attitude towards Plato's ideas, notably psyche–body dualism.[53] Thus, I suggested earlier, Galen's adoption of the Platonic tripartite psyche in *PHP,* rather than the Stoic unitary psyche, is likely to have been based on the belief that it matched his brain-centred anatomical theory, and not on doctrinal allegiance.[54]

It was, presumably, the embodied tripartite psyche of *Timaeus* 69–72 that he saw as most serviceable for this purpose, although he conflates this with the tripartite psychology of the *Republic,* eliding differences between these accounts.[55] In fact, as I have argued, the attempted combination of the Platonic tripartite psyche with the findings of Galen's anatomical inquiries gives rise to a whole series of difficulties in *PHP*;[56] but this is not how Galen sees the position. Galen's engagement with ethical psychology in *PHP* 4–5, in particular, with the question of the relationship between reason and emotion or desire arose as a by-product of his primary concern with psychophysiology.[57] Having already committed himself to the Platonic embodied tripartite psyche, rather than the Stoic unitary psyche, Galen aligns himself with the Platonic approach to ethical psychology, as he interprets this.[58] He adopts a part-based, non-holistic account of the psyche and a non-cognitive theory of emotion and desire. He also presupposes the Platonic (or Platonic–Aristotelian) view of ethical development, which is a corollary of part-based psychology, and rejects the Stoic

[52] See Ch. 2 above, text to nn. 40–4, Ch. 4 above, text to nn. 28–31.

[53] See Ch. 3 above, text to nn. 182–3, 238–40.

[54] See Ch. 4 above, text to nn. 28–31.

[55] See Ch. 3 above, text to nn. 120–38.

[56] See Ch. 3 above, text to nn. 72–91.

[57] See Ch. 4 above, text to nn. 8–13, 55–6.

[58] As highlighted in Ch. 4 above, text to nn. 178–84, there is much scope for debate about the proper way of interpreting the significance of Plato's ethical psychology in the *Republic,* and more cognitive readings of Plato's theory are possible. On this point and for a possible 'Chrysippean' reading of Plato's psychology, see Gill 2006: 309–22.

view, which is linked with holistic psychology.[59] Once these intellectual commitments are made in *PHP*, they reappear in subsequent ethical contexts, including *Mor.*, *Aff. Dig.*, and *QAM* ch. 11. This is so even though they are at odds with the broadly Stoic framework and objectives assumed in *Aff. Dig.*[60] The tenacity with which Galen maintains Platonic-style part-based psychology and ideas about development should not lead us to overlook the fact that Galen, probably, originally adopted these ideas in an indirect or *ad hoc* way, as a way of supplementing his anatomically based location of the control-centre in the brain.[61] Also, despite the vigour with which Galen maintains these positions, they do not derive from the exercise of a distinctive methodology or expertise in the same way as his medical technique and natural inquiry. Paradoxically, it seems to me, Galen looks for support in Platonic-style ethical psychology to substantiate a theory (about the location of the psychological control-centre) that does not really need this support and does not gain much from it either.

In the modern context, as highlighted earlier, we can find the combination of (1) brain-based psychophysiology, (2) a unitary psychological centre, and (3) a cognitive theory of emotions. As with the previous combination of ideas, one might hope that Galen's attitude might have changed if he had seen convincing versions of this combination. I can see no conceptual reason why Galen, if he had been presented with effective ancient analogues for this set of ideas, should not have recognized their force. More complex issues are raised by the third combination of ideas outlined here: that is, the integration of Stoic ethical principles with (brain-based) unitary and cognitive psychology. In the modern context, as noted earlier, it is harder to locate an equivalent for this combination. This aspect of Galen's response is more undeveloped and it is difficult to tell how far he is aware of the links between Stoic psychology and ethics, and of the implications of this linkage for their ideas about emotions and ethical development.[62] However, in the other two respects considered here, modern parallels serve, I think, to bring out the credibility and coherence of the

[59] See Ch. 4 above, text to nn. 185–221. [60] See 5.2 above.

[61] See Ch. 4 above, text to nn. 8–13, 55–6.

[62] The most explicit engagement with Stoic ethics comes in *PHP* V.589–600, 7.1.9–3 De Lacy, on the question of the unity or plurality of the virtues. But Galen attacks Stoic psychology and theory of development in *PHP* 4–5 and *QAM* ch. 11,

combination of ideas involved. My hypothesis is that Galen too might have seen this coherence, if the position had been presented to him in this form (at least that he would have had good reason to do so), and that he could have produced in this way a Galenic–Stoic synthesis of ideas on psychology that would have been consistent with the 'high naturalistic' approach he shares with Stoicism.

6.3 GALENIC AND STOIC PSYCHOTHERAPY AND MODERN PARALLELS

I now turn to the question of modern parallels for Galenic and Stoic approaches to the therapy of the emotions. How do the Chrysippean and Galenic essays discussed in Chapter 5 relate to anything we might call 'psychotherapy', in modern terms? In the light of discussion of modern parallels, I return to the issue raised at the end of Chapter 5, which is similar to that discussed in the preceding section (6.2).What scope was there—or could there have been—for a combination of Galenic medical technique and the Stoic approach to the therapy of the emotions? I begin by locating these questions in a much broader context, namely the relationship between ancient and modern practices or ideas as regards the treatment of mental or psychological illness. I then consider, more specifically, how Galenic and Stoic techniques relate to modern methods. Finally, I ask if this comparison makes more credible the possibility of combination or synthesis of Galenic and Stoic approaches in this area, thus complementing the possible linkages discussed in 6.2

If one compares, in a general way, ancient and modern approaches to the treatment of psychological or mental illness, one feature especially stands out. This is the expansion in the modern context of the role of medicine or medical approaches, in comparison with other types of treatment. In the Greco-Roman world of the second century AD, for instance, as in most periods of Classical Antiquity, doctors often found themselves in competition with priests

for instance, without giving any indication that he recognizes that these ideas reflect a distinctive approach to ethics. See further Ch. 3 above, text to nn. 282–3, and 4.2.

or philosophers, among others, in this respect.[63] Hence, in looking for ancient analogues for modern techniques of psychotherapy, promising areas include the interface between religion and medicine or medicine and philosophy.[64] In modern Western society, by contrast, medicine has consolidated its position, in relation to other approaches, in two main ways. One is that some of the standard methods of modern medicine, especially chemical drugs and, to a much more limited extent, brain surgery, have been applied extensively to the treatment of mental illness.[65] This means that modern medicine has access to methods not available in the ancient world, methods which seem to be relatively successful, at least in controlling behaviour. The other main difference is that techniques of therapeutic dialogue, of widely differing kinds, have been developed and applied in medical settings or from a medical standpoint. The most famous and pioneering method is Freudian-style psychoanalysis, originally developed within a medical framework, though now largely practised independently. The reputation of psychoanalysis has helped to promote the use of a wide range of types of therapeutic dialogue, falling under the general heading of 'psychotherapy', used either in conjunction with institutional medical treatment or separately.[66] Hence, medical approaches, broadly understood, have been extended to a type of response to psychological illness, namely therapeutic dialogue, that was dominated in the ancient world by philosophy. These changes mean that the overall 'map' of types of treatment and expertise for psychological illness is very different from that in any period or type of ancient culture, including that of second-century AD Greco-Roman elite society.

In discussing ancient types of therapy, I considered how far they were directed at the body, the psyche, or a combination (or

[63] An interesting marginal case, important both from the religious and the medical standpoint, is the cult of Asclepius, god of medicine, which is still very significant for Galen. See Lloyd 2003: chs. 3 and 8, on the interface of medicine and religion; also M. Frede 2003, on Galen's theology.

[64] See further Gill 1985*a*, with discussion of specific material on these borderlines; also Pigeaud 1981 on the interface between medicine and philosophy regarding psychotherapy.

[65] On these treatments, see the surveys on 'psychopharmacology' and 'psychosurgery' in Gregory 2004, also on surgery on the brain, Damasio 1994: chs. 1–4. The use of surgery in cases of psychological illness is ethically problematic except in special cases, such as localized brain damage.

[66] On types of psychotherapy, see text to nn. 77–80 below.

synthesis) of both. In broad terms, I suggested, there was a clear distinction between ancient medical technique directed at the body and philosophical method (mostly in dialogue form) directed at the psyche. This generalization applies, I argued, to Stoic therapeutic methods, even though Stoic theory presupposes that people are psychophysical wholes.[67] In the modern context, a comparable distinction can be drawn within the two main types of (broadly) medical treatment for psychological illness. Drug-based or surgical treatment is applied to people as bodies, though the objective, of course, is to modify their psychological states in the short or long term. Psychotherapy, by contrast, is directed to people as, in various ways, psychological agents or minds, although the treatment may issue in changes that affect physical health. This distinction applies, I think, to most conventional medical or medical-type therapy in a modern Western culture such as Great Britain. However, there has also emerged in recent years, in Britain and elsewhere, an active 'alternative' movement, offering a range of therapies that are more 'holistic' in various ways, and are directed at the person as a psychophysical whole. Some of these, including reflexology or aromatherapy, are physically based, but aim to affect the whole person, in mood and attitude as well as bodily state. Others, such as the 'journey-work' therapy developed by Brandon Bays, use dialogue or 'scripts' to explore the psychological roots of mental or physical problems. A related development, with very wide influence, is a focus on diet, life-style, and attitude, treated as factors with a major impact on psychological as well as physical health. The explicit aim of much of this therapy is to break down what is seen as a rigid mind–body distinction in much conventional health-care, in the case of both physical and psychological illness. These movements have started to have a significant impact on some aspects of conventional medical practice, for instance in the treatment of cancer.[68]

How do Galenic or Stoic forms of therapy appear, if we consider them against the background of the modern map of treatments? In

[67] See Ch. 5 above, text to nn. 242–89.

[68] See further Bays 1999; also (on diet) McKeith 2004. Rosie Daniel, formerly at the independent Bristol Cancer Clinic, has developed a 'Health Creation Package'

Galen's case, to take this first, there are some rather striking implications. One is that Galen's standard medical approach, like that of ancient medicine generally, emerges as relatively broad, and to a degree at least, 'holistic', in comparison with conventional modern medical treatment. The part of Galen's medical treatment that bears most directly on psychological states is 'hygiene' or treatment of 'regime' (*diaita*), including diet, environment, and to some extent attitude and life-style as well.[69] By comparison with much modern Western medicine, focused on extensive use of chemical drugs and surgery, even in the treatment of psychological illness, ancient medicine (including Galen's) appears close to some strands in modern 'alternative' medicine. However, in some ways, I think this impression of breadth is rather misleading, as far as Galen is concerned. If we consider what is distinctive in Galen's medical technique, it consists in a highly systematic and research-based method of treating *the body*, rather than the person as a whole.[70] The emphasis on 'hygienic', and on what we might see as preventive medicine, is a feature shared with ancient medicine generally, which reflects its relative lack of resources for interventionist treatments rather than expressing a programmatic focus on the person as a whole.[71] Also, certain of Galen's special emphases might predispose him towards the characteristic modern medical approach to mental illness. His stress on the importance of the 'mixtures' of elements in the body as a determinant of psychological, as well as physical, capacities and qualities, expressed most strongly in *QAM*, might make modern drug-based treatment of psychic illness very attractive to Galen.[72]

including diet and psychological support for cancer. (I owe these references to my late wife Karen.)

69 See Ch. 5 above, text to nn. 299–305.

70 See van der Eijk 2008, and Ch. 5 above, text to nn. 290–8.

71 Pharmacology formed an important part of ancient medicine, and is treated extensively by Galen e.g. in *On the Properties of Simple Drugs* (*SMT*); see further Vogt 2008. But these are not drugs produced by chemical means; and, from a modern standpoint, ancient pharmacology overlaps with dietetics.

72 See further Ch. 2 above, text to nn. 163–9; also Ch. 3 above, text to nn. 226–31. In *QAM* ch. 9, IV.807–8, *SM* 2.67.2–16 (trans. Singer 1997*a*: 169), Galen focuses esp. on regimen as exemplifying his body-based method of treating psychic states. But the underlying logic of *QAM* points towards the use of drugs to improve the body's 'mixtures' of elements.

Also, his path-breaking anatomical work, especially on the brain and central nervous system, would render of special interest the possibility of treating certain mental illness by surgical intervention.[73] In these respects, Galen's distinctive methods and interests fit rather closely with the more narrowly medical, body-based, aspects of modern health-care for psychological illness, despite the fact that he shares the characteristically ancient awareness of the importance of regime.

Galen, of course, has broader objectives than is normal in modern medicine in one respect. He was also exceptional in the ancient context in that he aimed to be a doctor both of the body and the psyche, writing essays on the therapy of the emotions (*Aff. Dig.*, *Indol.*), as well as providing medical treatment.[74] In this respect, his work offers analogues for both of the main strands in modern medical therapy. However, this raises the question how we should understand the relationship between ancient and modern versions of therapy for the psyche, a question that also bears, of course, on the understanding of Stoic therapy. This question is more difficult than that raised by the relationship between ancient and modern medicine. Broadly speaking, we can see modern medicine as having similar objectives and, indeed, comparable methods to those of ancient medicine, even though modern technical resources are immensely richer and the institutional and socio-cultural frameworks are different. But, in the case of the therapy of the psyche, it is more difficult to know whether we are comparing like with like. Is there really such a practice as 'ancient psychotherapy'[75] or does the modern shift, relocating this type of therapy from the realm of philosophy to medicine, mean that the project has become radically different? After all, although ancient therapy is sometimes addressed to people who are in distress and need help, its more revisionist forms, especially those of Stoicism and Epicureanism, are directed to people in general, who may not regard themselves as psychologically sick at all.[76] However, it is worth pursuing the question

[73] On this side of his work, see Rocca 2003 and Ch. 2 above, text to nn. 101–10, 137–40. [74] See 5.2 above.

[75] For this question, see e.g. Gill 1985*a*: also Pigeaud 1981: 525–39, and, as far as Galen is concerned, Ballester 1988: 118–21. Sorabji 2000: part 2 offers a full and interesting review of ancient philosophical therapies with some modern parallels.

[76] On Stoic–Epicurean approaches to psychic 'illness' and therapy, see Ch. 5 above, text to nn. 3–5, 14–16, also 5.3–4. On this point of difference between modern

of the relationship between ancient and modern therapy of the psyche, since this is revealing, I think, for both sides of the comparison.

A useful initial move is to distinguish some of the main strands in modern therapy and then to see how far these correspond to aspects of the ancient therapy of emotions. In the modern context, we can distinguish between (1) counselling, (2) cognitive therapy, and (3) psychotherapy, which covers a diverse range of techniques. Counselling is offered, normally, by trained non-medics to people suffering from situational problems, such as bereavement or difficulties with interpersonal relationships. Cognitive therapy, as I understand this, is provided by psychologists (not doctors) and is used, typically, to respond to relatively determinate psychological problems. including phobias, eating disorders, and certain types of anxiety.[77] 'Psychotherapy' is a very broad category, practised by people trained in psychology, psychiatry, or types of analysis (such as Freudian), as well as those using 'alternative' methods.[78] Although it is difficult to identify a single common quality, psychotherapy tends to be marked by a more extended series of sessions and a developing relationship between therapist and patient or client. Also, at least some forms of therapy employ methods such as free-association, meditation, or interpretation of dreams, which are designed to explore the underlying, unconscious roots of psychological (or physical) problems, rather than addressing them explicitly as is more normal in the case of counselling and cognitive therapy. None of these methods is usually deployed as the primary response to people in acute states of mental illness (psychosis or schizophrenia), who are, typically, treated with drugs.[79] They may form part of the long-term, rehabilitative, response to such acute

and (much) ancient therapy, see Gill 1985*a*: 321–3. See also Sorabji 2000: ch. 11, responding on pp. 159–60 to Williams's critique of ancient philosophical therapy on this score (Williams 1997). For the suggestion that ancient philosophical therapy *is* sometimes directed at what we would call 'neurosis', see Pigeaud 1981: 512–18.

[77] On modern cognitive therapy, and its targets and methods, see Sorabji 2000: 153–5.

[78] For a useful general account, see Storr 1979, used as the starting-point for Gill 1985*a*, which tries to correlate ancient and modern practices.

[79] Only exceptionally is psychotherapy used for acute mental illness; this approach is advocated by Karon and VanDenBos 1981 and was taken as fundamental by the radical British psychoanalyst R. D. Laing.

states, but are also, more normally, deployed in the case of people with relatively mild states of psychological illness or problems.[80]

This bare outline of modern methods highlights some of the differences that arise when the therapy of emotions is located within a medical or quasi-medical framework. Any attempt to correlate this set of practices with ancient ones needs also to take account of the nature of our ancient sources and of divergences within these. Most of the relevant texts are what one might call exemplary exercises in therapy. They are texts (letters or essays) offering advice addressed to a particular addressee but more broadly directed to readers in similar situations.[81] Seneca's letters, and in a different way, Marcus Aurelius' meditations, are unusual in providing a sequence of such communications addressed to the same person; in Seneca's case, his friend and contemporary Lucilius and in Marcus' case, himself.[82] Of the two works mainly discussed here, Chrysippus' 'therapeutic' book is a highly theoretical work, though it seems to have included some discussion about the practical application of this type of therapy. Galen's essays (*Aff. Dig.* and *Indol.*), and also Seneca's *On Anger*, which was influenced by Chrysippus' book, constitute works of exemplary therapy, though they also incorporate more theoretical elements.[83]

Correlating this kind of ancient material with modern practices is, of course, quite difficult. However, I think, one can make some general comments which meet the needs of the present inquiry. The context and approach envisaged in most works of ancient philosophical therapy is closer to that of modern counselling than to cognitive therapy or psychotherapy. The psychological states addressed are mostly emotional reactions to external situations, such as bereavement or other situational problems, rather than the kinds of phobias or delusions typically tackled by cognitive therapy or the (often long-term)

[80] On modern psychiatric practice, see also Lloyd 2003: 243–4, referring to Kaplan and Sadock 1996, for an outline of modern methods, and Luhrmann 2000, which underlines sharp diversities in modern pathology and treatment.

[81] See e.g. Sen. *Ira*, a three-book essay addressed to his brother Novatus and *On Peace of Mind* (*De Tranquillitate Animi*), presented as a dialogue between Seneca and Serenus.

[82] See further, on texts of this type, as forms of therapeutic discourse (and as exercises in practical ethics), Nussbaum 1994, Hadot 1995, 1998, Gill 2003: 40–50, 2008*d*, Griffin 2007, Sellars 2003, 2007.

[83] See 5.2–3 above.

neurosis or anxiety addressed by psychotherapy.[84] Also, as in modern counselling, and also cognitive therapy, as I understand these practices, the methods are essentially rational, appealing to the subject as a psychological agent, rather than using free association or other methods designed to probe unconscious sources of illness or distress. On the other hand, unlike most modern counselling and cognitive therapy, but like some modern psychotherapy, ancient therapeutic method is supported by highly developed theories about the nature of psychological illness and cure. There is also a strongly revisionist dimension in some ancient therapy, especially Stoic, in relation to conventional ideas about psychology and ethics, which has parallels with some modern versions of psychotherapy, including Freud's. Hence, although there is a general difficulty in knowing whether the term, 'psychotherapy', or therapy of the psyche, means anything like the same thing in ancient and modern contexts, there are some specific points of comparison and contrast that are worth exploring.

I now pursue these points in rather more detail, focusing initially on the implications for understanding the Stoic therapy of emotions. In correlating ancient and modern ideas and practices, it is important to distinguish between (1) therapeutic contexts, (2) therapeutic methods, and (3) implied or underlying psychological theories. (1) In the case of Stoic therapy, for instance, as with ancient therapy generally, the context envisaged is more like that of modern counselling, enabling people to confront specific problems and the reactions they produce, such as bereavement or material loss, rather than responding to phobias or tackling neuroses. (2) The therapeutic method employed is that of rational argument or persuasion, rather than techniques of free association designed to recover buried or unconscious memories. In this respect, at least, we can say that Stoic therapy is 'cognitive' in approach, though in its targets and approach it is not very similar to modern 'cognitive therapy'.[85] (3) Stoic

[84] On the contrast with modern cognitive therapy, see Sorabji 2000: 152–5. On Stoic therapy as a response to (what is normally regarded as) disaster, Sorabji 2000: 173–80, and, on ancient therapeutic techniques generally, see his ch. 15.

[85] This difference is brought out in Sorabji 2000: 153–5. Although he repeatedly characterizes Stoic therapy as 'cognitive' (his chs. 10–11), this is, presumably, because it assumes a cognitive approach to the emotions, rather than because its aims are like those of modern cognitive therapy.

therapy, especially as expressed in Chrysippus' 'therapeutic' book, is supported by a strong theoretical basis. As highlighted earlier, the core of Chrysippus' therapeutic method consists in conveying key features of Stoic theory.[86] As in some modern psychotherapeutic approaches, notably Freud's, Stoic therapy is closely linked with well-elaborated theories about human psychology and development, which are highly revisionist, considered in relation to conventional ideas of their day. In particular, Stoic therapy, again like much modern psychotherapy, rests on a distinctive theory about what causes and constitutes psychological breakdown or collapse of personality and how the personality can be reconstructed, or properly constructed for the first time. Much of Stoic thinking on emotions, and emotional dispositions, as forms of 'feverish' sickness, and on ethical development as progress towards wholeness and 'health', can be understood in these terms and seen as analogous to modern psychotherapeutic therapy.[87] In these respects, Stoic therapy at least is closer in its theoretical framework to modern psychotherapy or psychoanalysis than to counselling or cognitive therapy, even though its methods of therapeutic dialogue are substantially different from those of most modern psychotherapy.

The main features of Stoic thinking about psychology and about the collapse and rebuilding of the personality are, of course, strikingly different from much modern psychotherapeutic theory, especially Freud's. Freud's therapeutic method is based on bringing to consciousness repressed, mostly sexual, memories and desire, as well as on a radical new theory about the partition of the personality between conscious and non-conscious (or partly conscious) elements.[88] Stoic theory does not have an analogous concern with uncovering repressed sexual experiences; and Stoic unified or holistic psychological theory is, on the face of it, in sharp contrast with Freudian partition of the self. On the other hand, Stoic

[86] See Ch. 5 above, text to nn. 146–56.

[87] See further Ch. 4 above, text to nn. 116–54, Ch. 5 above, text to nn. 271–85. On these, core, aspects of Stoic therapy, see Nussbaum 1994: chs. 9–10, and (from a rather critical standpoint) Sorabji 2000: 159–93.

[88] See further (in outline) Gregory 2004: 356–60, also 353–5 (on free association). On Freud's philosophy of mind, see Wollheim and Hopkins 1982, and, for comparison with Platonic partition of the personality, Santas 1988, Price 1990.

therapy has in common with Freudian and other modern psychotherapeutic approaches the belief that progressive self-knowledge and the understanding of the nature of human psychology play a key role in helping people to cure psychological illness and reconstruct their personality. Earlier, I stressed that, in spite of the Stoic unified or holistic psychological framework, Chrysippus offers some very striking and illuminating analyses of internal conflict, as in the case of Medea and the explanation why grief reduces over time while (some) beliefs remain intact.[89] The overall aim of presenting these and other analyses of psychological conflict and collapse is, surely, to promote (what the Stoics see as) a correct understanding of what constitutes a sound or healthy personality and its opposite, and thus to help people gain self-knowledge by relating their states to these paradigms. In this sense, Stoicism too, like Freudian analysis, aims at extending the boundaries of one's consciousness or self-understanding with a view to effecting psychological cure, even though the conception of consciousness or self-knowledge in each of the two theories is very different. A further point of similarity, noted earlier, is that Stoic theories of psychology and development, like those of some modern psychotherapeutic approaches, are radically revisionist, in relation to conventional, or earlier theoretical, thinking. Indeed, for Chrysippus, as for Freud, conveying the force of his innovative ideas about psychology and about what constitutes psychic health and sickness, was central for his therapeutic strategy.[90]

These points of resemblance between the ancient therapy of the emotions and modern psychotherapy apply more strongly to Stoic (and Epicurean) theory,[91] than to the Galenic therapy of emotions.

[89] See Ch. 4 above, text to nn. 138–45, Ch. 5 above, text to nn. 194–203.

[90] On Chrysippus' core strategy, see Ch. 5 above, text to nn. 146–75; on Freud, see refs. in n. 88 above, also Trilling 1971: 140–59, which locates Freud's revisionist approach to psychology in the history of modern ideas about sincerity and authenticity.

[91] Similar points could be made about Epicurean therapy, which depends on showing people that an unconscious or unrecognized fear of death (together with other 'empty') desires makes their state of mind anxious and disturbed. See e.g. Lucr. 3. 31–93, 1053–75, Epicur. *Ep. Men.* 124–7 (LS 24 E(5)); also Gill 2008*d*: 374–7. On the parallel with Freud's thinking about the unconscious (and differences between them), see Nussbaum 1994: 196–201, Warren 2004: 21 n. 3, 219. On therapeutic tactics in Philodemus, and their theoretical assumptions, see Tsouna 2007: 74–87.

Indeed, within Stoic thinking about therapy, they apply more strongly to the core, theoretically informed, aspects of Chrysippus' approach than to the more pragmatic considerations, about timing and about how to address different people, which also formed part of Chrysippus' ideas.[92] Galen's essays (*Aff. Dig.* and *Indol.*), like some earlier eclectic therapeutic writings, such as Plutarch's *On Peace of Mind*,[93] are less theoretical in focus than Chrysippus' book seems to have been. Galen's essay, again like much earlier therapeutic writings, apart from those written from a Stoic or Epicurean standpoint, is also less revisionist in relation to conventional or earlier philosophical thought. Even so, Galen's essay too contains theoretically informed discussion about psychological structures and about ethical development, though in *Aff. Dig.*, at least, this is not altogether consistent with the therapeutic method being applied.[94] To this extent, Galen's essays might seem to be more like modern counselling or cognitive therapy in approach. Although Galen also aims to promote self-knowledge and a grasp of what constitutes a sound psychological structure, this side of his objectives is less fully grounded in theory as well as less revisionist than Stoic therapy or (at least) some modern psychotherapy.[95]

In the light of this comparison between Stoic and Galenic modes of therapy of the psyche and modern approaches, I return to the question raised earlier, about how far it would have been conceptually possible to combine Galen's approach to medical therapy and the Stoic therapy of the emotions. I suggested that this combination might have seemed fairly straightforward from a Stoic standpoint, though less so for Galen, mainly because of his reservations about—or limited understanding of—the objectives of Stoic therapy of the emotions, especially in its more revisionist aspects. The rationale for this combination is that each represents, arguably, the best and most influential ancient example of its type; and so the combination of the two (if they are indeed compatible)

[92] See Ch. 5 above, text to nn. 177–93.

[93] On the therapeutic strategy of this essay, see Gill 1994: 4624–31.

[94] See 5.2 above, text to nn. 56–76.

[95] See further 5.2 above; also Ch. 5, text to nn. 223–30, on the more practical side of Seneca's *On Anger*; and Sorabji 2000: ch. 15 on the kind of practical advice offered in ancient therapy.

would constitute an especially powerful one.[96] In connection with the Stoic–Galenic combinations considered in the preceding section (6.2), I suggested that the implication of modern parallels was to make the combinations seem more credible. What is the effect of approaching the question raised here against the background of modern practices and concerns?

I think that there are several features of the modern situation that might make one inclined to look positively on *any* attempt to integrate body-based and psychological approaches to illness (both mental and physical illness). By contrast with the ancient position, as brought out earlier, there has been a huge expansion of methods of treatment of mental illness, both in the form of body-based treatment, especially drugs, and of types of psychotherapy and counselling. However, I think there is a rather general view (not just confined to 'alternative' movements) that these methods could and should be more closely linked and integrated than they usually are. Also, I think there is a growing recognition that treatment of physical illness, for instance, cancer, should be handled in a more 'holistic' way, which complements drug-based or surgical treatment with attention to psychological factors including life-style and attitude.[97] From this modern standpoint, at least, certain aspects of ancient medical or social practice take on an added interest and suggestiveness. This applies, for instance, to the substantial role given in ancient medicine to regime (*diaita*), embracing factors such as diet, environment, and mode of life, and giving scope, as illustrated earlier in Galen's writings, for exploration of the interface between physical and psychological factors in health and treatment.[98] Also striking, in this connection, is the fact that a major medical practitioner such as Galen finds it appropriate to write essays on the therapy of emotions as well as on body-based treatment, though we might hope for a more complete integration between these two sides of his work than we find in Galen.[99] So,

[96] See Ch. 5 above, text to nn. 230–1. [97] See text to nn. 65–8, 77–80 above.

[98] See Ch. 5, text to nn. 299–305. Works such as Galen's *On the Preservation of Health* and Plutarch's *Advice on Healthcare* (*Mor.* 122 B–137 E), on which see Van Hoof 2010, take on new interest in this connection. This emerged in a seminar on these texts at Exeter involving Classical scholars and medical researchers.

[99] See Ch. 5 above, text to nn. 90–8.

from this modern perspective, exploring the implications of the combination of what are, arguably, the most impressive examples of ancient medical and psychological treatment (Galenic body-based medicine and Stoic psychological therapy) is, in principle at least, a highly suggestive one.

In the preceding section, it was a relatively straightforward matter to identify modern parallels for the combination being considered here (Stoic unified or 'holistic' psychology and Galenic brain-centred psychophysiology). Indeed, it was possible to find modern work, both in research on the brain and in the philosophy of mind (for instance, Nussbaum's) that could be seen as exploring the modern equivalent of this kind of combination. However, it is less clear to me quite where one would look in the modern Western context for analogues of the combination of Galenic-style body-based medicine and Stoic-style psychological therapy, especially bearing in mind the strongly revisionist assumptions of Stoic therapy, both in psychology and ethics. A precondition of such a combination would be that the methods and objectives of each side of the technique are recognized as valid and effective from the standpoint of the partner discipline. In the modern, as well as the ancient, context this is a rather demanding precondition; and there is often quite a wide methodological gap between body-based and psychological medicine (or between subdivision of these practices). For instance, the scientific credentials of Freudian-style psychoanalysis (which I have suggested is in some respects the closest modern parallel to Stoic psychological therapy) have been widely questioned.[100] On the other side, from a more 'holistic' (whole-person) standpoint, questions are often raised about the heavy reliance on drugs in modern Western medicine, including the treatment of psychological illness. In these and other respects, the gap between the modern analogues of the two ancient approaches under consideration remains potentially wide, though one would hope that the modern response to this gap is less combative and polemical than it often is in Galen's case.

[100] On analogous features of Freudian and Stoic psychotherapy, see text to nn. 86–90 above. For scientific evaluation of Freudian theories and therapy, see e.g. Fisher and Greenberg 1978.

Overall, the question whether this type of combination looks more or less viable, if we view it from a modern standpoint, remains an open one, though the answer is not obviously negative. I think there would be broad assent to the idea that the best type of treatment, both for mental and physical illness, is one which balances the formidable resources of modern (scientifically based) medicine with an ethically informed and psychologically sophisticated approach to people as psychological agents. There is, of course, much room for argument about how closely such a modern synthesis would resemble the combination of Galenic medicine and Stoic psychological therapy envisaged here. As regards Stoicism, at least, I think that their ethical approach merits more serious consideration, in the modern context, than it has received even from some of its recent scholarly advocates.[101] Since Stoic psychological theory is already being taken seriously by a number of modern thinkers,[102] I think we have the basis for a positive reappraisal of their ideas about psychological health, sickness, and therapy, and of the contribution that Stoic ideas could make to the kind of ideal synthesis of body-based and psychological approaches just suggested. However, thinking through the implications of the last suggestion would form the subject matter of a different kind of inquiry.[103] At any rate, I hope this book as a whole has given a better understanding of Galenic and Stoic thinking on psychology and therapy and of how and how far they could have been combined, in a way that can usefully inform modern reflection on psychophysical health and on how this can best be achieved.

[101] Nussbaum 2001: chs. 1–2, is presented as offering a 'Neo-Stoic' psychological theory, but marks dissent from key features of Stoic ethics (e.g. in 11–12); Becker 1998 is more unequivocal in his support for Stoic ethics; but I would want to place Stoic ethics more firmly within stoic theory as a whole than he does.

[102] Nussbaum 2001 is again a clear example; she highlights links with comparable modern cognitivist treatments of emotions in chs. 1–2.

[103] This is a line of inquiry I hope to pursue elsewhere.

References

ALGRA, K., BARNES, J., MANSFELD, J., and SCHOFIELD, M. (1999) (eds.). *The Cambridge History of Hellenistic Philosophy.* Cambridge: Cambridge University Press.

ALLEN, J. (2001). *Inference from Signs.* Oxford: Oxford University Press.

ANNAS, J. (1981). *An Introduction to Plato's Republic.* Oxford: Oxford University Press.

—— (1992). *Hellenistic Philosophy of Mind.* Berkeley: California University Press.

—— (1993). *The Morality of Happiness.* Oxford: Oxford University Press.

—— (1999). *Platonic Ethics, Old and New.* Ithaca: Cornell University Press.

—— (2004). 'Marcus Aurelius: Ethics and its Background', *Rhizai* 2: 103–19.

—— (2007). 'Ethics in Stoic Philosophy', *Phronesis* 52: 58–87.

ARMSTRONG, D. (2008), '"Be Angry and Fear Not": Philodemus versus the Stoics on Natural Bites and Natural Emotions', in J. T. Fitzgerald (ed.), *Passions and Moral Progress in Greco-Roman Thought.* London: Routledge, 79–121.

ARNIM, H. VON (1903–5). *Stoicorum Veterum Fragmenta.* 4 vols. Leipzig: Teubner. Reprint (2004), Munich: Sauer (*SVF*).

ASMIS, E. (1999). 'Epicurean Epistemology', in Algra *et al.*, 260–94.

BABUT, D. (1969). *Plutarque et le Stoicisme.* Paris: Presses Universitaires de France.

BALLESTER, L. G. (1988). 'Soul and Body, Disease of the Soul and Disease of the Body in Galen's Medical Thought', in Manuli and Vegetti, 117–52.

BARNES, J. (1991). 'Galen on Logic and Therapy', in Kudlien and Durling, 50–102.

—— (2003). 'Proofs and Syllogisms in Galen', in Barnes and Jouanna, 1–24.

—— and JOUANNA, J. (2003) (eds.). *Galien et la philosophie.* Entretiens vol. 49. Vanoeuvres-Geneva: Fondation Hardt.

BASTIANINI, G., and LONG, A. A. (1992). 'Hierocles', in *Corpus dei papiri filosofici greci e latini 1.1***. Florence: Olschki, 268–451.

BAYS, B. (1999). *The Journey.* London: Element.

BECCHI, F. (1990). 'La nozione di *orgē* e di *aorgēsia* in Aristotele e in Plutarco', *Prometheus* 16: 65–87.

BECKER, L. C. (1998). *A New Stoicism.* Princeton: Princeton University Press.

BLAKEMORE, C., and JENNETT, S. (2001) (eds.). *The Oxford Companion to the Body.* Oxford: Oxford University Press.

BOBZIEN, S. (1998). *Determinism and Freedom in Stoic Philosophy.* Oxford: Oxford University Press.

—— (1999). 'Chrysippus' Theory of Causes', in Ierokiadonou, 196–242.

BONAZZI, M., and HELMIG, C. (2007) (eds.). *Platonic Stoicism and Stoic Platonism: The Dialogue between Platonism and Stoicism in Antiquity.* Leuven: Leuven University Press.

BONHÖFFER, A. (1890, repr. 1968). *Epictet und die Stoa: Untersuchungen zur Stoischen Philosophie.* Stuttgart: Frommann.

BOUDON-MILLOT, V. (2007*a*). *Galien: tome 1: Introduction générale, Sur l'order de ses propres livres, Sur les propres livres, Que l'excellent médecin est aussi philosophe.* Edition, translation, and notes. Paris: Les Belles Lettres.

—— (2007*b*). 'Un traité miraculeusement retrouvé, *Sur l'inutilité de se chagriner*: texte grec et traduction française', in V. Boudon-Millot, A. Guardasole, and C. Magdelaine (eds.), *La Science médicale antique: nouveaux regards: études réunies en l'honneur de Jacques Jouanna.* Paris 2007, 73–124.

—— (2009). 'Galen's *Bios* and *Methodos*: From Ways of Life to Paths of Knowledge', in Gill, Whitmarsh, and Wilkins, 175–89.

—— and PIETROBELLI, A. (2005) (eds.). 'Galien ressuscité: Édition *princeps* du texte grec du *de propriis placitis*', *Revue des Études Grecques* 118: 168–213.

BOYS-STONES, G. (2001). *Post-Hellenistic Philosophy: A Study of its Development from the Stoics to Origen.* Oxford: Oxford University Press.

BRAUND, S. M., and GILL, C. (1997) (eds.). *The Passions in Roman Thought and Literature.* Cambridge: Cambridge University Press.

BRENNAN, T. (1998). 'The Old Stoic Theory of Emotions', in Sihvola and Engberg-Pedersen, 21–70.

—— (2003). 'Stoic Moral Psychology', in Inwood, 257–94.

—— (2005). *The Stoic Life: Emotions, Duties, and Fate.* Oxford: Oxford University Press.

BRITTAIN, C. (2001). *Philo of Larissa: The Last of the Academic Sceptics.* Oxford: Oxford University Press.

BROCK, A. J. (1916). *Galen: On the Natural Faculties.* Text, translation, and notes. Loeb Classical Library. Cambridge, Mass.: Harvard University Press.

BRUNSCHWIG, J., and NUSSBAUM, M. C. (1993) (eds.). *Passions and Perceptions: Studies in Hellenistic Philosophy of Mind.* Cambridge: Cambridge University Press.

CHIARADONNA, R. (2009). 'Galen and Middle Platonism', in Gill, Whitmarsh, and Wilkins, 243–60.

Colombetti, C. (2007). 'Enactive Appraisal', *Phenomenology and the Cognitive Sciences* 6: 527–46.
—— (2008). 'The Feeling Body: Towards an Enactive Approach to Emotion', in W. F. Overton, U. Müller, and J. L. Newman (eds.), *Developmental Perspectives on Embodiment and Consciousness.* New York: Lawrence Erlbaum, 45–68.
Cooper, J. M. (1984). 'Plato's Theory of Human Motivation', *History of Philosophy Quarterly* 1: 3–21. Reprinted in (1999), 118–37.
—— (1997) (ed.). *Plato: Complete Works.* Indianapolis: Hackett.
—— (1998). 'Posidonius on Emotions', in Sihvola and Engberg-Pedersen, 71–111. Reprinted in (1999), 449–84.
—— (1999). *Reason and Emotion: Essays on Ancient Moral Psychology and Ethical Theory.* Princeton: Princeton University Press.
—— (2004). *Knowledge, Nature and the Good: Essays on Ancient Philosophy.* Princeton: Princeton University Press.
—— and Procopé, J. (1995). *Seneca: Moral and Political Essays.* Translation with introduction and notes. Cambridge Texts in the History of Political Thought. Cambridge: Cambridge University Press.
Damasio, A. (1994). *Descartes' Error.* London: Vintage Books.
Debru, A. (1994). 'L'Expérimentation chez Galien', in Haase and Temporini II.37.2: 1718–56.
—— (2008). 'Physiology', in Hankinson (2008*c*), 263–82.
De Lacy, P. (1972). 'Galen's Platonism', *American Journal of Philology* 93: 27–39.
—— (1988). 'The Third Part of the Soul', in Manuli and Vegetti, 43–63.
—— (1992) (ed.). *Galeni: De Semine* (*Galen: On Semen*). Edition, translation, and commentary. *CMG* V 3,1. Berlin: Akademie Verlag.
—— (1996). *Galeni: De Elementis ex Hippocratis Sententia* (*Galen: On the Elements According to Hippocrates*). Edition, translation, and commentary. *CMG* V 1,2. Berlin: Akademie Verlag.
—— 2005 (ed.). *Galeni: De Placitis Hippocratis et Platonis* (*Galen: On the Doctrines of Hippocrates and Plato*), 3 vols. Edition, translation, and commentary. 3rd edn., vols. 1–2 unrevised, vol. 3 revised and augmented (1st edn. 1978–84). *CMG* V 4,1,2. Berlin: Akademie Verlag.
Diller, H. (1970, 2nd edn. 1999) (ed.). *Hippocratis: De Aere, Aquis, Locis.* Edition, translation, and commentary. Akademie *CMG* I 1,2. Berlin: Verlag.
Dillon, J. (1977, 2nd edn. 1995). *The Middle Platonists.* London: Duckworth.
—— (1983). '*Metriopatheia* and *Apatheia*: Some Reflections on a Controversy in Later Greek Ethics', in J. P. Anton and A. Preus (eds.), *Essays in Ancient Greek Philosophy*, vol. 2. Albany, NY: State University of Albany Press, 508–17.

DILLON, J. (1993). *Alcinous: The Handbook of Platonism*. Translation with introduction and commentary. Clarendon Later Ancient Philosophers. Oxford: Oxford University Press.

——(2003). *The Heirs of Plato: A Study of the Old Academy* (347–274 BC). Oxford: Oxford University Press.

——and LONG, A. A. (1988) (eds.). *The Question of 'Eclecticism': Studies in Later Greek Philosophy*. Berkeley: University of California Press.

DODDS, E. R. (1951). *The Greeks and the Irrational*. Berkeley: University of California Press.

DONINI, P. (1974). *Tre studi sull'aristotelismo nel II secolo d. C.* Toronia: G. B. Paravia.

——(1988). 'Tipologia degli errori e loro correzione secondo Galeno', in Manuli and Vegetti, 65–116.

——(1992). 'Galeno e la filosofia', in Haase and Temporini II.36.5: 3484–3504.

——(1995). 'Struttura delle passione e del vizio e loro cura in Crisippo', *Elenchos* 16: 305–29.

——(2008).'Psychology', in Hankinson (2008*c*), 184–209.

DORANDI, T. (1999). 'Chronology', in Algra *et al.*, 31–54.

DUFF, T. E. (1999). *Plutarch's Lives: Exploring Virtue and Vice*. Oxford: Oxford University Press.

DYCK, A. (1981). 'On Panaetius' Conception of *megalopsuchia*', *Museum Helveticum* 38: 153–61.

EDELSTEIN, L., and KIDD, I. G. (1972, 2nd edn. 1989) (eds.). *Posidonius I: The Fragments*. Classical Texts and Commentaries 13.1. Cambridge: Cambridge University Press.

ENGBERG-PEDERSEN, T. (1990). *The Stoic Theory of Okeiosis: Moral Development and Social Interaction in Early Stoic Philosophy*. Aarhus: Aarhus University Press.

EVERSON, S. (1991*a*), 'Introduction' in (1991*b*), 1–12.

——(1991*b*) (ed.). *Psychology: Companions to Ancient Thought, 2*. Cambridge: Cambridge University Press.

——(1999). 'Epicurean Psychology', in Algra *et al.*, 542–59.

FEYERABEND, P. (1975). *Against Method: Outline of an Anarchistic Theory of Knowledge*. London: NLB.

FILLION-LAHILLE, J. (1984). *Le 'De Ira' de Sénèque et la philosophie stoïcienne des passions*. Paris: Klincksieck.

FISHER, S., and GREENBERG, R. P. (1978) (eds.). *The Scientific Evaluation of Freud's Theories and Therapy: A Book of Readings*. Hassocks: Harvester Press.

FLASHAR, H. (1966). *Melancholie und Melancholiker in den medizinischen Theorien der Antike*. Berlin: De Gruyter.

FLEMMING, R. (2008). 'Commentary', in Hankinson (2008*c*), 323–54.
——(2009). 'Demiurge and Emperor in Galen's World of Knowledge', in Gill, Whitmarsh, and Wilkins, 59–84.
FÖLLINGER, S. (1997) (ed.). *Aristotelische Biologie: Intentionen, Methoden, Ergebnisse.* Stuttgart: Kullmann.
FOUCAULT, M. (1990). *The Care of the Self*, trans. M. Hurley. London: Penguin.
FREDE, D. (2003). 'Stoic Determinism', in Inwood, 179–205.
FREDE, M. (1985). 'Introduction', in Walzer and Frede, ix–xxxvi.
——(1987). *Essays in Ancient Philosophy.* Oxford: Clarendon Press.
——(1995). 'Introduction', in Frede and Striker, 1–28.
——(1999*a*). 'Epilogue', in Algra *et al.*, 771–97.
——(1999*b*). 'On the Stoic Conception of the Good', in Ieradiakonou, 71–94.
——(1999*c*). 'Stoic Epistemology', in Algra *et al.*, 295–322.
——(2003). 'Galen's Theology', in Barnes and Jouanna, 73–129.
——and STRIKER, G. (1995) (eds.). *Rationality in Greek Thought.* Oxford: Oxford University Press.
GERSON, L. (2002). *Knowing Persons in Plato.* Oxford: Oxford University Press.
GILL, C. (1983). 'Did Chrysippus Understand Medea?', *Phronesis* 28: 136–49.
——(1985*a*). 'Ancient Psychotherapy', *Journal of the History of Ideas* 46: 307–25.
——(1985*b*). 'Plato and the Education of Character', *Archiv für Geschichte der Philosophie* 67: 1–26.
——(1991). 'Is there a Concept of Person in Greek Philosophy?', in Everson (1991*b*), 166–93.
——(1994). 'Peace of Mind and Being Yourself: Panaetius to Plutarch', in Haase and Temporini II.36.7: 4599–4640.
——(1996). *Personality in Greek Epic, Tragedy, and Philosophy: The Self in Dialogue.* Oxford: Oxford University Press.
——(1998). 'Did Galen Understand Platonic and Stoic Thinking on Emotions', in Sihvola and Engberg-Pedersen, 113–48.
——(2000). 'The Body's Fault? Plato's *Timaeus* on Psychic Illness', in M. Wright (ed.), *Reason and Necessity: Essays on Plato's Timaeus.* London: Duckworth and the Classical Press of Wales, 59–84.
——(2003). 'The School in the Roman Imperial Period', in Inwood, 33–58.
——(2005). 'Competing Readings of Stoic Emotions', in Salles, 445–70.
——(2006). *The Structured Self in Hellenistic and Roman Thought.* Oxford: Oxford University Press.
——(2007*a*). 'Galen and the Stoics: Mortal Enemies or Blood Brothers?', *Phronesis* 52: 88–120.

Gill, C. (2007*b*). 'Marcus Aurelius', in Sorabji and Sharples, vol. 1, 175–87.

—— (2007*c*). 'Marcus Aurelius' *Meditations*: How Stoic and How Platonic?', in Bonazzi and Helmig, 189–207.

—— (2008*a*). 'Die antike medizinische Tradition: Die körperliche Basis emotionaler Dispositionen', trans. D. Caluori, in H. Landweer and U. Renz (eds.), *Klassische Emotionstheorien: Von Platon bis Wittgenstein.* Berlin: De Gruyter, 97–120.

—— (2008*b*). 'The Ancient Self: Issues and Approaches', in P. Remes and J. Sihvola (eds.), *Ancient Philosophy of the Self*, New Synthese Historical Library. Berlin: Springer, 35–56.

—— (2008*c*). 'The Ancient Self: Where Now?', *Antiquorum Philosophia* 2: 77–99.

—— (2008*d*). 'The Self and Hellenistic-Roman Philosophical Therapy', in A. Arweiler and M. Möller (eds.), *Vom Selbst-Verständnis: Notions of the Self in Antiquity and Beyond.* Berlin: De Gruyter, 359–95.

—— (2009).'Galen and the Stoics: What Each Could Learn from the Other about Embodied Psychology', in D. Frede and B. Reis (eds.), *Leib und Seele in der antiken Philosophie / Body and Soul in Ancient Philosophy.* Berlin: De Gruyter, 234–41.

—— (2010). 'Stoicism and Epicureanism', in Goldie, 143–65.

—— Whitmarsh, T., and Wilkins, J. (2009) (eds.). *Galen and the World of Knowledge.* Cambridge: Cambridge University Press.

Glucker, J. (1988). 'Cicero's Philosophical Affiliations', in Dillon and Long, 34–69.

Goldie, P. (2010) (ed.). *Oxford Handbook of Philosophy of Emotion.* Oxford: Oxford University Press.

Gotthelf, A. (1985) (ed.). *Aristotle on Nature and Living Things.* Pittsburgh.

—— and Lennox, J. G. (1987) (ed.). *Philosophical Issues in Aristotle's Biology.* Cambridge: Cambridge University Press.

Gourinat, J.-B. (2005). 'Le Traité de Chrysippe *Sur l'âme*', *Revue de Métaphysique et de Morale* 4: 557–78.

Graver, M. (1999). 'Philo of Alexandria and the Origins of the Stoic *propatheia*', *Phronesis* 44: 300–25.

—— (2002). *Cicero on the Emotions: Tusculan Disputations 3 and 4.* Translation with introduction and commentary. Chicago: Chicago University Press.

—— (2007). *Stoicism and Emotion.* Chicago: University of Chicago Press.

Gregory, R. L. (2004) (ed.). *The Oxford Companion to the Mind.* Oxford: Oxford University Press.

Griffin, M. (2007). 'Seneca's Pedagogic Strategy: *Letters and De beneficiis*', in Sorabji and Sharples, vol. 1, 89–113.

Gundert, B. (2000). 'Soma and Psyche in Hippocratic Medicine', in Wright and Potter, 13–35.

Haase, W., and Temporini, H. (1972–) (eds.). *Aufstieg und Niedergang der römischen Welt (Rise and Decline of the Roman World)* (multi-volume series). Berlin: De Gruyter.

Hadot, P. (1995). *Philosophy as a Way of Life*, trans. M. Chase, ed., with introduction by A. I. Davidson. Oxford: Blackwell.

—— (1998). *The Inner Citadel: The Meditations of Marcus Aurelius*, trans. M. Chase. Cambridge, Mass.: Harvard University Press.

Hankinson, R. J. (1987*a*). 'Causes and Empiricism: A Problem in the Interpretation of Later Greek Medical Method', *Phronesis* 32: 329–48.

—— (1987*b*). 'Evidence, Externality and Antecedence: Inquiries into Later Greek Causal Concepts', *Phronesis* 32: 80–100.

—— (1988). 'Galen Explains the Elephant', in M. Matthen and B. Linksy (eds.), *Philosophy and Biology*, *Canadian Journal of Philosophy* Supplementary Volume 14, 135–57.

—— (1989). 'Galen and the Best of All Possible Worlds', *Classical Quarterly* 39: 206–27.

—— (1991*a*). 'Galen's Anatomy of the Soul', *Phronesis* 36: 197–233.

—— (1991*b*). 'Galen on the Foundations of Science', in López Féres, 15–29.

—— (1991*c*) (ed.). *Galen: On the Therapeutic Method, Books I and II.* Translation with introduction and commentary. Oxford: Oxford University Press.

—— (1992). 'Galen's Philosophical Eclectism', in Haase and Temporini II.36.5: 3505–22.

—— (1993). 'Actions and Passions: Affection, Emotion and Moral Self-Management in Galen's Philosophical Psychology', in Brunschwig and Nussbaum, 184–222.

—— (1994). 'Galen's Theory of Causation', in Haase and Temporini II.37.2: 1757–74.

—— (1997). 'Natural Criteria and the Transparency of Judgement: Antiochus, Philo and Galen on Epistemological Justification', in B. Inwood and J. Mansfeld (eds.), *Assent and Argument.* Leiden: Brill, 161–216.

—— (1998) (ed.). *Galen on Antecedent Causes.* Translation with introduction and commentary. Cambridge Classical Texts and Commentaries. Cambridge: Cambridge University Press.

—— (1999). 'Explanation and Causation', in Algra *et al.*, 479–512.

—— (2003). 'Causation in Galen', in Barnes and Jouanna, 31–66.

—— (2006). 'Body and Soul in Galen', in King, 232–58.

—— (2008*a*). 'Epistemology', in Hankinson (2008*c*), 157–83.

—— (2008*b*). 'Philosophy of Nature', in Hankinson (2008*c*), 210–41.

Hankinson, R. J. (2008*c*) (ed.). *The Cambridge Companion to Galen*. Cambridge: Cambridge University Press.

—— (2008*d*). 'The Man and his Work', in Hankinson (2008*c*), 1–33.

—— (2009). 'Galen on the Limitations of Knowledge', in Gill, Whitmarsh, and Wilkins, 206–42.

Harkins, P. W., and Riese, W. (1963). *Galen on the Passions and Errors of the Soul*. Translation, with introduction and interpretation. Columbus: Ohio State University Press.

Harris, W. V. (2001). *Restraining Rage: The Ideology of Anger Control in Classical Antiquity*. Cambridge, Mass.: Harvard University Press.

Harte, V. (2002). *Plato on Parts and Wholes: The Metaphysics of Structure*. Oxford: Oxford University Press.

Helmreich, G. (1907–9) (ed.). *Galeni De Usu Partium, Libri XVII*, 2 vols. Leipzig: Teubner.

Ierodiakonou, K. (1999) (ed.). *Topics in Stoic Philosophy*. Oxford: Oxford University Press.

Ilberg, J. (1889–97). 'Über die Schriftstellerei des Klaudios Galenos', *Rheinisches Museum* 44 (1889), 207–39; 47 (1892), 489–514; 51 (1896), 165–96; 52 (1897), 591–623.

Indelli, G. (1988) (ed.). *Filodemo: L'ira*. Edition and translation, with introduction and commentary. Naples: Bibliopolis.

Inwood, B. (1984). 'Hierocles: Theory and Argument in the Second Century AD', *Oxford Studies in Ancient Philosophy* 2: 151–83.

—— (1985). *Ethics and Human Action in Early Stoicism*. Oxford: Oxford University Press.

—— (1993). 'Seneca and Psychological Dualism', in Brunschwig and Nussbaum, 150–83.

—— (2003) (ed.). *Cambridge Companion to the Stoics*. Cambridge: Cambridge University Press.

—— (2005). *Reading Seneca: Stoic Philosophy at Rome*. Oxford: Oxford University Press.

—— and Donini, P. (1999). 'Stoic Ethics', in Algra *et al.*, 675–738.

—— and Gerson, L. (1997, 2nd edn.). *Hellenistic Philosophy: Introductory Readings*. Indianapolis: Hackett.

—— —— (2008). *The Stoics Reader: Selected Writings and Testimonia*. Indianapolis: Hackett.

Irwin, T. (1977). *Plato's Moral Theory*. Oxford: Oxford University Press.

—— (1991). 'Aristotle's Philosophy of Mind', in Everson (1991*b*), 56–82.

—— (1995). *Plato's Ethics*. Oxford: Oxford University Press.

Jackson-McCabe, M. (2004). 'The Stoic Theory of Implanted Preconceptions', *Phronesis* 49: 323–47.

JOHANSEN, T. K. (2004). *Plato's Natural Philosophy: A Study of the Timaeus-Critias*, Cambridge: Cambridge University Press.

JOHNSON, M. R. (2005). *Aristotle on Teleology*. Oxford: Oxford University Press.

JOUANNA, J. (1999). *Hippocrates*, trans. M. B. DeBevoise. Baltimore: Johns Hopkins University Press.

——(2003). 'La Notion de nature chez Galien', in Barnes and Jouanna, 229–68.

——(2009). 'Does Galen Have a Medical Programme for Intellectuals and the Faculties of the Intellect?', in Gill, Whitmarsh, and Wilkins, 190–205.

JU, A. (2007). 'Chrysippus on Nature and Soul in Animals', *Classical Quarterly* 57: 97–108.

KAHN, C. H. (1987). 'Plato's Theory of Desire', *Review of Metaphysics* 41: 77–103.

KAPLAN, H. I., and SADOCK, B. J. (1996, 2nd edn.). *Pocket Handbook of Clinical Psychiatry*. Baltimore.

KARON, B. P., and VANDENBOS, G. V. (1981). *Psychotherapy of Schizophrenia: The Treatment of Choice*, New York.

KERFERD, G. (1983). 'Two Problems Concerning Impulses', in W. W. Fortenbaugh (ed.), *On Stoic and Peripatetic Ethics: The Work of Arius Didymus*. Rutgers University Studies in Classical Humanities, 1. New Brunswick: Transaction Books, 87–98.

KIDD, I. G. (1971). 'Posidonius on Emotions', in Long, 200–15.

——(1988). *Posidonius II: The Commentary*, 2 vols. Classical Texts and Commentaries 14A–B. Cambridge: Cambridge University Press.

——(1992) (ed.). *Plutarch:* Essays. Translation by R. Waterfield with introduction and notes by I. G. Kidd. Penguin Classics. London: Penguin.

KING, R. A. H. (2006) (ed.). *Common to Body and Soul: Philosophical Approaches to Explaining Living Behaviour in Greco-Roman Antiquity*. Berlin: De Gruyter.

KLIBANSKY, R., PANOFSKY, E., and SAXL, F. (1964). *Saturn and Melancholy: Studies in the History of Natural Philosophy, History, and Art*. London: Nelson.

KNUUTTILA, S. (2004). *Emotions in Ancient and Medieval Philosophy*. Oxford: Oxford University Press.

KOCH, K. *et al.* (1923) (eds.). *Galeni: De Sanitate Tuenda* etc. Edition, translation, and commentary. *CMG* V4,2. Berlin: Akademie Verlag.

KOLLESCH, J. (1988). 'Anschauungen von den *archai* in der *Ars medica* und ihre Voraussetzungen bei Galen', in Manuli and Vegetti, 215–29.

——and NICKEL, D. (1993) (eds.). *Galen und das hellenistische Erbe*. Stuttgart: Steiner.

KOLLESCH, J., and NICKEL, D. (1994). 'Bibliographia Galeniana: Die Beiträge des 20. Jahrhunderts zur Galenforschung', in Haase and Temporini II.37.2: 1351–1420.

KONSTAN, D. (2001). *Pity Transformed.* London: Duckworth.

——(2006). *The Emotions of the Ancient Greeks: Studies in Aristotle and Classical Literature.* Toronto: University of Toronto Press.

KOVAČIĆ, F. (2001). *Der Begriff der Physis bei Galen vor dem Hintergrund seiner Vorgänger.* Stuttgart: Steiner.

KRAUS, P. (1939) (ed.). 'Kitāb al-ahlāq li-Ğālīnūs', *Bulletin of the Faculty of Arts of the Egyptian University* 5: 1–51.

KUDLIEN, F., and DURLING, R. (1991) (eds.). *Galen's Method of Healing.* Leiden: Brill.

KHN, C. G. (1819–33). *Galeni Opera Omnia.* 20 vols. Leipzig: Carl Knobloch. Reprint (1965) Hildesheim: Georg Olms.

KUHN, T. S. (1962). *The Structure of Scientific Revolutions.* Chicago: University of Chicago Press.

KUPREEVA, I. (2004). 'Aristotelian Dynamics in the 2nd Century School Debates: Galen and Alexander of Aphrodisias on Organic Powers and Movements', *Bulletin of the Institute of Classical Studies* Supplement 83, vol. 1: 71–92.

LAÍN ENTRALGO, P. (1970). *The Therapy of the Word in Classical Antiquity.* New Haven: Yale University Press.

LARRAIN, C. J. (1992) (ed.). *Galens Kommentar zu Platons Timaios.* Beiträge zur Altertumskunde 29. Stuttgart.

LAZARUS, R. S. (1991). *Emotion and Adaptation.* New York: Oxford University Press.

LEDOUX, J. (1998). *The Emotional Brain: The Mysterious Underpinnings of Emotional Life.* London: Phoenix.

LEWIS, M. D., and TODD, R. M. (2007). 'The Self-Regulating Brain: Cortical-Subcortical Feedback and the Development of Intelligent Action', *Cognitive Development* 22: 406–30.

LITTRÉ, E. (1839–61) (ed.). *Oeuvres complètes d'Hippocrate,* 10 vols. Paris: Baillière.

LLOYD, G. E. R. (1979). *Magic, Reason and Experience: Studies in the Origin and Development of Greek Science.* Cambridge: Cambridge University Press.

——(1988). 'Scholarship, Authority and Argument in Galen's *Quod Animi Mores*', in Manuli and Vegetti, 11–42.

——(1991). *Methods and Problems in Greek Science.* Cambridge: Cambridge University Press.

——(1993). 'Galen on Hellenistics and Hippocrateans: Contemporary Battles and Past Authorities', in Kollesch and Nickel, 125–43.

——(2003). *In the Grip of Disease: Studies in the Greek Imagination.* Oxford: Oxford University Press.

——(2008). 'Galen and his Contemporaries', in Hankinson (2008*c*), 34–48.

Long, A. A. (1971, repr. 1996) (ed.). *Problems in Stoicism*. London: Athlone Press.

——(1996). *Stoic Studies*. Cambridge: Cambridge University Press.

——(1999). 'Stoic Psychology', in Algra *et al.*, 560–84.

——(2002). *Epictetus: A Stoic and Socratic Guide to Life*. Oxford: Oxford University Press.

——and Sedley, D. N. (1987). *The Hellenistic Philosophers*, 2 vols. Cambridge: Cambridge University Press (=LS).

López Féres, J. A. (1991) (ed.). *Galeno: Obra Pensiamento y Influencia*. Madrid: Universidad Nacional de Educación a Distancia.

Lorenz, H. (2004). 'Desire and Reason in Plato's *Republic*', *Oxford Studies in Ancient Philosophy* 27: 83–116.

Luhrmann, T. M. (2000). *Of Two Minds: The Growing Disorder in American Psychiatry*. New York.

McDonald, G. (2009). 'Concepts and Treatments of Phrenitis in Ancient Medicine', Ph.D. thesis, Newcastle University.

McKeith, G. (2004). *You Are What You Eat*. London: Michael Joseph.

Mackenzie, M. M. (1981). *Plato on Punishment*. Berkeley: University of California Press.

Manetti, D., and Roselli, A. (1994). 'Galeno Commentatore di Ippocrate', in Haase and Temporini II.37.2: 1529–1635.

Mansfeld, J. (1989). 'Chrysippus and the Placita', *Phronesis* 34: 311–42.

——(1990). 'Doxography and Dialectic: The *Sitz im Leben* of the Placita', in Haase and Temporini II.36.4: 3056–3229.

——(1991). 'The Idea of the Will in Chrysippus, Posidonius, and Galen', *Boston Area Colloquium in Ancient Philosophy* 7: 107–45.

——(1999). 'Sources', in Algra *et al.*, 3–30.

Manuli, P., and Vegetti, M. (1988) (eds.). *Le opere psichologiche di Galeno*. Naples: Bibliopolis.

Marquardt, I., Müller, I., and Helmreich, G. (1967) (eds.). *Claudii Galeni Pergameni: Scripta Minora*, 3 vols. Reprint of 1st edn. (Leipzig: Teubner, 1884). Amsterdam: Hakkert (=*SM*).

Mattock, J. N. (1972). 'A Translation of the Arabic Epitome of Galen's Book *peri ēthōn*', in S. M. Stern, A. Hourani, and V. Brown (eds.), *Islamic Philosophy and the Classical Tradition: Essays Presented by his Friends and Pupils to Richard Walzer on his Seventieth Birthday*. Oxford: Oxford University Press, 235–60.

May, M. T. (1968). *Galen: On the Usefulness of the Parts of the Body*. Translation with introduction and commentary, 2 vols. Ithaca: Cornell University Press.

Moraux, P. (1981). 'Galien comme philosophe: la philosophie de la nature', in Nutton, 87–116.

—— (1984). *Der Aristotelismus bei den Griechen von Andronikos bis Alexander von Aphrodisias* (2 vols.): vol. 2, *Der Aristotelismus im I und II Jh. n. Chr.* Berlin: De Gruyter.

—— (1985). 'Galen and Aristotle's *De partibus animalium*', in Gotthelf, 327–44.

Morison, B. (2008). 'Logic', in Hankinson (2008*c*), 66–115.

Nickel, D. (1989). *Untersuchungen zur Embryologie Galens.* Berlin: Akademie Verlag.

—— (1993). 'Stoa und Stoiker in Galens Schrift *De foetuum formatione*', in Kollesch and Nickel, 79–86.

—— (2001) (ed.). *Galeni: De Foetuum Formatione.* Edition, translation, and commentary. *CMG* V 3,3. Berlin: Akademie Verlag.

Nussbaum, M. C. (1994). *The Therapy of Desire: Theory and Practice in Hellenistic Ethics.* Princeton: Princeton University Press.

—— (2001). *Upheavals of Thought: The Intelligence of Emotions.* Cambridge: Cambridge University Press.

Nutton, V. (1979) (ed.). *Galeni De Praecognitione* (*Galen: On Prognosis*). Edition, translation, and commentary. *CMG* V 8,1. Berlin: Akademie Verlag.

—— (1981) (ed.). *Galen: Problems and Prospects.* London: Wellcome Institute for the History of Medicine.

—— (1999) (ed.). *Galeni: De Propriis Placitis* (*Galen: On My Own Opinions*). Edition, translation, and commentary. *CMG* V 3, 2. Berlin: Akademie Verlag.

—— (2004). *Ancient Medicine.* London: Routledge.

—— (2009). 'Galen's Library', in Gill, Whitmarsh, and Wilkins, 19–34.

O'Keefe, T. (2005). *Epicurus on Freedom.* Cambridge: Cambridge University Press.

Pembroke, S. (1971), '*Oikeiōsis*', in Long, 114–49.

Penner, T. (1990). 'Plato and Davidson: Parts of the Soul and Weakness of the Will', *Canadian Journal of Philosophy* 16: 35–74.

Pessoa, L. (2008). 'On the Relationship between Emotion and Cognition', *Nature* 9: 148–58.

Pigeaud, J. (1981). *La Maladie de l'âme: Étude sur la relation de l'âme et du corps dans la tradition médico-philosophique antique.* Paris: Les Belles Lettres.

—— (1988). 'La Psychopathologie de Galien', in Manuli and Vegetti, 153–83.

Pohlenz, M. (1959, 2nd edn.). *Die Stoa: Geschichte einer geistigen Bewegung*, 2 vols. Göttingen: Vandenhoeck und Ruprecht.

Price, A. W. (1990). 'Plato and Freud', in C. Gill (ed.), *The Person and the Human Mind: Issues in Ancient and Modern Philosophy.* Oxford: Oxford University Press, 247–70.

—— (1995). *Mental Conflict.* London: Routledge.

Price, A. W. (2005). 'Were Zeno and Chrysippus at Odds in Analysing Emotion?', in Salles, 471–88.

Reydams-Schils, G. (1999). *Demiurge and Providence: Stoic and Platonist Readings of Plato's Timaeus.* Turnhout: Brepols.

—— (2002). 'Human Bonding and *Oikeiōsis*', *Oxford Studies in Ancient Philosophy* 22: 221–51.

—— (2003) (ed.). *Plato's Timaeus as Cultural Icon.* Notre Dame: University of Notre Dame Press.

—— (2005). *The Roman Stoics: Self, Responsibility, and Affection.* Chicago: University of Chicago Press.

Robinson, T. M. (2000). 'The Defining Features of Mind–Body Dualism in the Writings of Plato', in Wright and Potter, 37–55.

Rocca, J. (2003). *Galen on the Brain.* Leiden: Brill.

—— (2008). 'Anatomy', in Hankinson (2008*c*), 242–62.

Rorty, A. O. (1980) (ed.). *Explaining Emotions.* Berkeley: University of California Press.

Rowe, C. (2007). *Plato and the Art of Philosophical Writing.* Cambridge: Cambridge University Press.

Salles, R. (2005) (ed.). *Metaphysics, Soul, and Ethics in Ancient Thought: Themes from the Work of Richard Sorabji.* Oxford: Oxford University Press.

Santas, G. X. (1988). *Plato and Freud.* Oxford.

Schofield, M. (2003). 'Stoic Ethics', in Inwood, 233–56.

Scott, D. (1995). *Recollection and Experience: Plato's Theory of Learning and its Successors.* Cambridge: Cambridge University Press.

Sedley, D. N. (1997). 'Plato's *Auctoritas* and the Rebirth of the Commentary Tradition', in J. Barnes and M. Griffin (eds.), *Philosophia Togata II: Plato and Aristotle at Rome.* Oxford: Oxford University Press, 110–29.

—— (2002). 'The Origins of Stoic God', in D. Frede and A. Laks (eds.), *Traditions of Theology: Studies in Hellenistic Theology.* Leiden: Brill, 41–83.

—— (2003). 'The School, from Zeno to Arius Didymus', in Inwood, 7–32.

—— (2007). *Creationism and its Critics in Antiquity.* Berkeley: University of California Press.

Sellars, J. (2003). *The Art of Living: The Stoics on the Nature and Function of Philosophy.* Aldershot: Ashgate.

—— (2007). 'Stoic Practical Ethics in the Imperial Period', in Sorabji and Sharples, 115–40.

Sherman, N. (1989). *The Fabric of Character: Aristotle's Theory of Virtue.* Oxford: Oxford University Press.

—— (1997). *Making a Necessity of Virtue: Aristotle and Kant on Virtue.* Cambridge: Cambridge University Press.

Sihvola, J., and Engberg-Pedersen, T. (1998) (eds.). *The Emotions in Hellenistic Philosophy.* Dordrecht: Kluwer.

Singer, P. N. (1991). 'Aspects of Galen's Platonism', in López Féres, 41–55.

——(1992). 'Galen on the Soul: Philosophy and Medicine in the Second Century AD', Cambridge University Ph.D. thesis.

——(1997*a*). *Galen: Selected Works.* Translation with introduction and notes. The World's Classics. Oxford: Oxford University Press.

——(1997*b*). 'Levels of Explanation in Galen', *Classical Quarterly* 47: 525–42.

——(forthcoming) (ed.). *Galen: Psychological Works.* Translation with introduction and commentary. Cambridge: Cambridge University Press.

Solmsen, F. (1961). 'Greek Philosophy and the Discovery of the Nerves', *Museum Helveticum* 18: 150–97.

Sorabji, R. (1997) (ed.). *Aristotle and After.* Bulletin of the Institute of Classical Studies, Supplement 68. London: Institute of Classical Studies.

——(2000). *Emotion and Peace of Mind: From Stoic Agitation to Christian Temptation.* Oxford: Oxford University Press.

——(2004). *The Philosophy of the Commentators 200–600 AD: A Sourcebook. Vol. 1: Psychology.* London: Duckworth.

——(2007). 'What is New on the Self in Stoicism after 100 BC?', in Sorabji and Sharples, 141–62.

——and Sharples, R. W. (2007) (eds.). *Greek and Roman Philosophy 100 BC–200 AD*, 2 vols. Bulletin of the Institute of Classical Studies, Supplement 94. London: Institute of Classical Studies.

Staden, H. von (1989). *Herophilus: The Art of Medicine in Early Alexandria.* Cambridge: Cambridge University Press.

——(1997*a*). 'Galen and the "Second Sophistic"', in Sorabji, 33–55.

——(1997*b*). 'Teleology and Mechanism: Aristotelian Biology and Early Hellenistic Medicine', in Föllinger, 183–208.

——(2000). 'Body, Soul, and Nerves: Epicurus, Herophilus, Erasistratus, the Stoics, and Galen', in Wright and Potter, 79–116.

——(2009). 'Staging the Past, Staging Oneself: Galen on Hellenistic Exegetical Traditions', in Gill, Whitmarsh, and Wilkins, 132–56.

Stalley, R. (2007). 'Persuasion and the Tripartite Soul in Plato's *Republic*', *Oxford Studies in Ancient Philosophy* 32: 63–89.

Steel, C. (2001). 'The Moral Purpose of the Human Body: A Reading of *Timaeus* 69–72', *Phronesis* 46: 105–28.

Stern, S. M. (1956). 'Some Fragments of Galen's *On Dispositions* (*peri ēthōn*) in Arabic', *Classical Quarterly* NS 6: 91–101.

Storr, A. (1979). *The Art of Psychotherapy.* London.

Straaten, M. van (1962, 3rd edn.). *Panaetii Rhodii Fragmenta.* Leiden: Brill.

STRIKER, G. (1996). *Essays on Hellenistic Epistemology and Ethics.* Cambridge: Cambridge University Press.

TECUSAN, M. (2004). *The Fragments of the Methodists*: vol. 1, *Methodism outside Soranus.* Leiden: Brill.

TIELEMAN, T. (1991). 'Diogenes of Babylon and Stoic Embryology. Ps. Plutarch, *Plac* V 15.4 Reconsidered', *Mnemosyne* 44: 106–25.

—— (1996). *Galen and Chrysippus on the Soul: Argument and Refutation in the De Placitis II–III.* Leiden: Brill.

—— (2002). 'Galen on the Seat of the Intellect: Anatomical Experiment and Philosophical Tradition', in T. Rihll and C. Tuplin (eds.), *Science and Mathematics in Ancient Greek Culture.* Oxford: Oxford University Press, 256–73.

—— (2003*a*). *Chrysippus' On Affections: Reconstruction and Interpretation.* Leiden: Brill.

—— (2003*b*). 'Galen's Psychology', in Barnes and Jouanna, 131–61.

—— (2008). 'Methodology', in Hankinson (2008*c*), 49–65.

—— (2009). 'Galen and the Stoics, or The Art of Not Naming', in Gill, Whitmarsh, and Wilkins, 282–99.

TRAPP, M. (2007). *Philosophy in the Roman Empire: Ethics, Politics and Society.* Aldershot: Ashgate.

TRILLING, L. (1971). *Sincerity and Authenticity.* London: Oxford University Press.

TSOUNA, V. (2007). *The Ethics of Philodemus.* Oxford: Oxford University Press.

VAN DER EIJK, P. (1999) (ed.). *Ancient Histories of Medicine.* Leiden: Brill.

—— (2000). 'Aristotle's Psychophysiological Account of the Soul-Body Relationship', in Wright and Potter, 57–77.

—— (2008). 'On Galen's Therapeutics', in Hankinson (2008*c*), 283–303.

—— (2009). 'Aristotle! What a Thing for You to Say!' Galen's Engagement with Aristotle and Aristotelians', in Gill, Whitmarsh, and Wilkins, 261–81.

VANDER WAERDT, P. A. (1985). 'Peripatetic Soul Division, Posidonius, and Middle Platonic Moral Psychology', *Greek, Roman and Byzantine Studies* 26: 373–94.

VAN HOOF, L. (2010). *Plutarch's Practical Ethics: The Social Dynamics of Philosophy.* Oxford: Oxford University Press.

VAN STRAATEN: see Straaten, M. van.

VEGETTI, M. (1986). 'Tradizione e verità: Forme della storiografia filosofico-scientifica nel *De Placitis* di Galeno', in G. Cambiano (ed.), *Storiografia e dossografia nella filosofia antica.* Turin: Tirrenia, 227–43.

—— (1999). 'Historiographical Strategies in Galen's Physiology', in van der Eijk, 383–95.

Vogt, S. (2008). 'Drugs and Pharmacology', in Hankinson (2008*c*), 304–22.

Von Arnim: see Arnim, H. von.

von Staden: see Staden, H. von.

Wachsmuth, C., and Hense, O. (1884–1912, repr. 1958) (eds.). *Ioannis Stobaei: Anthologium*, 5 vols. Berlin: Weidmann.

Walzer, R. (1949). 'New Light on Galen's Moral Philosophy', *Classical Quarterly* 43: 82–96. Reprinted as (1962), 142–63.

—— (1954). 'A Diatribe of Galen', *Harvard Theological Review* 47: 243–54. Reprinted as (1962), 164–74.

—— (1962). *Greek into Arabic: Essays on Islamic Philosophy.* Oxford: Oxford University Press.

—— and Frede, M. (1985). *Galen: Three Treatises on the Nature of Science*, translated with introduction. Indianapolis: Hackett.

Warren, J. (2004). *Facing Death: Epicurus and his Critics.* Oxford: Oxford University Press.

White, M. (2003). 'Stoic Natural Philosophy (Physics and Cosmology)', in Inwood, 124–52.

Williams, B. (1997). 'Stoic Philosophy and the Emotions: Reply to Richard Sorabji', in Sorabji, 211–13.

Wilson, M. (1997). 'The Subjugation of Grief in Seneca's *Epistles*', in Braund and Gill, 48–67.

Wollheim, R., and Hopkins, J. (1982) (eds.). *The Thread of Life.* Cambridge: Cambridge University Press.

Wright, J. P., and Potter, P. (2000) (eds.). *Psyche and Soma: Physicians and Metaphysicians on the Mind–Body Problem from Antiquity to Enlightenment.* Oxford: Oxford University Press.

Index of Ancient Passages

Entries for each author are arranged by alphabetical order of Latin titles (or abbreviations) even if English titles are also given. For full details of editions cited by editor's name alone see References or Note on Conventions.

General Index

The manufacturer's authorised representative in the EU for product safety is Oxford University Press España S.A. of el Parque Empresarial San Fernando de Henares, Avenida de Castilla, 2 – 28830 Madrid (www.oup.es/en or product.safety@oup.com). OUP España S.A. also acts as importer into Spain of products made by the manufacturer.

www.ingramcontent.com/pod-product-compliance
Lightning Source LLC
LaVergne TN
LVHW101443200926
848483LV00001B/37
* 9 7 8 0 1 9 9 5 5 6 7 9 3 *